DATE DUE

Unless Recalled Earlier

JUN - 4 1991			
JUN - 7 1994			
ILL 4-2-96			

DEMCO 38-297

HANDBOOK OF
BIOLOGICAL
CONFOCAL MICROSCOPY

HANDBOOK OF BIOLOGICAL CONFOCAL MICROSCOPY

Edited by
James B. Pawley

Integrated Microscopy Resource for Biomedical Research
University of Wisconsin–Madison
Madison, Wisconsin

REVISED EDITION

PLENUM PRESS • NEW YORK AND LONDON

ISBN 0-306-43538-1

Based on papers given at a confocal microscopy workshop, supported
by the National Science Foundation and held at the Electron
Microscopy Society of America meeting, August 8–9, 1989,
in San Antonio, Texas

© 1990, 1989 Plenum Press, New York
A Division of Plenum Publishing Corporation
233 Spring Street, New York, N.Y. 10013

Printed in the United States of America

Authors

David A. Agard
Department of Biochemical Science
The Howard Hughes Medical Institute
University of California, San Francisco
San Francisco, CA 94143-0448

Jonathan Art
Department of Physiology
University of Chicago
947 East 58th Street
Chicago, IL 60637

Robert Bacallao
Division of Nephrology
University of California, Los Angeles
Department of Medicine
Center for the Health Sciences
10833 LeConte Avenue
Los Angeles, CA 90064-1736

Morgane Bomsel
Cell Biology Program
European Molecular Biology Laboratory
Postfach, 10.2209
D-6900, Heidelberg
Federal Republic of Germany

Alan Boyde
Department of Anatomy & Embryology
University College London
Gower Street
London WC1E 6BT, UK

G. J. (Fred) Brakenhoff
Department of Molecular Cell Biology
Section of Molecular Cytology
University of Amsterdam
Plantage Muidergracht 14
1018 TV Amsterdam
Amsterdam, Netherlands

Walter A. Carrington
Physiology Deptartment
University of Massachusetts
Medical School
55 Lake Avenue North
Worcester, MA 01655

Hans Chen
Department of Biochemical Science
The Howard Hughes Medical Institute
Universtiy of California, San Francisco
San Francisco, CA 94143-0448

Victor Chen
K.H.C. Associates
P.O. Box 21
Amherst, NY 14226–0021

Ping-Chin Cheng
Advanced Microscopy Laboratory for
  Biomedical Sciences
Deptartment of Anatomical Sciences
317 Farber Hall
State University of New York
Buffalo, NY 14214

Jan De Mey
Cell Biology Program
European Molecular Biology Laboratory
Postfach, 10.2209
D-6900, Heidelberg
Federal Republic of Germany

C. Kathleen Dorey
Eye Research Institute of Retina
  Foundation
20 Staniford Street
Boston, MA 02114

Fredric S. Fay
Physiology Deptartment
University of Massachusetts
Medical School
55 Lake Avenue North
Worcester, MA 01655

Kevin E. Fogarty
Physiology Deptartment
University of Massachusetts
Medical School
55 Lake Avenue North
Worcester, MA 01655

Enrico Gratton
Physics Department
University of Illinois, Urbana-Champaign
Laboratory for Fluorescence Dynamics
1110 West Green Street
Urbana, IL 60637

Shinya Inoué
Marine Biology Laboratory
Woods Hole, MA 02543

H. Ernst Keller
Carl Zeiss Incorporated
One Zeiss Drive
Thornwood, NY 10594

Gordon S. Kino
Edward L. Ginzton Laboratory
Stanford University
Stanford, CA 94305-4085

Charles J. Koester
Department of Opthalmology

Columbia University
635 West 165th Street
New York, NY 10032

Larry Lifschitz
Physiology Deptartment
University of Massachusetts
Medical School
55 Lake Avenue North
Worcester, MA 01655

James B. Pawley
Integrated Microscopy Resource
1675 Observatory Drive
University of Wisconsin
Madison, WI 53706

David R. Sandison
Developmental Resource for Biophysical
  Imaging and Optoelectronics
Applied Engineering and Physics
Clark Hall
Cornell University
Ithaca, NY 14853

John W. Sedat
Department of Biochemical Science
The Howard Hughes Medical Institute
University of California, San Francisco
San Francisco, CA 94143-0448

Ernst H. K. Stelzer
Light Microscopy Group
European Molecular Biology Laboratory
Postfach, 10.2209
D-6900, Heidelberg
Federal Republic of Germany

James Strickler
Developmental Resource for Biophysical
  Imaging and Optoelectronics
Applied Engineering and Physics
Clark Hall
Cornell University
Ithaca, NY 14853

Robert G. Summers
Department of Anatomical Sciences
317 Farber Hall
State University of New York
Buffalo, NY 14214

Roger Y. Tsien
Department of Pharmacology M-036
School of Medicine
University of California, San Diego
LaJolla, CA 94720

H.T.M. van der Voort
Department of Molecular Cell Biology

Section of Molecular Cytology
University of Amsterdam
Plantage Muidergracht 14
1018 TV Amsterdam
Amsterdam, Netherlands

Martin J. vandeVen
Physics Department
University of Illinois, Urbana-Champaign
Laboratory for Fluorescence Dynamics
1110 West Green Street
Urbana, IL 60637

K. Visscher
Department of Molecular Cell Biology
Section of Molecular Cytology
University of Amsterdam
Plantage Muidergracht 14
1018 TV Amsterdam
Amsterdam, Netherlands

Alan Waggoner
Resident Biologist, Department
    of Biological Sciences and
Center for Fluorescence Research in the
    Biomedical Sciences
Carnegie-Mellon University
4400 5th Avenue
Pittsburgh, PA 15213

Robert Webb
Eye Research Institute of Retina
    Foundation
20 Staniford Street
Boston, MA 02114

Watt Webb
Developmental Resource for Biophysical
    Imaging and Optoelectronics
Applied Engineering and Physics

Clark Hall
Cornell University
Ithaca, NY 14853

K. Sam Wells
Developmental Resource for Biophysical
    Imaging and Opto-electronics
Applied Engineering and Physics
Clark Hall
Cornell University
Ithaca, NY 14853

Tony Wilson
Department of Engineering Science
University of Oxford
Oxford, OX1 3PJ
United Kingdom

Preface

In 1987 the Electron Microscopy Society of America (EMSA) under the leadership of J. P. Revel (Cal Tech) initiated a major program to present a discussion of recent advances in light microscopy as part of the annual meeting. The result was three special LM sessions at the Milwaukee meeting in August 1988: The LM Forum, organized by me, and Symposia on Confocal LM, organized by G. Schatten (Madison), and on Integrated Acoustic/LM/EM organized by C. Rieder (Albany). In addition, there was an optical micro-analysis session emphasizing Raman techniques, organized by the Microbeam Analysis Society, for a total of 40 invited and 30 contributed papers on optical techniques.

Following this successful meeting, discussions among the participants revealed support for a slightly more focussed approach at the next meeting. The benefits of confocal techniques were now felt to be widely appreciated and it seemed time to really evaluate the actual performance of the various instruments and to compare this with theoretical benchmarks and so produce a consensus on where major improvements were likely to be possible in the future. It was felt important to shift from the assertion that "Confocal Works" to the matter of how to make it work better.

Because of the rapid pace of development in the field, we recognized that we were unlikely to be able to be totally definitive on all matters affecting the confocal microscope, but we also felt that the field would benefit from access to a good list of questions and as many answers as time permitted. To do this, it was decided to try to elicit a series of talks in which each one covered a single instrumentational feature unique to confocal microscopy (particularly biological confocal microscopy). The initial list included 12 topics ranging from laser and conventional sources through scanning systems, objective lenses, chromophors, "the pinhole", photon detectors and 3D data display, as well as three overviews on the genesis of the confocal approach, its fundamental limitations and its quantitative capabilities.

In parallel with these developments at EMSA, Drs. J. Wooley and S. Pierce of the Instrumentation and Instrument Development Program at the National Science Foundation had followed a similar path. The Instrumentation and Instrument Development Program is responsible for supporting the purchase of major items of multi-user instrumentation for the conduct of basic research in the life sciences, particularly that which is supported by the NSF Divisions of Behavioral and Neural sciences, Cellular Biosciences, Molecular Biosciences, and BIOTIC Systems and Resources. For the past five years, the Program had emphasized three areas of activity: 1) New instruments that either extend current sensitivity or resolution, or provide new techniques for detection, quantification or observation of biological phenomena. 2) New computer software to enhance current or new instrumentation, and 3) Sponsored workshops in emerging areas of instrumentation or instrument development. They believed that it was clear that confocal microscopy and other new microscopical instrumentation was going to drive important scientific discoveries across wide areas of physiology, cellular biology and neurobiology. They had been looking for a forum in which they could advance the state of the art of confocal microscopy, alert manufacturers to the limitations of current instruments, and catalyze progress toward new directions in confocal instrument development.

These goals were so close to those of the EMSA project that the two groups decided to join forces with EMSA to provide the organization and the venue for a Confocal Workshop and NSF to provide the financial support for the speakers expenses and for the publication of extended abstracts.

The abstracts were initially envisioned as each being about 10–15 pages of camera-ready manuscript but, because of the generous and enthusiastic response of the many leaders of the confocal LM community who agreed to participate, the manuscripts actually submitted were up to fifty pages in length. In addition, scissions and additions increased the list of the topics covered to a total of 19, plus an annotated bibliography.

As the aim of the volume was to discuss the instrument rather than to describe specific applications, the biological emphasis emerges in most chapters as the need to use photons efficiently at every stage of the imaging process and thereby reduce the effects of bleaching and photo-damage to the specimen. In this context, several chapters in this volume emphasize for the first time limitations imposed by everything from fluorescence saturation and sub-optimal signal digitization to specimen preparation.

On a more general level, chapters were added on related instrumentation and on the often unrecognized limitations imposed by the process of pixelating the data contained in digitally recorded images. Several months of frenzied activity got the final mock-ups to the printer in early July.

The nineteen papers were presented at a two day workshop on August 8–9, 1989 at the EMSA Meeting in Houston, TX where the first, soft-cover edition of the Handbook was distributed at that time under the convenient but largely fanciful imprimatur of the IMR Press.

The response was so enthusiastic that it was decided to produce a second, hard-cover edition with an established publisher. This would permit wider distribution and would allow us to correct the errors associated with the short preparation time of the first edition. In addition, extra paragraphs and figures were added to fill gaps in the original or to take note of recent developments.

Taken as a whole, I believe these papers constitute the most complete consideration on the topic available at this time. I am sure that all of the other authors join me in the hope that it will prove to be a catalyst in the development of yet better instrumentation and techniques in the field of biological confocal microscopy. Indeed, improvements evident in the design of the Biorad MRC-600 and of the Leitz CLSM show some evidence of this trend.

Many people have contributed to the production of this volume starting with Drs. Pierce and Wooley and all of the authors.

In addition, I should like to single out R. and C. Moen and K. Hamele for their editorial assistance and C. Thomas, C. Ewing, K. Morgan and P. Henderson for help in retyping some of the manuscripts, A. Freidman and L. Moberly of University of Wisconsin-Madison Publications and W. Kasdorf and N. MacMiller of Impressions for their patience with the typesetting. Special thanks are also due to G. Benham of the Biorad Corporation, and V. Argiro of Vital Images who, when rising costs threatened to delay publication of the first edition, stepped in to fund the printing of the colored cover. This gesture is noted here because, due to a printing mix-up, no mention of the source of the cover images or of the support was included in that edition.

My heartfelt thanks to you all.

James Pawley
Editor
12/89

Contents

CHAPTER 15: DIRECT RECORDING OF
STEREOSCOPIC PAIRS OBTAINED DIRECTLY
FROM DISK SCANNING CONFOCAL LIGHT
MICROSCOPES   163–168
Alan Boyde

CHAPTER 16: FLUOROPHORES FOR CONFOCAL
MICROSCOPY: PHOTOPHYSICS AND
PHOTOCHEMISTRY   169–178
Roger Y. Tsien and Alan Waggoner

CHAPTER 17: IMAGE CONTRAST IN CONFOCAL
LIGHT MICROSCOPY   179–195
P.C. Cheng and R.G. Summers

CHAPTER 18: GUIDING PRINCIPLES OF
SPECIMEN PRESERVATION FOR CONFOCAL
FLUORESCENCE MICROSCOPY   197–205
Robert Bacallao, Morgane Bomsel, Ernst H.K. Stelzer and
Jan De Mey

Chapter 1

Foundations of Confocal Scanned Imaging in Light Microscopy

Shinya Inoué

Marine Biological Laboratory, Woods Hole, MA 02543
The preparation of this article was supported in part by NIH grant R37 GM 31617–07 and NSF grant DCB 8518672

Seldom has the introduction of a new instrument generated as instant an excitement among biologists as the laser-scanning confocal microscope. With the new microscope one can slice incredibly clean, thin optical sections out of thick fluorescent specimens; view specimens in planes running parallel to the line of sight; penetrate deep into light-scattering tissues; gain impressive 3-dimensional views at very high resolution; and improve the precision of microphotometry.

While the instruments that engendered such excitement mostly became commercially available in 1987, the optical and electronic theory and the technology that led to this sudden emergence had been brewing for several decades. The development of this microscope stems from several roots, including light microscopy, confocal imaging, video and scanning microscopy, and coherent or laser-illuminated optics (see historic overview in Table 1). In this chapter, I will review these developments as they relate to the principles and use of the confocal microscope, and then end with some general remarks regarding the new microscope.

LIGHT MICROSCOPY

Lateral Resolution

The foundation of light microscopy was established, a century ago, by Ernst Abbe (1873, 1884). He demonstrated how the diffraction of light by the specimen and by the objective lens determined image resolution, defined the conditions needed to design a lens whose resolution was diffraction limited (rather than limited by chromatic and spherical aberrations), and established the role of objective lens and condenser numerical apertures on image resolution (Equation 1). Thus,

$$d = 1.22 \times \lambda_o / (NA_{obj} + NA_{cond}) \qquad (1)$$

where d is the minimum distance that the diffraction images of two points in the specimen can approach each other laterally before they merge and can no longer be resolved as two separate points (in accordance with Rayleigh's criterion for visually resolving two nearly equally bright points). d is expressed as distance (within the focused plane) in the specimen space; λ_o is the wavelength of light in vacuum; and NA_{obj} and NA_{cond} the numerical apertures (NA)s of the objective and condenser lenses respectively. The NA is the product of 'the sine of the half angle of the cone of light either acceptable by the objective lens or emerging from the condenser lens' and 'the refractive indexes of the imbibition medium between the specimen and the objective or condenser lens, respectively.' [The impact of the quality and NA of the condenser lens on image resolution are considered from a more precise, theoretical standpoint by Zernicke and Hopkins (see Born and Wolf 1980). Their derivations lead to a more complex relationship which is somewhat at variance with Equation (1) or with the alternate Sparrow criterion.]

Using the Rayleigh criterion for resolution, the value for d equals the radius of the Airy disk, namely the radius of the first minimum of a unit diffraction image. The unit diffraction image is the diffraction pattern (produced in the image plane under the particular conditions of observations) of an infinitely small point in the specimen space.

In addition to the wavelength and NA of the objective and condenser lenses, three additional factors or conditions affect the unit diffraction image and image resolution in the microscope. The first factor is the degree of coherence of the light waves. Equation (1) assumes that one is dealing with points (or periodic objects) in the specimen that emit or scatter light waves whose coherence varies with the condenser NA. For objects that are illuminated fully coherently (a condition that pertains when NA_{cond} approaches 0, namely when the condenser iris is closed down to a pinhole), the minimum resolvable distance becomes 2d; in other words, the resolution decreases by a factor of two compared to the case when adjoining specimen points are illuminated incoherently. As the condenser iris is opened up and NA_{cond} becomes larger, the illumination becomes progressively less coherent. [Note, however, that laser beams tend to illuminate objects coherently even when the condenser iris is not closed down (see "LASERS AND MICROSCOPY").]

The second factor is the field size. Equation (1) holds true only when the field of view is not extremely small. When the field of view is extremely small, as in confocal microscopy, the resolution can in fact be greater than when the field of view is not limited. We shall return to this point later.

The third, and equally important, condition is that the resolution criterion applies only to objective lenses used under conditions in which the image is free from significant aberrations. This implies several things: a well-corrected, clean objective lens is used within the wavelengths of light and diameter of field for which the lens was designed (in many cases in conjunction with specific oculars); the refractive index, dispersion, and thickness of the immersion media and cover slip are those specified for the particular objective lens; the correct tube length and ancillary optics are used and the optics are axially aligned; the full complement of image-forming rays and light waves leaving the objective aperture converge to the image plane without obstruction; the condenser aperture is homogeneously and fully illuminated; and the condenser is properly focused (see Chapters 6, 7, 8, 9, and 11; also Inoué, 1986, Chapter 5).

TABLE 1 HISTORIC OVERVIEW

Confocal Microscopy	Microscopy	Video (Microscopy)
	Abbe (1873, 1884)[a]	Nipkow (1884)
	Berek (1927)[d]	
	Zernicke (1935)[a,c]	Zworykin (1934)
	Gabor (1968)[a]	
	H.H. Hopkins (1951)[a]	Flory (1951)
	Linfoot & Wolf (1953)	Young/Roberts (1951)
	3-D diffraction by annul. apert.[a,d]	Flying spot[c]
	Tolardo di Francia (1955)	Montgomery et al (1956)
	Limited field[b]	Flying spot UV[c]
	Nomarski (1955)[c]	
	Linfoot & Wolf (1956)	
	3-D diffraction pattern[a,d]	
	Ingelstam (1956)	
	Resolution and info. theory[a]	
Minsky Patent (1957)		
Insight[a,b,c,d]		
Stage scanning[f]	Kubota & Inoué (1959)[a]	
	Smith & Osterberg (1961)[a]	
	Harris (1964)[a,b]	Freed & Engle (1962)
		Flying spot[c]
	Ellis (1966)	
	Holomicrography[c,d]	
Petráň et al (1968)		
Tandem scanning[d]		
Davidovits & Egger		
(1971)		
Laser illumination,		
Lens scan[d]	Hoffman & Gross (1975)	
	Modulation contrast[c]	
Sheppard & Choudhury		
(1977)		
Theory[a,b,d]		
Sheppard et al (1978)	Ellis (1978)	
Stage scanning	Single sideband edge	
	enhancement microscopy[c]	
Brakenhoff et al (1979)		Castleman (1979)
Specimen scan[e]		Digital image
(1985)		processing[a,c,e]
Koester (1980)	Quate (1980)	
Scanning mirror[d]	Acoustic microscopy[a,c]	
		Inoué (1981)[a,c]
		Allen et al (1981a,b)[a,c]
		Fuchs et al (1982)[f]
		Agard & Sedat (1983)[a,c,d]
Boyde (1985a)		
Nipkow type[d,e]		
Cox & Sheppard (1983)		
Digital recording[d,e]		
Åslund et al (1983)		
2-mirror laser scanning[d]		
Hamilton et al (1984)		
Differential phase[c,d]		
Wilson & Sheppard (1984)		Sher & Barry (1985)[f]
Extended depth		
of field[c,d,e,f]		
Carlsson et al (1985)		Inoué (1986)
Laser scan		Overview, how to[a,c,e,f]
Stacks of confocal images[d,e]		
Wijnaendts van Resandt	Ellis (1985)	Fay et al (1985)[a,c,d]
et al (1985)	Light scrambler[d]	
x-z view[d,e]		
Suzuki-Horikawa (1986)	Cox & Sheppard (1986)[b]	Castleman (1987)[a]
Video rate laser scan,		
Acousto optical modulator,		
No exit pinhole		
Xiao & Kino (1987)		
Nipkow type[d]		
McCarthy & Walker (1988)		
Nipkow type[d]		
Amos et al (1987)[c,d,e]	Ellis (1988)	
	Scanned aperture phase contrast[a,c,d]	

a—Diffraction theory; b—Superresolution; c—Contrast modes; d—Optical sectioning/depth of field; e—Stereo; f—3-D in objective space

Axial Resolution

We now turn to the axial (z-axis) resolution, measured along the optical axis of the microscope, i.e., perpendicular to the plane of focus.

In the case of lateral resolution, i.e., the resolution in the plane of focus, we defined resolution in terms of the minimum distance that the diffraction images of two point sources in the specimen could approach each other and still visually be distinguished as two. Using the Rayleigh criterion, this minimum distance equaled the radius of the first minimum of the unit diffraction image.

Similarly, axial resolution can be defined using two criteria, either the minimum distance that the diffraction images of two points can approach each other along the axis of the microscope and still be seen as two, or by the radius of the first minimum of the diffraction image of an infinitely small point object. I shall now expand on the latter point.

The precise distribution of energy in the image-forming light above and below focus, especially for high NA objective lenses, cannot be deduced by geometric ray tracing, but must be derived from wave optics. The wave optical studies of Linfoot and Wolf (1956) show that the image of a point source produced by a diffraction-limited optical system (such as a properly constructed and used microscope) is not only periodic around the point of focus in the focal plane, but is also periodic above and below the focal plane along the axis of the microscope. [Such 3-dimensional diffraction images (including those produced in the presence of lens aberrations) are presented photographically by Cagnet et al. (1962). The intensity distribution calculated by Linfoot and Wolf for an aberration-free system is reproduced in Born and Wolf (1980); also in Inoué (1986, Fig. 5–21). The 3-dimensional pattern of a point source formed by a lens possessing an annular aperture was calculated by Linfoot and Wolf (1953).]

Near the plane of focus, the axial magnification of the microscope rises as the square of the lateral magnification, and the distance from the center of the diffraction image to the first minimum along the microscope axis turns out to be approximately twice as far as it is to the first minimum in the plane of focus (again both translated into dimensions measured in the specimen space). The central zone of the unit diffraction image is thus stretched along the z-axis of the microscope like an American football, whose major radius is twice as long as its minor radius.

For an incoherent source or scatterer, the cross section through the middle of the football (transverse to its axis of elongation) yields the familiar Airy disk. Therefore, the minimum distance that one can resolve axially is twice as large as the minimum distance that one can resolve transversely. In other words, the axial resolving power is approximately one half of the lateral resolving power.

The axial resolution of the microscope also gives rise to its "axial setting accuracy." The axial setting accuracy is defined as the distance that one has to shift the fine focus of the microscope before the image of an infinitely thin object changes perceptibly. According to Françon (1961), the axial setting accuracy (2ζ) is given by:

$$2\zeta = \lambda / \{4n \times \sin^2(u/2)\} \qquad (2)$$

where, λ is the wavelength of light, n the refractive index of the immersion medium, and u the half angle of the cone of light that is captured by the objective lens. Françon points out that

measurements of the axial setting accuracy is influenced by several factors, and that a value as small as 2ζ is seldom achieved in practice.

Regardless of whose equation is chosen for calculating the axial resolution, it is important to note that the axial resolution (and the related axial-setting accuracy and the shallowness of depth of field) rises with the square of the NA, in contrast to the lateral resolution which rises with the first power of the NA [cf. Eqs. 2, 1].

Depth of Field

The depth of field of a microscope is the depth of the image (measured along the microscope axis translated into distances in the specimen space) that appears to be sharply in focus at one setting of the fine focus adjustment. In bright field microscopy, this depth should be approximately equal to the axial resolution, at least in theory. The actual depth of field has been measured, and the contribution of various factors that affect the measurement have been explored by Berek (1927).

According to Berek, the depth of field is affected by several factors, including (a) the geometric spreading, above and below the plane of focus, of the light beam that arose from a single point in the specimen; (b) accommodation of the observer's eye; and (c) the final magnification of the image. The second factor becomes irrelevant when the image is not viewed directly through the ocular but is instead focused on a thin detector (in the absence of an auto-focusing device). The third factor should also disappear once the total magnification is raised sufficiently so that the unit diffraction image becomes significantly larger than the resolution unit of the detector (see e.g., Castleman, 1987; Hansen in Inoué, 1986).

Many other authors have calculated the depth of field, but unlike Equation (1) that specifies the lateral resolution, no equation is generally accepted as specifying the depth of field. One reason that several equations have been proposed for the depth of field is that different criteria have been used for what is "in focus."

In conventional fluorescence and dark field microscopy, the light that makes up each point of the image spreads in a solid cone that can reach a significant distance above and below focus (as seen in the point spread functions for these modes of microscopy; see e.g., Streibl, 1985, and also Chapters 8, 9, 10, 11, 13 and 14). The spreading cone of light blurs the focused image of the specimen. Also, fluorescent (or light-scattering) objects that are out of focus can inject unwanted light and further reduce the contrast of the specimen region in focus.

For these reasons, the depth of field may be difficult to measure or even to define precisely in fluorescence and dark field microscopy. Or, one could say that the apparent depth of field is very much greater than the axial resolution when objects that are not infinitely thin are observed in conventional fluorescence and dark-field microscopy.

The unwanted light that expands the apparent depth of field is exactly what confocal imaging eliminates. Thus we can view only those fluorescent and light-scattering objects that lie within the depth that is given by the axial resolution of the microscope and attain the desired shallow depth of field.

As mentioned earlier, the lateral resolution of a microscope is a function of the size of the field (observed at any one instant). Tolardo di Francia (1955) suggested, and Ingelstam (1956) argued on the basis of information theory that one gains lateral resolution by a factor of $\sqrt{2}$ as the field of view becomes diminishingly small. These theoretical considerations set the stage for the development of confocal imaging.

CONFOCAL IMAGING

As a young postdoctoral fellow at Harvard University, Marvin Minsky applied for a patent in 1957 for a microscope that uses a stage-scanning confocal optical system. Not only was the conception far sighted, but his insight into the potential application and significance of confocal microscopy was nothing short of remarkable. [See the delightful article by Minsky (1988) that shows even greater insight into the significance of confocal imaging than do the following extracts culled from his patent application.]

In Minsky's embodiment of the confocal microscope, the conventional microscope condenser is replaced by a lens identical to the objective lens. The field of illumination is limited by a pinhole, positioned on the microscope axis. A reduced image of this pinhole is projected onto the specimen by the "condenser." The field of view is also restricted by a second (or exit) pinhole in the image plane placed confocally to the illuminated spot in the specimen and to the first pinhole (Fig. 1). Instead of trans-illuminating the specimen with a separate "condenser" and objective lens, the confocal microscope could also be used in the epi-illuminating mode, making the single objective lens serve both as the condenser and objective lens (Fig. 2).

Using either transmitted- or epi-illumination, the specimen is scanned through a point of light by moving the specimen over short distances in a raster pattern. (The specimen stage is supported on two orthogonally vibrating "tuning forks" that are driven by electromagnets.) The variation in the amount of light, modulated by the specimen and passing the second pinhole, is captured by a photoelectric cell. The photoelectric current is amplified and modulates the beam intensity of a long-persistence cathode-ray oscilloscope. The image of the specimen is displayed on the oscilloscope by scanning its electron writing beam synchronously with the specimen, however, over a greatly expanded distance. The ratio of scanning distances between the electron beam and the specimen provides an image magnification which is variable and can be very large.

With this stage scanning confocal microscope, Minsky says, "Light scattered from parts other than the point of specimen illuminated is rejected from the optical system [by the exit pinhole] to an extent never before realized." As pointed out in the patent application, the advantages of such an optical system are several fold:

- "Reduced blurring of the image from light scattering;
- Increased effective resolution;
- Improved signal to noise ratio;
- Permits unusually clear examination of thick and light scattering objects;
- x-y scan can be made over wide areas of the specimen;
- Inclusion of a z-scan is possible;
- The magnification can be adjusted electronically;
- Especially well-suited for making quantitative studies of the optical properties of the specimen;
- Essentially an infinite number of aperture planes are available for modulating the aperture with dark field stops, annuli, phase plates, etc.;
- Complex contrast effects can be provided with comparatively simple equipment;
- Less complex objective lenses can be used, including those for long working distance, UV or infrared imaging, since they need to be corrected only for a single axial point."

[The high resolution acoustic microscope developed by Quate and coworkers (Quate, 1980), and the laser disk video and audio recorder/players are object-scanning-type confocal microscopes. The designers of these instruments take advantage of the fact that only a single axial point is focused or scanned (see e.g., Inoué, 1986, Sects. 8.9 and 11.5).]

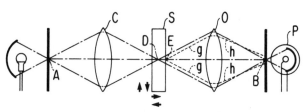

FIG. 1 Optical path in simple confocal microscope. The condenser lens (C) forms an image of the first pinhole (A) onto a confocal spot (D) in the specimen (S). The objective lens (O) forms an image of (D) onto the second (exit) pinhole (B) which is confocal with (D) and (A). Another point, such as (E) in the specimen, would not be focused at (A) or (B), so that the illumination would be less and in addition most of the light g-h scattered from (E) would not pass the exit pinhole. The light reaching the phototube (P) from (E) is thus greatly attenuated compared to that from the confocal point (D). In addition, the exit pinhole could be made small enough to exclude the diffraction rings in the image of (D), so that the resolving power of the microscope is improved. The phototube provides a signal of the light passing through points D_1, D_2, D_3, etc. (not shown), as the specimen is scanned. D_1, D_2, D_3, etc., can lie in a plane normal to the optical axis of the microscope (as in conventional microscopy), or parallel to it, or at any angle defined by the scanning pattern, so that optical sections can be made at angles tilted from the conventional image plane. Since, in the stage scanning system, (D) is a small spot that lies on the axis of the microscope, lenses (C) and (O) can be considerably simpler than conventional microscope lenses. (After Minsky, 1957.)

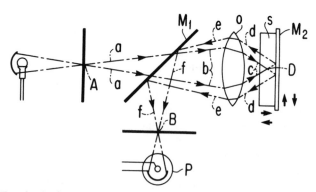

FIG. 2 Optical path in epi-illuminated confocal microscope. The entrance pinhole (A), point (D) in the specimen (S), and exit pinhole (B) are confocal points as in Fig. 1. A partial, or dichroic, mirror (M_1) transmits the illuminating beam a-b-c, and reflects the beam d-e which passed (D) and was reflected by the mirror (M_2) on which the specimen is lying. Only the reflected beam which passes point (D) focuses onto the exit pinhole and reaches the photocell (P). The single lens (O) replaces the condenser and objective lenses in Fig. 1. (After Minsky, 1957.)

IMPACT OF VIDEO

The Nipkow Disk

Just about the same time that Abbe in Jena laid the foundation for modern light microscopy, a young student in Berlin, Paul Nipkow (1884) figured out how to transfer a 2-dimensional optical image into an electrical signal that could be transmitted as a one-dimensional or serial, time-dependent signal (as in a Morse code) over a single cable. Prior to Nipkow, attempts at electrical transmission of optical images involved the use of multiple detectors and as many cables.

Nipkow dissected the image by scanning the image in a raster pattern, using a spinning opaque wheel perforated by a series of rectangular holes. The successive holes, placed at a constant angle apart around the center of the disk but on a constantly decreasing radius, i.e., arranged as an Archimedes spiral, generated the raster scanning pattern (Fig. 3). The brightness of each image element, thus scanned as a raster, was picked up by a photocell. The output of the photocell, reflecting the brightness of the sequentially scanned image elements, drove a neon bulb that, viewed through another (part of the) Nipkow disk, produced the desired picture.

The same type of scanner disk (but with multiple sets of spirally placed holes) was used by Mojmir Petráň (pronounced Petrah'nyu) and coworkers at Prague and New Haven to develop their tandem scanning confocal microscope (Egger and Petráň, 1967; Petráň et al., 1968). In Petráň's microscope, holes on a portion of the spinning disk placed in front of the light-source collector lens, are imaged onto the specimen by the objective lens. Each point of light, reflected or scattered by the specimen thus illuminated, is focused by the same objective lens onto a centro-symmetric portion of the "Nipkow disk." The pinholes at this region exclude the light originating from points in the specimen not illuminated by the first set of pinholes, thus giving rise to confocal illumination.

The tandem scanning microscope, as with Nipkow's initial attempt at television, tends to suffer from the low fraction of light that is transmitted through the source pinholes. Also, very high mechanical precision is required for fabricating the "Nipkow disk" and for spinning it exactly on axis. Some of the advantages pointed out by Minsky for the stage-scanning type confocal optics are also lost, since the objective lenses are no longer focusing a single axial point of light. But, for biological applications the tandem scanning system provides the decided advantage that the specimen remains stationary.

Unlike the stage-scanning system, the specimen in the tandem scanning confocal microscope does not have to be moved. Instead, the stationary specimen is scanned by the focused, flying spots of light. In addition, with the tandem scanning type, the speed of raster scan is not limited by the mass of the specimen support as in the stage scanning type described earlier. Nor is the raster scan limited by the speed, accuracy, and efficiency of the scanning devices, as it is in the laser scanning types. Thus, with a tandem scanning confocal microscope, one can observe objects that reflect or scatter light moderately strongly in real time, using either a television camera, or by observing the image directly through the eyepiece.

In addition to Petráň and coworkers, Alan Boyde (1985a) in London has taken advantage of the good axial discrimination and light penetrating capability of the tandem scanning confocal microscope. He pioneered the use of this type of microscope for biological objects, in particular for penetrating hard tissue such as bone and teeth to visualize the cells and lacunae found in these light scattering tissues (see Lewin, 1985). Boyde also provides striking stereoscopic images obtained with the tandem scanning confocal microscope (1985b, 1987, and Chapter 15).

More recently, Gordon Kino and his coworkers at Stanford University have designed a confocal microscope using a Nipkow disk in a manner that differs somewhat from the Petráň type (Kiao and Kino, 1987; also see Chapter 10, this volume). In the Kino type, the rays illuminating the specimen and those scattered by the specimen traverse the *same* set of pinholes on the spinning Nipkow disk rather than those which are centrosymmetric. By using a special, low-reflection Nipkow disk, somewhat tilted to the optic axis of the microscope, and crossed polarizers and a quarter-wave birefringent plate to further reduce the spurious reflections, they are able to use only one side of the disk, thus alleviating some of the alignment difficulties of the Petráň type. The confocal images shown by Kino at the 1989 EMSA conference were impressive indeed.

Electron-Beam Scanning TV

While Nipkow's invention laid the conceptual groundwork for television, raster scanning based on a mechanical device was simply too inefficient for practical television. Thus it was not until five decades after Nipkow, following the advent of vacuum tube and electronic technology, that Zworykin (1934) and his colleagues at RCA were able to devise a practical television system. They developed the image iconoscope, an image storage type, electron-beam scanning image pickup tube. The image iconoscope, coupled with a cathode ray tube for picture display, provided very rapid, "inertialess" switching and scanning of the image and picture elements. With these major breakthroughs, television not only became practical for broadcasting, but it emerged as a tool that could be applied to microscopy (see Inoué, 1986, Sect. 1.1 and 1.2).

An early application of video (the picture portion of television) was the flying spot UV microscope of Young and Roberts (1951). With this microscope, the specimen remains stationary and single object points are scanned serially by the reduced image of a spot of light (UV), flying in a raster pattern on the face of a special, high-intensity cathode ray tube. The brightness of the flying spot of light modulated by the specimen

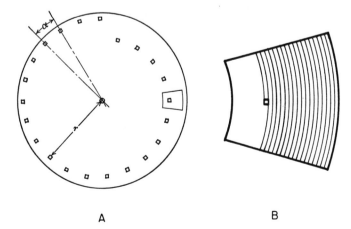

A   B

FIG. 3 Nipkow disk. The perforations in the opaque disk (A, which is rotating at a constant velocity), scan the image in a raster pattern as shown in (B). (From Inoué, 1986.)

is picked up by a phototube and the signal is amplified before it is displayed on another cathode ray tube scanned in synchrony with the source cathode ray tube.

Young and Roberts point out that by illuminating only a single specimen point at a time with a flying spot microscope, flare is reduced and the image becomes a closer rendition of the specimen's optical properties compared to that obtained with a non-scanning type microscope. They also point out that for these same reasons—and because a photoelectric detector can provide a sequential, linear output of the brightness of each specimen point—quantitative analysis becomes possible with a flying spot microscope. Additionally, they note that the electronic light detector raises the sensitivity of image capture by perhaps two orders of magnitude compared to photography.

It should be noted that the flare that would otherwise arise from the unilluminated parts of the specimen is significantly reduced with a flying spot microscope (see legend to Fig. 1; also Sheppard and Choudhury, 1977), even though the exit pinhole used in a confocal microscope is not present. Thus, for example, Wilke et al (1983) and Suzuki and Hirokawa (1986) developed laser scanning flying spot microscopes (coupled with digital image processors) to raise image contrast (at video rate) in fluorescence, DIC, and bright field microscopy. Naturally the exit pinhole in a confocal system very much more effectively excludes the unwanted light arising from different layers or portions of the specimen not currently illuminated by the source "pinhole", albeit at considerably reduced image brightness, speed of scanning, and at increased instrument complexity and price.

While the flying spot, or beam-scanning, microscope was developed and applied in UV microscopy for about a decade after Young and Roberts developed it, its further development as an imaging device was eclipsed for some time by the need and the opportunity to develop automated microscopy for rapid cell sorting and diagnosis. Here, the aim was not the imaging of cell structures as such, but rather the rapid and efficient classification of cells based on their biochemical characteristics and taking advantage of the emerging power of high-speed digital computers. The size, shape, absorbance, light scattering, or light emission of cells [labeled with specific (fluorescent) markers] was used either to classify the cells by scanning the slide under a microscope or to sort the cells at very high rates as the cells traversed a monitoring laser beam in a flow cell.

Impact of Modern Video

Meanwhile, starting in the late 1970s, the introduction of new solid state devices, especially large scale integrated circuits and related technology, led to dramatic improvements in the performance, availability, and price of industrial grade video cameras, video cassette recorders, and display devices. Concurrently, ever more compact and powerful digital computers and image processing systems appeared in rapid succession. These advances led to the birth of modern video microscopy, which in turn brought about a revitalized interest in the power and use of the light microscope (for reviews see Allen, 1985; Inoué 1986, 1989b).

In brief, dynamic structures in living cells could now be visualized with a clarity, speed, and resolution never achieved before in DIC, fluorescence, polarized light, dark field, and other modes of microscopy; the gliding motion, growth and shortening of individual molecular filaments of microtubules and f-actin could be followed in real time, directly on the monitor screen; and the changing concentration and distribution of ions and specific protein molecules could be followed, moment by moment, in physiologically active cells.

In addition to its immediate impact on cellular and molecular biology, video microscopy and digital image processing also stimulated the exploration of other new approaches in light microscopy along several fronts. These include the development of ratio imaging and new reporter dyes for quantitative measurement of local intracellular pH, calcium ion concentration, etc. (Bright et al., 1989; Tanasugarn et al., 1984; Tsien, 1989 and Chapter 16); the computational extraction of pure optical sections from whole-mount specimens in fluorescence microscopy (based on deconvolution of multi-layered images utilizing the microscope's point-spread function; Agard and Sedat, 1983; Agard et al., 1989; see also Chapters 13 and 14); 3-dimensional imaging including stereoscopy; (Åslund et al., 1987; Brakenhoff et al., 1986, 1989; Inoué, 1986, Sects. 11.5 and 12.7; Inoué and Inoué, 1986); and, finally, the further development of laser scanning microscopy, and confocal microscopy.

LASERS AND MICROSCOPY

Holography

In 1960, Maiman announced the development of the first operative laser. However, "his initial paper, which would have made his findings known in a more traditional fashion, was rejected for publication by the editors of *Physical Review Letters*—this to their everlasting chagrin." (For historic accounts including this quotation and a comprehensive discussion of the principles and application of lasers and holography, see Sects. 14.2 and 14.3 in Hecht, 1987.) Shortly thereafter, two types of applications of lasers were sought in microscopy. One took advantage of the high degree of monochromaticity and the attendant long coherence length, the distance over which the laser waves could be shifted in path and still remain coherent enough to clearly display interference phenomena (note that, in fact, this reflects a very high degree of temporal coherence). This high degree of monochromaticity and extremely long coherence length, or temporal coherence, made the laser an ideal source for holography (Leith and Upatnieks, 1963, 1964).

To explore the use of holography with the microscope, Ellis (1966) introduced a conventional light microscope into one arm of the split beam from a laser. When this beam was combined with another beam passing outside of the microscope, the two beams could be made to interfere in a plane above the ocular. The closely spaced interference fringes were recorded on very fine grained photographic film to produce the hologram.

What Ellis found was that the coherence length of the laser beam was so long that the hologram constructed as described above could be viewed not only to reconstruct an image of the specimen being magnified by the microscope, but also to reconstruct images of the inside of the microscope. Indeed, in the hologram one could see the whole optical train and interior of the microscope, starting with the substage condenser assembly, the specimen, the objective lens and its back aperture, the interior of the body tube, and up to the ocular and even the light shield placed higher. This made it possible for Ellis to view the hologram through appropriately positioned stops, phase plates, etc., and to generate contrast of the specimen in imaging modes such as darkfield illumination, oblique illumination, phase contrast, etc., after the hologram itself was recorded. In other words, the state of the specimen at a given point of time could be reconstructed and viewed after the fact in contrast modes different from the one present when the hologram was recorded.

In principle, holomicrography presents many intriguing possibilities including 3-dimensional imaging. But the very virtue of the long coherence length of the laser beam means that the hologram also registers all the defects and dirt in the microscope. Without laser illumination, these defects, or optical noise, would be far out of focus. With the laser illuminating the whole field of view of the microscope, the interference fringes from these out-of-focus defects intrude on the holographic image of the specimen where they are prominently superimposed. Because of this problem, holomicrography has so far not been widely used. (However, see Sharnoff et al, 1986, who have figured out how to obtain holomicrograms that display only the changes taking place in the specimen over an interval of time, and thus eliminate the fixed-patterned optical noise.)

Laser Illumination

Another practical application of lasers in microscopy is its use as an intense, monochromatic light source. Lasers can produce light beams with very high degree of monochromaticity, which implies a high degree of coherence. Some lasers also generate beams with very high intensity. Thus an appropriate laser could serve as a valuable light source in those modes of microscopy where monochromaticity and very high intensity and/or high degree of coherence of illumination are important.

However, to use the laser as an effective light source for microscopy, three conditions must be satisfied: (a) the field of view and the condenser aperture must appropriately be filled; (b) the coherence length of the laser beam (i.e., the temporal coherence) must be reduced to eliminate interference from out-of-focus defects; and (c) the coherence at the image plane must be reduced to eliminate laser "speckles" and to maximize image resolution. (In fact, these are not three totally independent conditions since they are interrelated, but they do specify the conditions that must be met.)

One of the four following approaches can be used to fulfill these conditions (See also Chapter 6):

1. The laser beam, expanded to fill the desired field, is passed through a spinning groundglass diffuser placed in front of the beam expander lens (Hard et al., 1977). The ground glass diffuses the light so that the condenser aperture is auto-

matically filled. If the ground glass were not moving, small regions of its irregular surface would act as coherent scatterers and the field would be filled with laser speckles; spinning or vibrating the ground glass diffuser cuts down the temporal coherence of each of the coherent scatterers to periods shorter than the integration time of the image sensor. Thus the field becomes uniformly illuminated. This approach, while simple to understand, can result in considerable light loss by the use of the diffuser. Also, inhomogeneity of the diffuser's texture can give rise to concentric rings of varying brightnesses which traverse the field.

2. The laser beam is focused onto the entrance end of a single-stranded optical fiber whose output end lies at the focal point of a beam expanding lens. The lens projects an enlarged image of the fiber tip to fill the condenser aperture. The fiber, which is fixed at both ends, is vibrated at some point along its length. The field and aperture are then uniformly filled with incoherent light without loss of intensity (Ellis, 1979). If the fiber were not vibrated, the simple fact that the light beam is transmitted through the fiber could make the laser beam highly multimodal; that would reduce the lateral coherence of the beam at the aperture plane. But the field would still be filled with speckles. The vibration reduces the temporal coherence of the beam below the integration time of the image sensor and integrates out the speckles without loss of light.

3. The field is scanned by a minute focused spot (the diffraction image) of a single-mode laser beam which has been expanded to fill the condenser aperture (as in a laser scanning confocal microscope). Since the field is scanned point by point (sequentially in a raster pattern), the temporal and spatial coherence of the laser beam is reduced at the field plane. In the laser scanning confocal microscope, the field is generally scanned by deviating the laser beam with a "scanner" placed at the conjugate of the aperture plane (Figs. 4, 5); thus the beam essentially remains coherent at the aperture plane while it is made incoherent in the field plane (see Chapter 5).

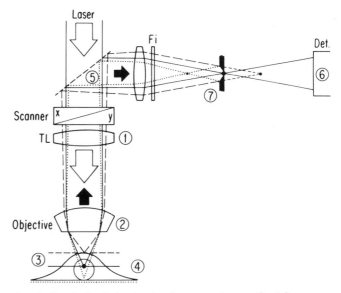

FIG. 5 Depth discrimination in a laser scanning, confocal fluorescent microscope. Compare with Fig. 2. (Courtesy of Dr. H. Kapitza, Carl Zeiss, Oberkochen.)

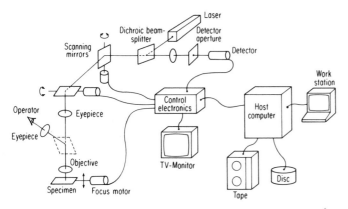

FIG. 4 Schematic of laser scanning confocal microscope. (From Åslund et al., 1987.)

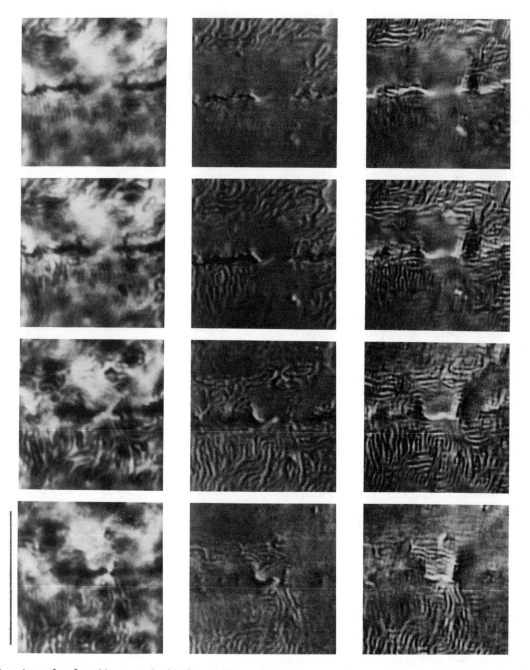

FIG. 6　Optical sections of surface ridge on oral epithelial cell. These ultrathin optical sections were obtained without confocal imaging in phase contrast (left), rectified DIC (middle), and rectified polarized light microscopy (right). The foci for the successive frames in each contrast mode were incremented 0.2 μm. Scale bar 10 μm. (See text and original article for details. From Inoué, 1988.)

4. The condenser aperture is scanned by the minute diffraction image of a single-mode laser, focused by the beam expander which fills the field of the microscope. The specimen at any instant of time is thus illuminated by a collimated (tilted) beam of light emerging from the condenser and originating at the illuminated aperture point. Selected regions of the aperture are filled in rapid succession by the scanning spot, so that the whole field is continuously illuminated by collimated coherent beams at successively changing tilt and azimuth angles. The rapid scan of the aperture reduces the temporal coherence of illumination at the field to less than the response time of the image detector. Nevertheless, the lateral coherence is maintained for each instantaneous beam that illuminates the specimen (Ellis, 1988).

Ellis has argued the theoretical advantage provided by the fourth approach, i.e., aperture scanning microscopy, and has demonstrated its practical attractiveness. With aperture scanning, one gains new degrees of freedom for optical image proccessing, since the aperture function, or image transfer function of the microscope, can be regulated dynamically for each point of the aperture. As discussed later in connection with Fig. 6, the image resolution and the shallow depth of field that can be achieved with aperture-scanning phase-contrast microscopy is most impressive.

The third approach leads to field scanning microscopy. A focused spot of the laser beam can be made to scan the field as in a flying spot microscope, or the specimen can be moved and scanned through the fixed focus of the laser beam. Alternatively, an exit pinhole and scanners could be added to generate a laser scanning confocal microscope.

Laser-illuminated Confocal Microscopes

In the early 1970s, Egger and his coworkers at Yale University developed a laser-illuminated confocal microscope in which the objective lens was oscillated in order to scan the specimen. Davidovits and Egger obtained a U.S. patent on this microscope in 1972 (see review by Egger, 1989).

A few years later, Sheppard and Choudhury (1977) provided a thorough theoretical analysis on various modes of confocal and laser scanning microscopy. The following year Sheppard et al. (1978) and Wilson et al. (1980) described an epi-illuminating confocal microscope of the stage scanning type, equipped with a laser source, a photomultiplier as the detector, and with a novel specimen holder. The specimen holder, supported on four taut steel wires running parallel to the microscope axis, allows precise, z-axis positioning as well as fairly rapid, voice-coil-actuated scanning of the specimen in the x-y plane. Using this instrument, Sheppard et al. demonstrated the utility of the confocal system particularly for examining integrated circuit chips. By confocal imaging, optical sections and profile images could be displayed on the (slow-scan) monitor, over areas very much larger than can be covered in the field of view of the same objective lens by conventional microscopy.

These authors capitalized on the fact that the signal falls off extremely sharply, and the image is therefore completely dark, for regions of the specimen that are not in focus in the confocal system. For example, with a tilted integrated circuit chip, the portion of the surface within the shallow depth of field (at any selected z value) alone could be displayed, as a strip-shaped region elongated parallel to the axis of tilt. The background would be dark and devoid of structure. Conversely, by combining the x-y scan with a slow z-scan, they could bring the whole tilted surface into view simultaneously, since the image can then be built up as the sum of all of the strips in focus (Wilson and Sheppard, 1984; Wilson, 1985).

This was true even when the specimen surface was not a single tilted plane but was wavy or consisted of complex surfaces. In their monograph on Scanning Optical Microscopy, Wilson and Sheppard (1984) show shallow optical sections of insect antennae shining on a dark background. They also show (stereo-paired images of) the same object with the x-y scan summed over the z axis to provide an image with the depth of field vastly increased over that obtainable with the same NA objective lens without confocal imaging. In other words, the confocal system can either decrease or increase the depth of field without loss of resolution. In fact, the lateral resolution is actually improved by using confocal optics as mentioned earlier (see also Chapter 8). In addition, lacking the extraneous light contributed by out-of-focus objects, the contrast is dramatically improved and the image is brilliantly sharp.

Sheppard et al also managed to display different regions on the surface of an integrated circuit chip in intensity or pseudocolor corresponding to the height of the region. This is possible because the amount of light reflected by an (untilted) step on the surface of the chip and passing the second pinhole varies with the distance of the reflecting surface from the focal plane. The authors also showed, by processing the photoelectric signal electronically, how the edges of the steps alone could be outlined, or the gradient of the steps could be displayed in a differential-interference-contrast (DIC)-like image (Hamilton and Wilson, 1984). (For the basics of digital image processing, see, Castleman (1979), Baxes (1984), Gonzales and Wintz (1987), and Chapter 10 in Inoué (1986).)

The integrated circuit chip could also be displayed with contrast reflecting the nature of the local circuit elements, for example, with the variation in photon-induced current in the circuit superimposed on the confocal image of the chip.

LASER SCANNING CONFOCAL MICROSCOPE

The pioneering work of the Oxford electrical engineering group described above were followed in succession by Brakenhoff et al. (1979, 1985), Wijnaendts van Resandt et al. (1985) and Carlsson et al. (1985) in several European laboratories. These investigators developed the stage-scanning confocal microscope further, verified the theory of confocal imaging, and expanded its application into cell biology. (I shall defer further discussions on these important recent contributions to authors of the other chapters of this volume). In the meantime, video microscopy and digital image processing were also advancing at a rapid rate.

These circumstances culminated in the development of the laser scanning confocal microscope (Figs. 4, 5; Åslund et al., 1987) and publication of its biological application by Carlsson et al. (1985), Amos et al. (1987), and White et al. (1987). The publications were followed shortly by introduction of laser scanning confocal microscopes to the market by Sarastro, Biorad, Olympus, Zeiss, and Leitz.

With the exquisite and convincing illustrations of the power of the laser-scanning confocal microscope, White, Amos, and Fordham of the Cambridge group immediately enraptured the world's biological community. Here at last was a microscope that could generate clear, thin optical sections of fluorescence microscope images, totally free from out-of-focus fluorescence, from whole embryos and cells at NAs as high as 1.4. Not only could one obtain such remarkable optical sections of fluorescence images in a matter of several seconds, but x-z sections (providing views at right angles to the normal direction of observation) could also be captured and displayed on the monitor quite rapidly. A series of optical sections (stored in the memory of the built-in digital image processor) could be converted into, and displayed as, stereo pairs. The confocal, fluorescent optical sections could also be displayed side by side, with a (non-confocal) bright-field or phase-contrast image acquired concurrently using the transmitted, scanning laser beam. These images could also be displayed superimposed on top of each other, e.g., with each image coded in different pseudocolor. The two images would appear in exact register and would show no parallax, since (unlike in conventional epi-illuminating fluorescence microscopes) the same scanning spot generates both images.

IS LASER SCANNING CONFOCAL MICROSCOPY A CURE ALL?

With the impressively thin and clean optical sections that are obtainable, and the x-z sections and stereoscopic images that can neatly be displayed or reconstructed, one can be tempted to consider the laser scanning confocal microscope as a cure all. One may even think of the instrument as the single microscope that one should use in modern cell biology or embryology. How valid is such a statement, and what in fact are the limitations of the current instruments?

The latter topic will be covered from the standpoint of the fundamental limits of confocal imaging by Pawley in the next Chapter. Here I will comment on three topics: the speed of image or data acquisition, the depth of field in phase-dependent imaging, and some optical and mechanical factors affecting confocal microscopy.

Speed of Image or Data Acquisition

Several factors affect the time needed to acquire a usable image with a confocal microscope. Those include the type of confocal system used; the optical magnification and numerical aperture of the system; the desired quality of the image (lateral and axial resolution, levels of image gray scale, degree of freedom from graininess, etc.); and the amount of light reaching the sensor, etc. Here we will survey a few general points relating to the choice of instruments, specifically as applied to biology.

Among the different confocal systems, the stage-scanning type requires the longest time (ca. ten seconds) to acquire a single image because the massive specimen support has to be translated very precisely. For biological specimens that often are bathed in a liquid medium, the movement, if allowed, may have to be even slower (even with the specimen chamber completely sealed and with gas phase excluded to minimize the inertial effects of stage scanning). The alternative lens-scanning system could be even worse. In addition, structures in the biological specimens are often moving or changing dynamically at rates incompatible with very slow scan. Thus, despite the many virtues of the stage-scanning system recognized by Minsky (1957) and by Wilson and Sheppard (1984), there is little chance that the stage scanning microscope would be used widely in biology. An exception might be with large area, 3-dimensional scanning of fixed and permanently mounted specimens that require or take advantage of those virtues of the stage-scanning system not provided by other types of confocal microscopes.

In the tandem-scanning (Petráň-type) or the Kino type confocal microscope, the disk can be spun rapidly enough to provide video-rate (30 frames/second) or near video-rate imaging. When speed of image acquisition is of paramount importance, as in the study of moving cells, living cells at high magnification, or microtubules growing in vitro, the type of speed provided by the Nipkow disk type system may be indispensable. For example, the Brownian motion of microtubules (even those many μm long) is sufficiently active at the approximately 10,000 times magnification needed for clear visualization, that image acquisition or integration time of 0.1 seconds or greater blurs the image beyond use.

As discussed earlier, the downside of the Nipkow disk type system is that the efficiency of light transmission is low, light tends to be reflected by the spinning disk, and the image may suffer from intrusive scan lines. Also, imaging would be by direct viewing through the ocular, via video imaging devices, or photography, rather than through a photomultiplier. Video imaging does have its own many advantages, but most video sensors (excepting chilled CCDs and special return-beam-type pickup tubes) operate within a limited dynamic range; conventional video pickup devices seldom respond linearly to light over a range beyond 100:1 and more commonly somewhat less (for example, see Inoué, 1986). In contrast, a photomultiplier tube can have a dynamic range of 10^6 or greater. When exceedingly weak signals need to be detected from among strong signals, or when image photometry demands dynamic ranges and precision beyond those attainable with video, an imaging system using chilled CCDs or photomultiplier detectors may have to be used. Modern stage-scanning and laser-scanning type confocal microscopes use photomultipliers as detectors.

The speed of acquiring a full frame image (or the sampling rate) of the laser-scanning confocal microscope falls somewhere between that of the stage-and tandem-scanning types. With the laser scanning confocal microscope, a single image scan is completed in 1 to 2 seconds. Note, however, that this sampling rate is the minimum time required by the mirror galvanometers (that are used to scan the illuminating and return beam) to produce a fully scanned image made up of about 512×512 picture elements. This limitation of scanning speed relates to the absolute time required for scanning along the fastest axis (usually the x, or horizontal-scan), and cannot be reduced without cost, for example to image resolution or confocal discrimination, by opening up the exit pinhole to increase the amount of light reaching the detector.

The scanning speed can be raised, e.g., by using a resonance galvanometer, a spinning mirror or an acousto-optical modulator instead of the linear mirror galvanometers that are commonly used (see Chapter 9). However, one sacrifices scan flexibility and efficiency of light use (per scan cycle). Furthermore, in a scanning confocal system used for fluorescence microscopy, the same acousto-optical (or any other diffraction-based electro-optical modulator) could not be used to scan both the exciting beam and the emitted beam, since the modulator would deviate (diffract) the two beams by different amounts.

Of even greater importance, the image captured by a laser scanning confocal microscope in a single scan time of 1 to 2 seconds is commonly too noisy; the image forming signal is simply not made up of enough photons. The image generally has to be integrated electronically over several frame times to reduce the noise, just as when one is using a very high sensitivity video camera. Thus, with a laser-scanning confocal microscope, it often requires several seconds to tens of seconds to acquire a well-resolved, high-quality fluorescence image.

If, in an attempt to reduce the number of frames that must be integrated, one tries to increase the flux reaching the photomultiplier, e.g., (for instance by raising the source brightness, by opening up the exit pinhole, or by increasing the concentration of fluorochrome), each alteration introduces new problems of its own. In fact, in laser-scanning confocal microscopes used for fluorescence imaging, one wants, if anything, to reduce the light reaching the specimen in order to avoid significant bleaching or other excitation-light-induced damage. There is almost an indeterminacy principle operating here: one simply cannot achieve high temporal resolution, combined at once with high spatial resolution, large pixel numbers, and large depth of gray scale simultaneously.

While the sampling rate for obtaining whole images with the laser scanning confocal microscope is limited, this does not imply that the temporal resolution of the detector system is inherently low. One can, for example, measure relatively high speed events with the laser scanning confocal microscope, if one decides to sacrifice pixel numbers, or the scanned area, and instead choose a line scan. In fact, Steve Smith at Yale (personal communication) has succeeded in obtaining line scans of fluorescence intensities in 2 msec, repeated every 6 msec with the Biorad instrument. He hopes to reduce the scan repeat time down to 2 msec in the near future. In addition to the high spatial resolution along the scan line that is retained, Smith notes a significant reduction in fluorochrome bleaching and photodynamic damage when the scan is restricted to a single line.

Another alternative for gaining speed is to use a slit instead of a pinhole for confocal scanning. This approach is said to be surprisingly effective in suppressing the contribution of out-of-focus objects (personal communication from Dr. Jeff Lichtman of Washington University; see also Chapter 19). Seth Goldstein of NIH (1989) and Watt Webb of Cornell University (personal communications) have used linear photodiode arrays as linear detectors to achieve similar results.

Depth of Field in Phase-Dependent Imaging

The depth of field measured for a confocal microscope with epi-fluorescence imaging is reported to be ca. 0.7 μm with an NA 1.4 objective lens at a wavelength of 488 nm or 514 nm (Amos et al., 1987), and not very much greater with an NA 1.3 objective lens used at a wavelength of 632.8 nm (Brakenhoff et al., 1979). These measurements are more or less in agreement with Equation (2), and the height of the 3-dimensional diffraction image discussed earlier. While confocal microscopes can also be used with differential phase imaging (e.g., Wilson and Sheppard, 1984, Sect. 4.4), I was unable to locate a report on the exact depth of field in this contrast mode.

How does the shallow depth of field attainable with a confocal microscope compare with that obtainable in the absence of confocal imaging? While I could come up with no hard numbers for fluorescence microscopy without confocal imaging, it is well known that the fluorescence from out-of-focus objects substantially blurs the image in focus. On the other hand, for contrast generated by phase-dependent methods such as phase-contrast, differential interference contrast, and polarized-light microscopy, I and Gordon Ellis have obtained data that show remarkably thin optical sections in the absence of confocal imaging.

Thus, using an $\times$100/1.4 NA Nikon Plan Apo objective lens, combined with an 1.35 NA rectified condenser [whose full aperture was uniformly illuminated through a light scrambler with 546 nm light from a 100 Watt high-pressure mercury arc source (as described in Ellis, 1985, and in Inoué, 1986, Appendix 3)], I obtained depth of fields of ca. 0.2, 0.25, and 0.15 μm respectively for phase-contrast, rectified DIC, and rectified polarized light-microscopy.

These values were obtained by examining video images of surface ridges that were present on a tilted portion of a human buccal epithelial cell. The video signal was contrast enhanced digitally but without spatial filtration. The change in image detail that appeared with each 0.2 μm shift of focus (brought about by incrementing a calibrated stepper motor) was inspected in the image, enlarged to ca. 10,000 times on a high resolution video monitor. As shown in Fig. 6, the fine ridges on the cell surface are not contiguous in the succeeding images stepped 0.2 μm apart in the polarized light and phase contrast images, but they are just contiguous in the differential interference contrast images. From these observations, the depth of field in the rectified polarized light image is estimated to be somewhat below, and the differential interference contrast image just above, the 0.2 μm step height. [The phase contrast images here should not be compared literally with the images in the two other contrast modes, since the diameter of the commercially available phase annulus was rather small, and the out-of-focus regions intruded obtrusively into the image. With Ellis' aperture scanning phase contrast microscope, where the illuminating points scan the outmost rim of the objective lens aperture, and where, essentially, the full NA of the objective lens is available to transmit the waves diffracted by the specimen, the high resolution optical section is even cleaner than with the two other contrast modes shown here (Ellis, 1988, and personal communication).]

We do not yet quite understand why the depth of field of phase-dependent images (of specimens which scatter light only slightly) should be so much thinner than the depth of field observed with fluorescence images in the confocal microscope or than the height of the unit 3-dimensional diffraction image [which is calculated for a point source imaged through an aberration-free lens with a uniform circular aperture; however, see the z-axis point spread function measured by Agard which also shows a much better contrast transfer function along Z than predicted by calculation (see Chapter 13)]. It may well be that contrast generation in phase dependent imaging involves partial coherence even at very high NAs, and that an effect similar to the one proposed elsewhere for half-wave masks (Inoué, 1989a) is giving us increased lateral as well as axial resolution. Whatever the theoretical explanation turns out to be, our observations show that for phase-dependent imaging of relatively transparent objects, even in the absence of confocal optics, one can obtain optical sections that are about three times thinner than for fluorescence imaging in the presence of confocal optics.

SOME OTHER OPTICAL AND MECHANICAL FACTORS AFFECTING CONFOCAL MICROSCOPY

Lens Aberration

With stage-, or object-, scanning confocal microscopes, we saw earlier that high NA lenses with simplified design and long working distances could be used because the confocal image points (source pinhole, illuminated specimen point, and second, or exit, pinhole) all lie along the axis of the microscope optics. This principle is now widely used in the design of optical disk recorder/players.

In contrast to the stage-scanning type, in the tandem-scanning and laser-scanning confocal microscopes, a sharp image of the source "pinhole(s)," focused by a stationary lens, must scan the specimen for a relatively large distance away from the lens axis. In addition, the objective lens and the scanner must bring images of the illuminated spot(s) and the source pinhole(s) into exact register with the exit pinhole(s) (and at different wavelengths for fluorescence microscopy).

For these systems to function efficiently, the microscope objective lens has to be exceptionally well corrected. The field must be flat over an appreciable area; axial and off axis aberrations must be well corrected for the expanse of the field; and lateral and longitudinal chromatic aberrations must be well corrected both for the illuminating and emission wavelengths. As far as is possible, the aberrations should be corrected within the objective lens without the need to use a complimentary ocular (see Chapters 7, 8 and 9). Finally, the lens and other optical components must have good transmission over the needed wavelength range.

These combined conditions place a strenuous requirement on the design of the objective lens. Fortunately, with the availability of modern glass stocks and high speed computer-optimized design, a series of excellent quality, high NA Plan Apo lenses have appeared in the last two years. The CF series Nikon ×60 and ×100/1.4 NA and the infinity-focused Zeiss ×63/1.4 NA, oil-immersion objectives are particularly impressive [the latter used with the proper "tube lens," which corrects the lateral chromatic aberration of the objective lens (see Chapter 7)].

Even with such excellent lenses, however, the image loses its sharpness when one focuses into a transparent, live, or wet specimen by more than about 15 to 20 μm from the inside surface of the coverslip. The problem here is that microscope objective lenses are designed to be used under rather stringent optical conditions. Standard oil-immersion objective lenses are designed for use with homogeneous immersion in a medium with a refractive index of 1.51. When we use such a lens on live or wet specimens immersed in water or physiological saline solution, even with the coverslip properly oil-contacted to the objective lens, aberrations are no longer properly corrected once the image-forming rays traverse a significant distance in the lower refractive index, aqueous medium. This distorts the unit diffraction image and alters the point-spread function, and does so to varying degrees as one focusses to different depths!

One approach to overcoming these problems is to switch to a water-immersion objective lens (D.A. Agard, personal communication, 1986). Then the cumulative depth of the water layer between the objective lens and the focused portion of the specimen remains unchanged with focus. Whether the objective lens is designed for homogeneous water-immersion or for use in the presence of a coverslip does not matter, so long as, in the latter case, a coverslip with proper thickness, refractive index, and dispersion is used.

While this approach does overcome some of the aberration problems, water-immersion lenses are generally not available with Plan Apochromatic corrections and cannot be made with NAs of much above 1.25 (because of the 1.33 refractive index of water). Since Plan Apochromatic correction is desirable, and the depth of field is reduced by the square of the NA, one would hope that well-corrected 1.4 NA Plan Apo oil-immersion objective lenses with appropriate correction collars would become available (for use with water or homogeneously immersed specimens). Adjustment of the collar, as in dry- or variable-immersion objective lenses, could compensate for the relative thickness of the higher and lower refractive index layers. With the increasing use of electronic and electro-mechanical controls in confocal and other types of microscopes, might it not be possible to design a superior high NA lens with an auto-compensating correction collar that is electronically linked to the fine focus control?

Unintentional Beam Deviation

The intensity of each point in the final image of a confocal microscope is supposed to measure the amount of light trans-mitted by the exit pinhole for the corresponding point in the specimen as it is being scanned in a raster pattern. If the amount of light reaching the opening in the exit pinhole is modulated by factors not related to the interaction of the illuminating point of light and the specimen at that raster point, or if the confocality between the entrance pinhole, illuminated specimen point and the exit pinhole were to be transiently lost for any reason, one would obtain a false reading for the brightness of that point.

One such error could be introduced if a localized, lens- or prism-shaped region with refractive index different from the surrounding, were accidentally present in the path of the scanning beam, e.g., a short distance above the focused region of the specimen. The scanning beam would then be refracted or deviated and the intensity of light reaching the detector would be falsely modified. Such a false signal could be difficult to distinguish from a genuine signal arising from the focused specimen plane. Also, the level of focus may be shifted by the presence of such refracting regions, so that one may no longer be scanning a flat optical section through the specimen.

Clearly, vibration of the microscope, and even minor distortions of the mechanical components that support the optics or the specimen, would tend to introduce misalignment between the two pinholes and what was supposed to be the confocal point on the specimen. This could lead to short-term periodic errors or longer-term drift. Anti-vibration tables that isolate the instrument from building and floor vibrations are commonly used to support confocal microscopes. While such a support is useful, and may be essential in some building locations, it does not eliminate the influence of airborne vibration, which can in fact raise major havoc in microscopy (G.W. Ellis, personal communication, 1966). Nor does it eliminate the influence of thermal drift, or vibration arising from within the instrument.

Given the need to precisely maintain the alignment of the confocal points, and to use some form of mechano-optical scanning within the instrument, a confocal microscope is especially susceptible to vibration and problems of mechanical distortion. Indeed, the success of a particular type of confocal instrument over another may well depend on the immunity of the instrument to such factors, once the other complex set of optical, electro-optical, mechanical, and electronic systems have been appropriately designed.

NOTE ADDED IN PROOF

Jim Pawley has wondered how one could store and utilize the large volume of 3D data generated by through-focal sectioning with confocal microscopy [see Taylor R. (1989), Confocal microscopy sheds new light on the dynamics of living cells. Journ. NIH Res. 1: 113–115]. At a recent conference on video microscopy, I gave a progress report on our effort towards 4D display of high-resolution light microscope images (i.e., 3D images that vary as a function of time) that may partly answer Jim's concern (Inoué, 1989). In my talk, I demonstrated a dynamic stereo display of high-resolution optical sections of Golgi-stained mouse neurons. The stereo images were generated from a stack of optical section stored on a laser disk recorder (OMDR, Panasonic TQ-2028F, Secaucus, NJ, capacity 16,000 images; picture can be recorded at video-frame rate of 30 Hz). The stack was converted to a set of stereo pairs viewed from different angles with an Image-1 processor (Universal Imaging

Corp., Media, PA) residing in an IBM PC-AT compatible 80386/25 computer. The stereo pairs, recorded back to the OMDR for playback, was projected through a StereoGraphics projector (StereoGraphics Corp., San Rafael, CA) for viewing by a large audience. The projected stereo images dynamically rotated back and forth and displayed the detailed, three-dimensional arrangement of neuronal spines on the dendrites.

ACKNOWLEDGMENT

I would like to thank the following individuals for their valuable comments during the preparation of this article: Drs. Gordon W. Ellis and John Murray, University of Pennsylvania; Dr. Stephen Smith, Yale University; Dr. Jeff Lichtman, Washington University; Dr. Sture Wahlsten, Sarastro, Inc.; Dr. Rudolf Oldenbourg, Brandeis University; and Dr. James Pawley, University of Wisconsin; also Dr. H. Kapitza of Carl Zeiss, Oberkochen, and Dr. N. Åslund of the Royal Institute of Technology in Sweden for kindly permitting me to use the figures provided by them.

REFERENCES

Abbe E (1873): Beitrage zur Theorie des Mikroskops und der mikroskopischen Wahrnehmung. Schultzes Archiv f. mikr. Anat. 9, 413–468.

Abbe E (1884): Note on the proper definition of the amplifying power of a lens or a lens-system. J. Roy. Microsc. Soc. (2) 4, 348–351.

Agard DA, Sedat JW (1983): Three-dimensional architecture of a polytene nucleus. Nature 302, 676–681.

Agard DA, Hiraoka Y, Shaw P, Sedat JW (1989): Fluorescence microscopy in three dimensions. In: Fluorescence Microscopy of Living Cells in Culture, Part B (Taylor DL, Wang Y-L, eds), Methods in Cell Biology, Vol. 30, pp. 353–377. Academic Press, San Diego.

Allen RD, Travis JL, Allen NS, Yilmaz H (1981a): Video-enhanced contrast polarization (AVEC-POL) microscopy: A new method applied to the detection of birefringence in the motile reticulopodial network of *Allogromia laticollaris*. Cell Motil. 1, 275–289.

Allen RD, Allen NS, Travis JL (1981b): Video-enhanced contrast, differential interference contrast (AVEC-DIC) microscopy: A new method capable of analyzing microtubule-related motility in the reticulopodial network of *Allogromia laticollaris*. Cell Motil. 1, 291–302.

Allen RD (1985): New observations on cell architecture and dynamics by video-enhanced contrast optical microscopy. Annu. Rev. Biophys. Biophysical Chem. 14, 265–290.

Amos WB, White JG, Fordham M (1987): Use of confocal imaging in the study of biological structures. Appl. Opt. 26, 3239–3243.

Åslund N, Carlsson K, Liljeborg A, Majlöf L (1983): PHOIBOS, a microscope scanner designed for micro-fluorometric applications, using laser induced fluorescence. In: Proc. of 3rd Scand. Conf. on Image Analysis, p. 338. Studentliteratur Lund.

Åslund N, Liljeborg A, Forsgren P-O, Wahlsten S (1987): Three-dimensional digital microscopy using the PHOIBOS scanner. Scanning 9, 227–235.

Baxes GA (1984): Digital Image Processing: A Practical Primer. Prentice-Hall, Englewood Cliffs, New Jersey.

Berek M (1927): Grundlagen der Tiefenwahrnehmung im Mikroskop. Marburg Sitzungs Berichte 62, 189–223.

Born M, Wolf E (1980): Principles of Optics (6th ed.). Pergamon Press, Oxford, England.

Boyde A (1985a): The tandem scanning reflected light microscope. Part 2—Pre-micro '84 applications at UCL. Proc. Roy. Micros. Soc. 20(3), 131–139.

Boyde A (1985b): Stereoscopic images in confocal (tandem scanning) microscopy. Science 230, 1270–1272.

Boyde A (1987): Colour-coded stereo images from the tandem scanning reflected light microscope (TSRLM). J. Microscopy 146(2), 137–142.

Brakenhoff GJ, Blom P, Barends P (1979): Confocal scanning light microscopy with high aperture immersion lenses. J. Microscopy 117, 219–232.

Brakenhoff GJ, van der Voort HTM, van Spronsen EA, Linnemans WAM, Nanninga N (1985): Three-dimensional chromatin distribution in neuroblastoma nuclei shown by confocal scanning laser microscopy. Nature 317, 748–749.

Brakenhoff GJ, van der Voort HTM, van Spronsen EA, Nanninga N (1986): Three- dimensional imaging by confocal scanning fluorescence microscopy. In: Recent Advances in Electron and Light Optical Imaging in Biology and Medicine (Somlyo A, ed), Vol. 483, pp. 405–414. Ann. N.Y. Acad. Sci., New York.

Brakenhoff GJ, van Spronsen EA, van der Voort HTM, Nanninga N (1989): Three- dimensional confocal fluorescence microscopy. In: Fluorescence Microscopy of Living Cells in Culture, Part B (Taylor DL, Wang Y-L, eds), Methods in Cell Biology, Vol. 30, pp. 379–398. Academic Press, San Diego.

Bright GR, Fisher GW, Rogowska J, Taylor DL (1989): Fluorescence ratio imaging microscopy. In: Fluorescence Microscopy of Living Cells in Culture, Part B (Taylor DL, Wang Y-L, eds), Methods in Cell Biology, Vol. 30, pp. 157–192. Academic Press, San Diego.

Cagnet M, Françon, M, Thrierr, JC (1962): Atlas of Optical Phenomena. Springer Verlag, Berlin.

Carlsson K, Danielsson P, Lenz R, Liljeborg A, Majlöf L, Åslund N (1985). Three-dimensional microscopy using a confocal laser scanning microscope. Opt. Lett. 10, 53–55.

Castleman KR (1979): Digital Image Processing. Prentice-Hall, Englewood Cliffs, New Jersey.

Castleman KR (1987): Spatial and photometric resolution and calibration requirements for cell image analysis instruments. Appl. Opt. 26, 3338–3342.

Cox IJ, Sheppard CJR (1983): Scanning optical microscope incorporating a digital framestore and microcomputer. Appl. Opt. 22, 1474–1478.

Cox IJ, Sheppard CJR (1986): Information capacity and resolution in an optical system. J. Opt. Soc. Am. 3, 1152–1158.

Davidovits P, Egger MD (1971): Scanning laser microscope for biological investigations. Appl. Opt. 10, 1615–1619.

Davidovits P, Egger MD (1972): U.S. Patent #3,643,015, Scanning Optical Microscope.

Egger MD (1989): The development of confocal microscopy. Trends in Neurosci. 12, 11.

Egger MD, Petráň M (1967): New reflected-light microscope for viewing unstained brain and ganglion cells. Science 157, 305–307.

Ellis GW (1966): Holomicrography: Transformation of image during reconstruction a posteriori. Science 154, 1195–1196.

Ellis GW (1978): Advances in visualization of mitosis in vivo. In: Cell Reproduction: In Honor of Daniel Mazia (Dirksen E, Prescott D, Fox CF, eds), pp. 465–476. Academic Press, New York.

Ellis GW (1979): A fiber-optic phase-randomizer for microscope illumination by laser. J. Cell Biol. 83, 303a.

Ellis GW (1985): Microscope illuminator with fiber optic source integrator. J. Cell Biol. 101, 83a.

Ellis GW (1988): Scanned aperture light microscopy. In: Proceedings of the 46th Annual Meeting of EMSA, pp. 48–49. San Francisco Press, Inc., San Francisco.

Fay FS, Fogarty KE, Coggins JM (1985): Analysis of molecular distribution in single cells using a digital imaging microscope. In: Optical Methods in Cell Physiology (De Weer P, Salzberg BM, eds). Wiley, New York.

Flory LE (1951): The television microscope. Cold Spring Harbor Symp. Quant. Biol. 16, 505–509.

Françon M (1961): Progress in Microscopy. Row, Peterson, Evanston, Illinois.

Freed JJ, Engle JL (1962): Development of the vibrating-mirror flying spot microscope for ultraviolet spectrophotometry. Ann. N.Y. Acad. Sci. 97, 412–448.

Fuchs H, Pizer SM, Heinz ER, Bloomberg SH, Tsai L-C, Strickland DC (1982): Design and image editing with a space-filling 3-D display based on a standard raster graphics system. Proc. Soc. Photo. Opt. Instrum. Eng. 367, 117–127.

Gabor D (1948): A new microscope principle. Nature 161, 777–778.

Goldstein S (1989). In: Digitized Video Microscopy (Herman B, Jacobson K, eds). Alan R. Liss, New York.

Gonzales RC, Wintz P (1987): Digital Image Processing (2nd ed.). Addison-Wesley Publishing Co., Reading, Massachusetts.

Hamilton DK, Wilson T (1984): Two-dimensional phase imaging in the scanning optical microscope. Appl. Opt. 23(2), 348–352.

Hansen GL (1969): Introduction to Solid-State Television Systems: Color and Black and White. Prentice-Hall, Englewood Cliffs, New Jersey.

Hard R, Zeh R, Allen RD (1977): Phase-randomized laser illumination for microscopy. J. Cell Sci. 23, 335–343.

Harris JL (1964): Diffraction and resolving power. J. Opt. Soc. Am. 54, 931–936.

Hecht E (1987): Optics (2nd ed.). Addison-Wesley Publishing Co., Reading, Massachusetts.

Hoffman R, Gross L (1975): Modulation contrast microscopy. Appl. Opt. 14, 1169–1176.

Hopkins HH (1951): The concept of partial coherence in optics. Proc. Roy. Soc. A 208, 263.

Ingelstam E (1956): Different forms of optical information and some interrelations between them. Problem in Contemporary Optics, Istituto Nazionale di Ottica, Arcetri-Firenze, 128–143.

Inoué S (1981): Video image processing greatly enhances contrast, quality, and speed in polarization-based microscopy. J. Cell Biol. 89, 346–356.

Inoué S (1986): Video Microscopy. Plenum Press, New York.

Inoué S (1988): Progress in video microscopy. Cell Motil. Cytoskel. 10, 13–17.

Inoué S (1989a): Imaging of unresolved objects, supperresolution, and precision of distance measurement, with video microscopy. In: Fluorescence Microscopy of Living Cells in Culture, Part B (Taylor DL, Wang Y-L, eds), Methods in Cell Biology, Vol. 30, pp. 85–112. Academic Press, San Diego.

Inoué S (1989b): Video enhancement and image processing in light microscope. Part I—Video microscopy. Part II—Digital image processing. American Laboratory, April, 52–70.

Inoué S (1989c): Whither video microscopy? Towards 4D imaging at the highest resolution of the light microscope. In: Digitized Video Microscopy (Herman B, Jacobson K, eds). Alan R. Liss, New York.

Inoué S, Inoué TD (1986): Computer-aided stereoscopic video reconstruction and serial display from high-resolution light-microscope optical sections. In: Recent Advances in Electron and Light Optical Imaging in Biology and Medicine (Somlyo A, ed), Vol. 483, pp. 392–404. Ann. N.Y. Acad. Sci., New York.

Koester CJ (1980): Scanning mirror microscope with optical sectioning characteristics: Applications in ophthalmology. Appl. Opt. 19, 1749–1757.

Kubota H, Inoué S (1959): Diffraction images in the polarizing microscope. J. Opt. Soc. Am. 49, 191–198.

Leith EN, Upatnieks J (1963): Wavefront reconstruction with continuous-tone objects. J. Opt. Soc. Am. 53, 1377–1381.

Leith EN, Upatnieks J (1964): Wavefront reconstruction with diffused illumination and three-dimensional objects. J. Opt. Soc. Am. 54, 1295–1301.

Lewin R (1985): New horizons for light microscopy. Science 230, 1258–1262.

Linfoot EH, Wolf E (1953): Diffraction images in systems with an annular aperture. Proc. Phys. Soc. B 66, 145–149.

Linfoot EH, Wolf E (1956): Phase distribution near focus in an aberration-free diffraction image. Proc. Phys. Soc. B 69, 823–832.

McCarthy JJ, Walker JS (1988): Scanning confocal optical microscopy. EMSA Bulletin 18(2), 75–79.

Minsky M (1957): U.S. Patent #3013467, Microscopy Apparatus.

Minsky M (1988): Memoir on inventing the confocal scanning microscope. Scanning 10, 128–138.

Montgomery PO, Roberts F, Bonner W (1956): The flying-spot monochromatic ultra-violet television microscope. Nature 177, 1172.

Nipkow P (1884): German Patent #30,105.

Nomarski G (1955): Microinterféromètre différentiel à ondes polarisées. J. Phys. Radium 16, S9–S13.

Petráň M, Hadravsky M, Egger D, Galambos R (1968): Tandem-scanning reflected-light microscope. J. Opt. Soc. Am. 58, 661–664.

Quate CF (1980): Microwaves, acoustic and scanning microscopy. In: Scanned Image Microscopy (Ash EA, ed), pp. 23–55. Academic Press, New York.

Sharnoff M, Brehm L, Henry R (1986): Dynamic structures through microdifferential holography. Biophys. J. 49, 281–291.

Sheppard CJR, Choudhury A (1977): Image formation in the scanning microscope. Optica 24, 1051.

Sheppard CJR, Gannaway JN, Walsh D, Wilson T (1978): Scanning Optical Microscope for the Inspection of Electronic Devices. Microcircuit Engineering Conference, Cambridge.

Sher LD, Barry CD (1985): The use of an oscillating mirror for three-dimensional displays. In: New Methodologies in Studies of Protein Configuration (Wu TT, ed). Van Nostrand-Reinhold, Princeton, New Jersey.

Smith LW, Osterberg H (1961): Diffraction images of circular self-radiant disks. J. Opt. Soc. Am. 51, 412–414.

Streibl N (1985): Three-dimensional imaging by a microscope. J. Opt. Soc. Am. A 2(2), 121–127.

Suzuki T, Hirokawa Y (1986): Development of a real-time scanning laser microscope for biological use. Appl. Opt. 25, 4115–4121.

Tanasugarn L, McNeil P, Reynolds GT, Taylor DL (1984): Microspectrofluorometry by digital image processing: Measurement of cytoplasmic pH. J. Cell Biol. 89, 717–724.

Tolardo di Francia G (1955): Resolving power and information. J. Opt. Soc. Amer. 45, 497–501.

Tsien RY (1989): Fluorescent indicators of ion concentration. In: Fluorescence Microscopy of Living Cells in Culture, Part B (Taylor DL, Wang Y-L, eds), Methods in Cell Biology, Vol. 30, pp. 127–156. Academic Press, San Diego.

White JG, Amos WB, Fordham M (1987): An evaluation of confocal versus conventional imaging of biological structures by fluorescence light microscopy. J. Cell Biol. 105, 41–48.

Wijnaendts van Resandt RW, Marsman HJB, Kaplan R, Davoust J, Stelzer EHK, Strickler R (1985): Optical fluorescence microscopy in three dimensions: Microtomoscopy. J. Microscopy 138, 29–34.

Wilke V, Gödecke U, Seidel P (1983): Laser-scan-mikroskop. Laser and Optoelecktron. 15(2), 93–101.

Wilson T (1985): Scanning optical microscopy. Scanning 7, 79–87.

Wilson T, Sheppard C (1984): Theory and Practice of Scanning Optical Microscopy. Academic Press, London.

Wilson T, Gannaway JN, Johnson P (1980): A scanning optical microscope for the inspection of semiconductor materials and devices. J. Microscopy 118, 390–314.

Xiao GQ, Kino GS (1987): A real-time confocal scanning optical microscope. Proc. SPIE, Vol. 809, Scanning Imaging Technology (Wilson T, Balk L, eds.), 107–113.

Young JZ, Roberts F (1951): A flying-spot microscope. Nature 167, 231.

Zernicke VF (1935): Das Phasenkontrastverfahren bei der mikroskopischen Beobachtung. Z. Tech. Phys. 16, 454–457.

Zworykin VK (1934): The iconoscope—a modern version of the electric eye. Proc. IRE 22, 16–32.

Chapter 2

Fundamental Limits in Confocal Microscopy

JAMES PAWLEY

Integrated Microscopy Resource, 1675 Observatory Dr., Madison, WI 53706

INTRODUCTION

The previous chapter described how the confocal approach developed from conventional light microscopy and outlined the basic advantages to be gained by the use of confocal sampling techniques. In this chapter I will discuss the fundamental considerations that limit the performance of all confocal microscopes. Though at present no commercially available equipment approaches these limits, I will describe some simple tests to help the user assess how closely a given instrument approaches the ideal.

What Limits?

The task of the confocal light microscope is to measure the optical or fluorescent properties within a number of small, contiguous sub-volumes of the specimen (Fig. 1). The fundamental limits on this process therefore are related to the quantitative accuracy with which these measurements can be made (n_2/n_1), the size $(\delta x, \delta y, \delta z)$ and position (x, y, z) of the sub-volume to be sampled, limitations imposed on the rate at which these measurements can be made by the effects of photo-damage to the specimen, source brightness and fluorescence saturation, and limitations imposed by the fact that the continuous specimen must be measured in terms of discrete volume elements called voxels (a voxel is the 3D equivalent of a pixel, which is the smallest element of a 2D image). This chapter will try to define the factors that ultimately limit the accuracy with which these measurements can be made. As such, it will serve as an introduction to a number of the chapters that follow, in which the practical and theoretical aspects of these problems will be discussed in greater detail. The discussion should be applicable to a consideration of all types of confocal microscopes, though here, as elsewhere in the this volume, microscopes in which scanning is accomplished by moving the beams(s) rather than specimen will be emphasized because they are more easily applied to living specimens. In some cases, differences between the mirror-scanning and disk-scanning instruments (including both tandem and single-sided disks) will dictate a separate consideration.

The data recorded from a confocal microscope will, in the simplest case, be a set of intensity values for every voxel throughout a 3-dimensional volume within the specimen. Though the data may often be displayed as an image, it should always be remembered that the confocal microscope is intrinsically a serial or sampling instrument not a parallel-imaging instrument. While it is true that we may choose to sample a plane by sequentially scanning the illumination over all of the points in that plane and that by doing so, we may produce an image, given sufficiently flexible equipment, we could also use the same total sampling (imaging) time to measure either a single point at a great many different times, a small volume within the sample, or indeed any collection of points within the specimen several times.

The distinction between sampling and imaging is, of course, not absolute; after all, most of us will view the final result as some sort of image. However, the distinction is still useful because it requires one to explicitly confront many problems that are not always so obvious when images are viewed visually or after photographic recording.

The sampling approach, which is covered in more detail in Chapter 4, allows an image to be built up from a number of individual measurements that reflect properties within specific regions of the sample. In the case that the measured properties are optical, the measurements involve counting photons and

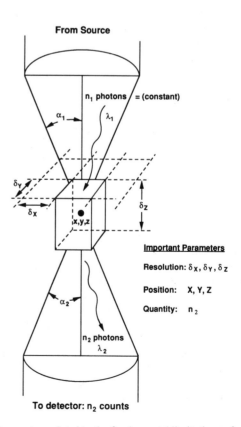

FIG. 1. Parameters related to the fundamental limitations of confocal microscopy.

this process implies limits on the accuracy and data rate usually not explicitly considered in normal microscopy. Factors that pose these limits are counting statistics, source brightness, and specimen response. These are discussed below.

Counting statistics

The accuracy of any specific measurement of fundamental quantum interactions is limited by Poisson statistics. Without going into the details, this means that if the same measurement is made repeatedly, and the average result of these measurements is N, the chance that any specific measurement is in the range of N $\pm$ $\sqrt{N}$ is 63%. For example, if N is 100, 63% of the measurements will be in the range from 100–$\sqrt{100}$ to 100 + $\sqrt{100}$ or between 90–110. Such a measurement is said to have 10% statistics. It can be seen that increasing the precision to 1% requires that N be increased to 100^2 or 10,000. While similar considerations limit the performance of all types of microscopical measurements, they are more explicit in their effect on confocal microscopy where photons are routinely counted individually.

Source brightness

There is a fundamental law of optics which states that the brightness of light in the image (measured in watts/cm²/steradian) can never be greater than that in the source. In the case of laser-scanning microscopes, the intrinsic brightness of the laser source is so high that this law does not present a practical limitation on performance (though degradation of the specimen may do so). However, it does pose a limitation on the performance of disk-scanning instruments, which currently use Hg arc sources and lose 99% of their intensity in passing through the disk. In the latter case, the source brightness and the optical design of the illuminating optics are crucial to being able to detect enough photons to produce a statistically well-defined fluorescence image in a reasonable amount of time. At present, narrow-band illumination emerging from the best disk-scanning instruments is at least an order of magnitude below that needed for them to compare with the laser instruments. Further improvement may require using large (5w), phase-randomized laser sources as described in Chapters 1 and 6.

Specimen response

In most cases it is safe to assume that photons interact with the specimen in a manner which is independent of the intensity of the illumination. However, this linear response may not be maintained at the high levels possible in laser-based confocal microscopes (see Chapter 16). Conceivable departures include the possibility that absorption in the specimen may cause sufficient warming to produce damage or that the electric field strength may become sufficient to produce a non-linear response, but the most obvious complication is the phenomenon of fluorescence saturation.

This phenomenon occurs when the flux of exciting illumination is so intense that, at any instant, a significant fraction of the fluorescent molecules are in the excited state. As excited molecules no longer absorb light at the usual wavelength, this has the effect of lowering the effective dye concentration and

reducing the fluorescent efficiency. This saturation threshold can easily be reached at the very high flux levels found in laser-scanning confocal microscopes (see Chapters 3, 5 and 16). The problem is more severe when using dye molecules with long fluorescent decay times or when the dye must be used at low concentration.

This fundamental limitation on the rate of fluorescent data acquisition can be side-stepped if the illuminating light is formed into more than one focussed spot on the specimen. However, to preserve confocal conditions, a separate pinhole and detector must be used for each spot, a condition present in the disk-scanning instruments. In addition to saturation limitations on data transfer rates, high light fluxes may effect the rate at which the fluorescent dye is bleached through a variety of complex mechanisms that while as yet imperfectly understood may in the end be sensitive to dose rate. (see Chapter 16).

A Typical Problem

To highlight the interactions between the limits imposed by counting statistics and more widely recognized limits such as spatial resolution, let us define a characteristic microscopical problem shown schematically in Fig. 2. The specimen is a cell in which some of the protein sub-units making up the cytoskeletal fibers have been replaced with fluorescent analogs. These fibers are very small, about ten times smaller than the resolution limit of light optics, and excitation of the fluorescent dye causes it to bleach, a process that is probably toxic to the cell. Because the object is to observe the formation and movement of the linear cytoskeletal elements within the living cell, we cannot take advantage of the higher spatial resolution of the electron microscope.

This example, though perhaps overly specific, is not uncharacteristic, and it has the advantage of highlighting most of the fundamental limitations that I wish to discuss. The important features of this example are as follows:

1) Observations will be improved by high spatial resolution.

2) Accuracy in measuring intensity will be important as it may permit determination of the number of linear polymers bundled together in each visible fiber.

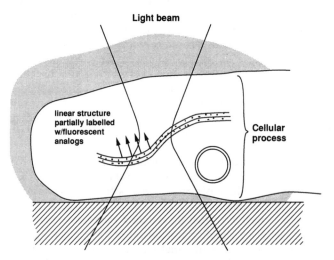

FIG. 2. Diagram of a notional specimen: a living cell process containing a filamentous structure smaller than the resolution limit and sparsely stained with fluorescent analog molecules.

3) A number of measurements will be necessary in order to show change and motion.

4) Each measurement will cause bleaching and cellular toxicity.

Clearly, these conditions contain an inherent contradiction: to obtain more quantitative temporal or spatial accuracy, we must pass more light through the sample but this will produce more fading and cytotoxicity, which will reduce the biological reliability of the measurement.

There are also other interactions between the parameters. High spatial resolution implies that the sampling points must be very close together or preferably partially overlapping. Because the measurement at each point can be reduced to the detection of some fraction of the small number of fluorescent excitations taking place while this point is illuminated, higher spatial resolution implies either a reduction in the average number of events counted per measurement (hence a reduction in the statistical accuracy of each measurement) or an increase in the total dose delivered to the imaged region of the specimen by the probing beam. Changes in the required dose are not insignificant: maintaining the statistical accuracy of the measurements when the desired resolution increases by a factor of two will require four times more dose in order to image a single image plane and eight times more dose if a 3D volume is to be sampled.

This interaction of statistical accuracy and spatial resolution can be emphasized by refining and simplifying our experimental example. Suppose the sampling beam scans over a single fluorescent fiber and that, as it does so, a fixed number of photons (n) are emitted. The electronic signal resulting from the detection of these photons will approximate a noisy Gaussian pulse on a background signal produced by nonspecific fluorescence and dark current in the photomultiplier tube (PMT) Fig. 3a. The width of this pulse will depend on the optical performance of the system, while the area of the pulse above the background will be proportional to n. Fig. 3b shows the same situation except that, by better alignment or improved optical performance, the spatial resolution of the system has been increased by a factor of two. As a result, the Gaussian pulse is, of course, narrower. But of more interest is the fact that, as the pulse area remains the same, the peak is higher; hence it is more easily detected above the background signal level because the signal-to-noise ratio (S/N) is higher.

This implies that a lower total dose could have been used to detect the fiber in the high resolution instrument. While this is true in part, another problem becomes evident when we try to reduce the PMT signal to a series of numbers in the memory of a computer. To do so requires breaking the continuous PMT signal into a number of digitizing intervals, then determining and recording the average value of the PMT voltage during each interval. Clearly, the results of this procedure will depend on whether the peak of the light pulse arrives near the center of such an interval (Fig. 3c) or at the boundary between two intervals (Fig. 3d). The fiber will be detected above background more easily in the former case than in the latter. The only reliable way to avoid this sort of problem, (which is discussed in more detail in Chapter 4) is to make the sampling interval smaller and accept the concomitant $2\times$ increase in the dose required per line to maintain a given S/N. It is worth noting, however, that in this case the increased dose at least results in improved spatial resolution in the pixel data, but this effect

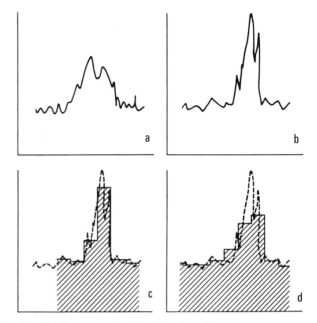

FIG. 3.   The fluorescent signal produced as a beam passes over a small ($< 0.1~\mu$m) feature, (a), changes as the beam diameter is reduced by a factor of two (b). The assumption is made that the illumination has been adjusted to elicit the same number of photons in each case. However, while the area under each curve is approximately the same, the peak in (b) is more readily distinguished from the noise background. Maintaining this easy distinction as the signal is digitized however, depends on whether the peak signal coincides with the center (c) or the boundary (d) of a digitizing interval.

decreases as the sampling interval becomes smaller than about one half of the optical resolution of the system.

Given the interrelated constraints highlighted by these examples, the two features needed for a confocal microscope to approach its ultimate performance are as follows:

1) *Photon Efficiency:* The system must count as many as possible of the photons transmitted or emitted by the sample.

2) *Spatial and Temporal Resolution*: The sampled volume should usually be as small as possible (though on occasion it may be advantageous to make this volume somewhat larger to avoid saturation or photodamage effects).

These two topics will now be discussed in more detail.

PRACTICAL PHOTON EFFICIENCY

Although photons can be lost both between the light source and the sample or between the sample and the detector, those lost before reaching the sample can usually be replaced with relative ease by an increase in source brightness. (As noted above, such an increase is more difficult when using the disk-scanning approach.) Those lost after leaving the sample represent a more fundamental loss, as they carry information obtained at the expense of radiation damage.

Current instruments waste photons in a number of straightforward ways, some of which are discussed in the remainder of this section. Two possibly less obvious ones are worthy of mention here.

Almost any specimen backscatters some light. In most present instruments used in the fluorescent mode, this light is reflected back to the source by the dichroic beam-splitter and thereby wasted. As pointed out in Chapter 9, a second (perhaps polarizing) beam-splitter between the source and the dichroic can selectively remove about 50% of this signal, thereby providing a simultaneous backscattered signal perfectly aligned with the fluorescent image(s). Most importantly, this image is obtained at no price in terms of radiation damage to the specimen (Fig. 4).

This second example of "unused light" is that elicited by the laser during line retrace in raster scanning instruments. As the results of the interaction between this light and sample are not detected, it represents a significant (30%) and unnecessary assault on the specimen. Fortunately, it can be eliminated by gating the light source during retrace using an acousto-optical modulator (K.S. Wells, personal communication). Unfortunately, such a feature is not yet available on commercial instruments (see also Gratton, Chapter 5).

Light can be effectively lost after the sample through several mechanisms:

1) absorption or scattering in either the objective lens, the medium that couples it to the specimen, or by the fixed and/or moving mirrors and transfer optics needed to scan the beam (see also Chapters 3 and 7 and 9).

2) incorrect alignment of the optical system resulting in the improper placement or orientation of the pinhole (see also Chapters 3, 8 and 11).

3) low quantum efficiency of the photon detector (see also Chapter 12).

4) imprecise digitization of the output of the photon detector (see also Chapter 12).

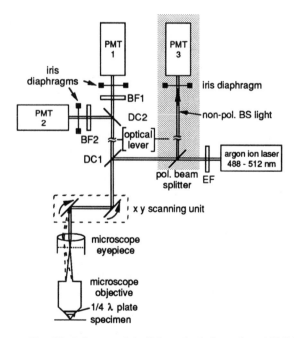

FIG. 4. Simplified diagram of the light path of a Lasersharp MRC-500 with the addition of a "permanent" channel for detecting backscattered light (stippled box). The polarizing beam-splitter (angle shown only schematically) permits polarized light from the laser to pass, but deflects scattered light from the specimen, because this light has passed twice through the ¼ wave plate incorporated into the objective. Regardless of the type of scattering in the specimen, at least some of this light is now at ~90° to the original laser light and is deflected to PMT-3. Such a system permits sensing the backscattered light signal whenever the specimen is illuminated without subjecting it to additional radiation.

While these subjects will be covered in much more detail in the chapters noted above, I wish to make a few points here as a background to descriptions of the practical tests of performance that I will describe.

Losses in the Optical System

Objectives

Although measuring the transmittance of objective lenses at full NA in absolute terms is far from simple (see Chapter 7), useful comparative measurements can be made on epi-illuminated instruments with significantly less trouble. All that is needed is a photo-diode light sensor, a sensitive current meter (or better, a basic photometer), and a front-surfaced mirror. After adjusting the instrument to measure backscattered (reflected) light and fitting objective lens A, measure the light emerging from it with the sensor (be sure to exclude stray light from the room and to couple the lens to the sensor with immersion oil if this is appropriate). This light reading is I_a. Now place the mirror, slightly tilted, on the specimen stage and set-up the microscope to image using backscattered (reflected) light. Be careful to keep the illumination level low so as not to damage the PMT or other detector. Focus on some dust on the mirror. Because of the slight tilt, the surface will only be near focus (bright) along a broad band. Use the computer controls to measure the peak brightness (B_a) of this band and that of some dark area (b_a) well away from the band. (b_a is a background reading to compensate for nonspecific reflections in the optical system, etc. A reading of zero indicates that the black level control is incorrectly adjusted.) Some microscopes produce severe specular reflection artifacts when used in the backscattered light mode: make your measurements in a part of the image field unaffected by these reflections. Also be sure to adjust the PMT gain so that you are well within the linear region of the digitizing system (about "half-full" or 128 counts in an 8-bit system).

Now change lenses and make a second set of measurements I_b, B_b and b_b without changing the PMT gain.

To a reasonable approximation, the comparative transmission (T) of the first lens as a fraction of the second will be the following:

$$T = \frac{I_b(B_a-b_a)}{I_a(B_b-b_b)}100\% \qquad (1)$$

Mirrors

A similar set-up can be used to test the performance of the internal mirrors on most microscopes. Again, the light intensity leaving the objective, I_a, is measured. Then the beam is stopped at the part of the scan when it is focussed on the mirror surface (brightest) and a second reading is made (after turning off the PMT!) with the photo-diode placed just in front of the pinhole (P_a) making sure that all of the light strikes the sensitive part of the sensor. P_a will often be a depressingly small fraction of I_a (10%) but the difference does cover losses at the various mirror surfaces, including the beam splitter (50–60% loss on each pass) and possibly at the eyepiece, and the various transfer lenses, as well as those in the objective.

Though indirect, such a measurement is useful for two reasons: 1) as a rough method of comparing the performance of different instruments (or different types of mirrors fitted to the same instrument) and 2) to monitor performance of an instrument over time. Performance can be degraded by the accumulation of dust on the mirrors by the slow deposition of hydrocarbon or other vapours from the atmosphere. In instruments having up to 11 reflective surfaces in the detector chain, a change in reflectance of even one or two percent can have marked effects on photon efficiency (see Chapter 3).

Pinhole

Is the confocal pinhole a "good thing?" It is argued by some, including the authors of Chapter 14, that the pinhole is the Achilles' heel of the confocal approach because it excludes photons which, while not originating from the plane of focus, do still carry relevant information regarding that plane because of the non-point nature of the focused optical probe. Leaving aside modifications to the detector (noted in the next segment) that would allow photons from nearby planes-of-focus to be separately collected in a confocal instrument, the contention that light from out-of-focus planes contains information deserves some consideration. (In the discussion that follows, all non-confocal images will be composed of light from both in-focus and out-of-focus planes while confocal images consist of light from *only* in-focus planes. The argument turns on when and to what extent the out-of-focus light can yield information regarding a 3D structure *beyond* that contained in the in-focus light.)

Let us take some examples. I think most will agree that an out-of-focus image of a point object will be a wider and less intense image than an in-focus one and furthermore, that a knowledge of the optical-transfer-function of the system, together with information from adjacent planes as to whether the actual plane of focus was above or below the plane containing the point object, will allow us to use computer signal-processing techniques to substantially improve the quality of the out-of-focus image. Supposing then that only this out-of-focus image was available, we might be justified in saying that this image had provided information as to the actual location of the object (i.e. in-focus information). But beyond that, would we be justified in saying that this would be a significant addition to the information present in an image of the plane containing the object (the in-focus image)? In other words, is the out-of-focus information useful only because we lack in-focus information?

Another aspect of measurement in which non-confocal techniques will give a more accurate estimate is, for instance, a measurement of the total fluorescence of the specimen. For a given dose to the specimen, the non-confocal technique can be more accurate simply because it will detect more total photons.

On the other hand, there must be some limit to the extent that light from sources outside the in-focus plane can provide information about that plane. For instance, suppose the specimen is 20μm (or 60 optical planes) thick and that the signal in a particular vertical column is confined to 10% of these voxels (six voxels equally spaced on planes 1, 12, 24, 36, 48 and 60). It is true that if we used a non-confocal microscope to focus on plane 30, equally spaced between the middle two bright voxels, we would obtain some information about the vertically adjoining voxels, and even some about those on planes 24 or 36. However, it seems unlikely that we can discern much about those on planes 1 and 60, especially in the presence of signal from the other four planes.

If we make the example more reasonable by putting only 50% of the total signal in the six voxels and distributing the remainder as background, it becomes more difficult for the non-confocal techniques to match the confocal approach even when images from all planes are collected and can be processed together. Assuming that the non-specific fluorescence is also present in neighboring columns of voxels, it will contribute a signal to the non-confocal image almost equal to that of a bright, in-focus voxel (the exact value will depend on the illuminating optics and the N.A.). Though processing can subtract the average value of this background signal from the non-confocal in-focus signal, the statistical photon noise associated with the remainder will still be higher than that associated with a measurement of the in-focus signal alone.

As a final example, consider a backscattered-light image of a tooth in which virtually every voxel scatters light. In such a dense specimen, the fraction of the signal originating from the in-focus plane is so small and so uniform that even detecting it using non-confocal imaging and signal processing would be extremely difficult, and the suggestion that the out-of-focus signal actually contributes information *beyond* that available in the in-focus or confocal image seems difficult to support.

The question then becomes: Up to what level of signal density or sparsity can information about the specimen (as distinct from signal) be gained from out-of-focus light? The answer will not be a simple one, as it depends on a number of practical factors apart from the sparsity of the staining, such as: How well one knows the optical response function of the microscope and how it changes with z; relative amounts of specific and non-specific staining and the exact effects of applying non-linear image processing algorithms such as non-negativity (see Chapter 14). Interesting results from the non-confocal/image-processing approach are also shown in there but, because of the relatively poor photon efficiency which characterized the first generation of commercial confocal microscopes, no meaningful side-by-side comparison has yet been possible.

My own feeling is that little, if any, additional, useful information will be gained from the out-of-focus light as long as: 1) bright voxels are each capable of producing at least 10 detectable photons when the voxel is in-focus in the confocal instrument, 2) both instruments are designed and adjusted in accordance with the sampling and photon-efficiency criteria proposed in this book, 3) the detector pinhole is kept at the size needed to demonstrate a lateral resolution equal to that of a non-confocal instrument with the same NA etc..

This will be increasingly true as the total number of planes sampled (or imaged) is reduced.

Features of the Confocal Pinhole In a confocal microscope the pinhole is present to prevent light originating from anywhere but the plane of focus from reaching the detector. It is mounted in an image plane and, if it is misaligned or if its size is reduced beyond that corresponding to a diffraction-limited spot on the sample, then it will severely reduce the number of photons reaching the detector while producing only a marginal improvement in X-Y or Z resolution. Making the pinhole larger than the diffraction-limited spot allows more photons to be detected at the expense of resolution. As will be explained in Chapters 8 and 11, choice of the proper size and shape for the pinhole is a sensitive function of the objective lens NA and magnification. However, even an "optimum" aperture will exclude at least some photons, (those present in the outer rings of the Airy disk) and this represents a fundamental cost of using the confocal pinhole.

Detection and Measurement Losses

The detector

The detector characteristics of most importance to photon efficiency are:

1) *Quantum efficiency:* the proportion of the photons arriving at the detector which actually contribute to its output signal. (This may be a strong function of the wavelength of the detected photons, Fig. 5.)

2) *Noise level:* This includes both additive noise, in the form of PMT dark current or amplifier electronic noise and multiplicative noise in the form of random variations in the actual digital output signals derived from identical input photons.

The PMT   Though the PMT is the most common detector used in the laser-scanning instrument, it is not necessarily the ideal detector. While the quantum efficiency of a PMT may be as high as 30% in the blue and green, this still means that 70% of the photons produce no signal. The quantum efficiency is much worse in the red and infrared and this may become more important if we must turn to long wavelengths in order to reduce phototoxicity.

The dark current of a PMT is low, but it is a strong function of the temperature and, in the heated confines of some commercial instruments, it may not always be small compared to the signal level of weakly fluorescent samples. Of more concern is the fact that output pulses from single photons may vary in size by an order of magnitude because of statistical effects on the small number of particles present in the early stages of the electron multiplier system (Fig. 6a). In addition, the digitizing circuitry found on many commercial instruments is poorly suited to quantitative applications in that identical pulses from a pulse generator are digitized as markedly different values depending on their time of arrival during the digitizing interval (Chapter 12 and Fig. 6b). Ideally, all photons should make an equivalent contribution to the output and as a result the output current would be exactly proportional to the number of photons. However, in practice, there is no way of knowing if the current sensed during a single digitizing interval corresponds to, for instance, one photon that happened to have made a large pulse or 3 photons that made smaller ones. This uncertainty

contributes to an equivalent noise term, called partition noise, and it can be a significant problem, particularly when only a few photons are counted per pixel.

This is true because the shape of the distribution of pulse sizes is fairly constant and as a result, the total summed area under say 100 pulses will probably demonstrate a variance which is small compared to that expected by statistical variations alone. (See Chapter 4.) On the other hand, images in which the brightest pixels represent only 10–30 counts, while the darkest vary between 1 and 0, can provide very useful information, and for such images pulse-counting as discussed below produces a significant improvement.

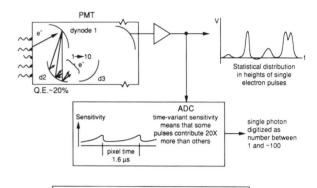

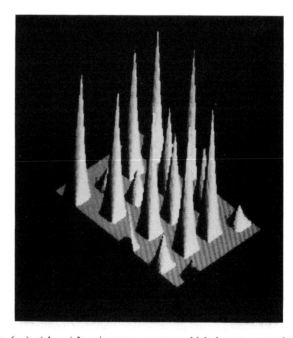

FIG. 6. a)   (above) In microscope systems which do not operate in the pulse-counting mode, two physical processes can add uncertainty to the measurement of the photon signal. Statistical variations in the number of secondary electrons produced during the early stages of electron multiplication in the PMT have the effect that identical photons can produce pulses which vary in height by a factor of 10. In addition, inappropriate design of the digitizing circuitry can have the result that even identical pulses from the PMT will be recorded as numbers that may vary by a factor of 20. Figure 6b (below) shows an intensity surface representing the pulse heights actually recorded by such a system when digitizing identical pseudo-guassian pulses from a signal generator. The overall result of both these processes is to add considerable uncertainty as to the actual intensity of the signal from the specimen.

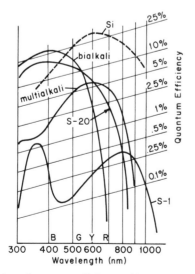

FIG. 5.   Variation of quantum efficiency with wavelength of some representative photo-cathode materials (solid lines) and of silicon photo-diodes (dashed line).

Finally, the PMT is a single channel device; it can give us a measure of only those photons that pass through the pinhole mask.

Solid-state photon detectors   The only practical alternative to the PMT is the solid-state detector, and this detector has both different capabilities and different problems. The quantum efficiency can be very high (70–80%) and extends well into the infrared (Fig. 5). Furthermore, each photon is recorded as an identical amount of current so there is no partition noise. Unfortunately, the detector must be cooled to −100°C and read out at the relatively low rate of 50k pixels/s to keep the noise level acceptably low (± 10 photons/measurement). This clearly is too high if the peak signal level is only 5 photons/pixel, as it is on many high-scan-speed laser instruments. It is less serious when the lowest signal is 100 photons/pixel because then statistical variations in this number are similar in size to the measurement noise. These features make the solid-state detector more suitable for slowly scanned images (100s/frame) producing high signal levels. Unfortunately, so far no solid-state detector has been optimized for this application.

In addition to high quantum efficiency, solid-state photon detectors have a variety of other potential practical advantages. As the sensitive element in such a detector is typically very small, selective use of only a few elements in a planar array could permit it to operate as a combination pinhole and detector. Pinhole alignment could be done electronically by simply searching for the detector element producing the most signal from a planar specimen. Likewise, the size of the pinhole could be adjusted on a size scale (5–20μm) compatible with operating at the intermediate image plane. Finally, a detector with concentric sensing elements could simultaneously acquire data at several effective pinhole sizes (see Chapter 11).

In the disk-scanning confocal microscopes, the image data emerges as a real image rather than as a sequence of intensity values from a single detector. This image can be detected photographically or by eye, but both of these sensors have very low quantum efficiency. Therefore, the only way for the disk-scanning instruments to approach the photon efficiency of the beam-scanning instruments is to incorporate a more efficient detector. This generally means either a sensitive vidicon camera or a cooled-CCD, solid-state image sensor having detection performance similar to that described in the last paragraph.

Digitization

As noted above, obtaining quantitative optical data is ultimately a question of counting photons. As intimated in the preceding section, this means not only using an electronic signal to which the largest fraction possible of the available photons have contributed, but also one to which the contribution of each photon is the same. In the case of the solid-state sensors, the uniformity condition is automatically met by the sensing process. This condition can also be met by the PMT if it is operated in a pulse-counting mode.

In pulse-counting, the object is not to measure the average level of the output current during the digitizing interval but rather to discriminate and actually count the output pulses resulting from the production of individual photo-electrons at the input surface of the PMT (Fig. 7). The problems arise when large numbers of photons must be counted in a short time. To reduce the effect of noise pulses generated from the dynodes of

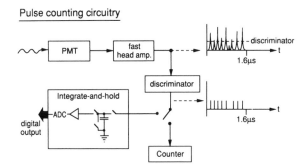

Pulse counting circuitry

FIG. 7.   Two alternative approaches to counting single photon pulses. In both the signal from a fast head amplifier is passed to a discriminator. Uniform pulses from the discriminator can either be counted with digital circuitry or integrated in a capacitor and then read-out through an analog-to-digital converter (ADC).

the PMT, photon pulses are passed through a discriminator; each time the PMT output goes above some preset threshold, one pulse is counted. Unfortunately, the PMT output does not immediately return to zero. If a second pulse arrives before the first one is over, the second or piled-up pulse, will be missed. Beyond the problem of pile-up there is the difficulty of actually counting the output from the discriminator at very high count rates (>5MHz).

Suppose a laser-scanning instrument scans a 512×512 raster in 40 seconds. Assuming 15 seconds for retrace, that leaves 100 μs/pixel. If we assume that each photon pulse takes $t_p = 0.5$μs, and that the brightest areas produce 200 photons/pixel (R), then the fraction of counts lost due to pulse pile-up (p) is

$$p = 1 - \exp\left(\frac{-Rt_p}{T}\right) = 1 - e^{-1} = 63\% \qquad (2)$$

Clearly this is unacceptable. Areas for improvement include the use of pulse counting PMT's, faster pulse amplifiers (shorter pulse widths) and improved counters. With regard to the latter, digital counters are not strictly mandatory. All that must be done in order to remove the multiplicative noise of the PMT is to integrate in a simple capacitor, a number of uniform pulses from the discriminator and then read out the capacitor voltage to an ADC and reset the capacitor voltage to zero (Fig. 7). It is also important to remember that piled-up losses are to some degree mathematically correctable and, furthermore, that they need not be reduced to zero, but merely made small, compared to the statistical noise.

Evaluating Photon Efficiency

All present instruments embody design compromises that prevent them from obtaining the ultimate in photon efficiency throughout the four processes discussed above. Mirror losses can be as much as 85% and the additional degradation imposed on the data by partition noise means that such systems may subject the specimen to 100× more exposure than should be necessary to produce a given image quality.

What is needed is a simple test of comparative performance to judge the effectiveness of various strategies for improvement. One possibility is to use luminescent uranyl glass as a test sample. Such a sample emits a low but constant flux of photons. If they are allowed to enter the objective lens of different instruments operating in the pulse-counting mode, differences in the

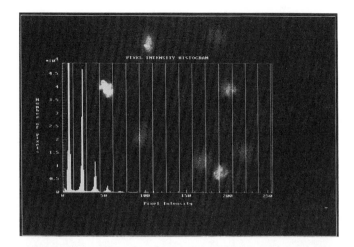

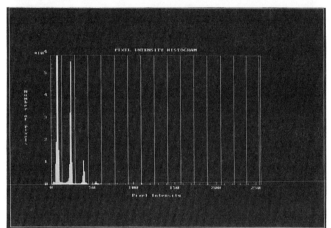

FIG. 8. Shows a histogram of counts vs pulse height from a MRC-600 operating in the new photon-counting mode. The digitizing intervals represented by the vertical lines can be adjusted to ensure that pulses representing 0,1,2, etc. photons are stored as distinct numbers. Initial versions of the system required that the PMT operate above its optimal voltage and this, plus a high level of stray light in the scanning box, had the effect that almost all the pulses counted represented noise pulses. This becomes evident if one compares the histogram in 8a (above) with that in 8b (below) which was made while the laser beam was obstructed as it left the mirror box. From the similarity of the histograms, it is evident that the majority of counted pulses do not represent photons elicited from the specimen. This problem is expected to be rectified in the near future.

mean count rate should give a measure of the relative efficiency of their internal mirrors and optics (the same objective lens should be used on all instruments). A comparison of the standard deviation of a number of such measurements made on a single instrument—first in the pulse-count mode and then in the analog mode—will give a measure of the quality of the detecting/digitizing system employed by the manufacturer. (An additional test is described in Chapter 12).

In response to this problem, BioRad has recently introduced its MRC-600 system. This system counts photons by discriminating the variable pulses from the PMT to produce 50 ns square pulses which are then integrated in a capacitor. The voltage on the capacitor is then read out into the ADC. The system is capable of counting 4–5 pulses per 1.6 μs pixel without significant pile-up losses. The digitizing intervals can be displayed, overlapped on a histogram of counts vs capacitor voltage

(Fig 8a) and then adjusted to separate pulses produced by 0,1,2,–- photons. Unfortunately, at the time of writing (12/89) the system requires the PMT to operate at a higher than optimal voltage (see Chapter 12, Fig. 8a) and there is a fairly high level of stray light present in the box. As a result, the majority of the pulses counted represent spurious signals. This technical problem is in no way fundamental and will undoubtedly be overcome in the near future. In any case, the MRC-600 represents a significant advance in the state of the art in photon counting in a confocal microscope.

RESOLUTION: HOW MUCH IS ENOUGH?

A peculiar feature of any properly aligned confocal microscope is that it is always "in focus," in that the exciting and detecting light paths are always focussed into a diffraction-limited spot. Details of the size and shape of the volume sampled in this way are dependent almost entirely on the design of the optical system (especially that of the objective lens), as is discussed below in Chapters 7 and 8. In addition, there is the trade-off between spatial resolution, statistical accuracy, and radiation damage, as outlined above.

Rather than continue with the straight-forward aspects of theoretical resolution, I will discuss in this section three other aspects that are perhaps less obvious, but which are both characteristic of confocal microscopy and which fundamentally limit the ability of the instrument to solve biological problems. These topics are:

1) Circumstances under which it may be desirable to reduce resolution,

2) The effect of image digitization on spatial and temporal resolution,

3) Practical considerations that may degrade resolution or produce distortion.

Can Resolution Be Too High?

Normally, the microscopist makes every effort to obtain the highest possible spatial resolution and, to the extent that the specimen is not degraded by being observed, this is entirely proper. Although, in the case of biological samples, the condition of non-degradation is never entirely met, such samples can be rendered very robust by treatment with anti-bleaching agents and fade-resistant dyes (Chapters 16 and 19). Agard and Sedat have used a cooled solid-state image sensor to record as many as 100 statistically well-defined, consecutive, non-confocal fluorescence images of a single nucleus without serious fading (Paddy et al, 1988, and see Chapters 8 and 13). Assuming similar photon efficiency, there seems to be no theoretical impediment to recording a similar series using confocal techniques. However, such fixed and chemically protected structures cannot be considered to be the general case and will be even less so as significant improvements are made in the photon efficiency of confocal instruments and they find more application on living specimens.

To determine when it may be advisable to intentionally reduce spatial resolution, it will be helpful to consider a second example: a living cell has been micro-injected with a substance which changes the spectral aspect of its fluorescent properties in response to the local concentration of certain ionic species.

The object of the experiment is to monitor changes in the concentration of these species as a function of time and experimental conditions. The major complication is that the dye is cytotoxic and this is especially true when it is excited by light. Furthermore, the fluorescence must be measured accurately at two different exciting wavelengths to determine the ion concentrations by ratioing the results. Significant changes in ion concentration are expected to occur on the scales of micrometers (or larger) and seconds (or longer).

How do we optimize the instrument to perform this experiment? Clearly the cytotoxicity problem implies 1) using a lens of large NA to collect as much light as possible, 2) using the lowest possible dye concentration, and 3) using a magnification such that, when referred to the specimen, a pixel is on the order of 1 micrometer square.

Yet undetermined are the amount of illuminating light that will be used and the number and accuracy of the measurements that are to be made. As we wish to measure changes, we can assume that the time available for each measurement is a constant, although the intensity of the illumination need not be. We know that both statistical accuracy and toxicity will increase with the intensity of the exciting beam. What we wish to know therefore, is how to arrange conditions to maximize the number of measurements that can be made before the cell is damaged. We will consider the case of a laser scanning instrument because this will bring into focus another important phenomenon: fluorescence saturation.

The need for ratio imaging implies a fairly short scan-time to avoid changes in the specimen between the two component images. The need for statistical accuracy implies an intensely illuminated spot to produce many countable photons, but saturation puts a limit on the maximum useful flux that can be used. Fortunately, the low spatial resolution required provides some flexibility. The flux of exciting illumination is highest at the neck of the cone formed by the objective lens and the diameter of this cone will be smaller (and the flux higher), when the full NA of the lens is used to form it. In the example we have described, however, the large NA was chosen only for high collection efficiency. As the pixel size is to be 1 micrometer, there is no need to focus the beam into a 0.2 micrometer spot. This would produce a maximum flux density 25 times greater than that present in a 1 micrometer spot and incur a proportionally greater risk of dye saturation. (Note: to insure that the signal is collected from the entire area of the larger spot, the pinhole size must also be enlarged.)

As is shown in Fig. 9, such an increase in spot size could be produced in two ways: 1) underfilling the aperture of the objective lens, thereby reducing its effective NA, or 2) using optics and apertures between the laser and the intermediate image plane to produce an effective source disk larger than a diffraction-limited spot. The former approach will reduce resolution in all directions while the effect of the latter is felt predominantly in the X-Y plane. In either case, considerable depth discrimination remains, and the confocal microscope retains all of the other desireable features, such as quantitative measurement accuracy and sampling flexibility, that make it ideal for studies of this kind.

The lesson here then is that because of the twin considerations of photo-damage and saturation it is often important to be able to adjust the image-forming properties of the instrument to produce a spot size appropriate to the experiment at hand.

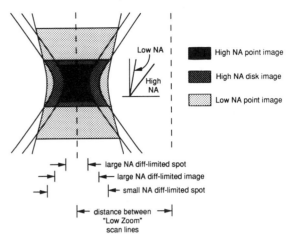

Control of Spot Size in CFM

High NA point image

High NA disk image

Low NA point image

large NA diff-limited spot

large NA diff-limited image

small NA diff-limited spot

distance between "Low Zoom" scan lines

FIG. 9. A schematic diagram of the way the volume most excited by a beam from a large NA, diffraction-limited lens (darkest stipple) can be expanded by either using a disk source rather than a point source (medium stipple) or by reducing the effective NA of the lens (lightest stipple).

At present this capability is only partially implemented on current commercial instruments.

Limitations Imposed by Spatial and Temporal Quantization

Although the image viewed in a disk-scanning confocal microscope is, in principle, as continuous as that from a nonconfocal microscope, this distinction from the other types of confocal microscopes is lost when the image is finally sensed using a video or a solid-state image sensor. The fact that the image must be recorded and treated in terms of measurements made within discrete pixels limits the effective resolution of the instrument in ways which may not be familiar to some who approach confocal microscopy for the first time. In a sense, these limits are more practical than fundamental because, if the microscope is operated in conformance to the rules of sampling theory as discussed in Chapter 4, they should not occur. At present, however, it is relatively easy to operate commercial instruments incorrectly, so a brief discussion of these limits is included here. They are mentioned under the heading "Resolution" because, although they do not involve the ability to discriminate two closely-spaced objects (δx, δy, δz), they do involve imprecision in the measurement of position (x, y, z).

Put simply, in a continuous image the edges of visible features can occur anywhere, but if this image is digitized, the edges are constrained to occur only at pixel boundaries. Normally the distortions produced by this process are not apparent in confocal images for two reasons: 1) such images tend to be oversampled—the size of the individual pixels (referred to the sample) is several times smaller than the optical resolution limit, and 2) the pixel intensities making up the images involve such a small number of quanta that statistical variations in the signal pose a greater limitation in measuring the position of the edge of a feature than does the quantization of the image in space.

Nonetheless, as applications of confocal technology more closely approach the absolute limits (for instance, by more closely matching the pixel size to that of the data deemed necessary and improving the photon efficiency to the point that the statistical noise is reduced) the costs of spatial (and temporal) quantizing will become more apparent.

These costs include

- *Aliasing effects*: The most easily understood limitation whereby spatial transitions in intensity are constrained to occur only at pixel boundaries, while the accuracy with which temporal changes can be detected is limited by the scan rate.
- *Mismatch of probe and pixel shape*: There is a mismatch in shape between the circularly symmetrical Airy disk of the probe and the square shape represented by a pixel in a rectangular raster.
- *Blind spots*: The design of the digitizer may leave the detector system dead for a significant and regular part of each digitizing interval and likewise the distance between scanned lines on the sample may be significantly more than the diameter of the probe. Both of these situations can lead to the signal from small features not being recorded.

Aliasing

The aliasing problem can be thought of as having both intensity and resolution components. The former, which was discussed in the first section, is associated with a reduction in the apparent intensity of a signal caused by its having been arbitrarily subdivided amongst two or more digitizing intervals. The resolution component, which is of interest in this section, has to do with imprecision in the measurement of the location (or motion) of the edges of objects associated with the process of quantizing the data in space and time.

In the case of a signal recorded by a cooled solid-state detector on a disk scanning system, I can make no suggestion that might simplify decisions regarding the optimal pixel size, beyond the optimal scanning theory of Crewe. (Crewe 1980) because the actual signal collection process spatially quantizes the signal in a manner entirely determined by the geometry of the planar detector and the total optical magnification. On the other hand, because the scanning mirrors in most laser-based systems follow ballistic rather than stepped trajectories, the output from the PMT of these instruments is, in principle, continuous in the horizontal direction. In other words, the signal from the PMT will increase exactly as the beam crosses the feature, regardless of whether this is later found to be at the edge of a pixel or not.

This fact provides some flexibility that might provide useful dividends. For instance, it is possible to digitize the signal twice using two clocks running at the original frequency but offset by one half of a pixel. The two sets of data would have to be stored in alternating locations of a memory having twice the original size and displayed on a monitor having higher resolution, but as the length of the digitizing interval of each measurement remains unchanged, the statistical accuracy of each data point would also remain unchanged. The effect of this system would be to allow more accurate localization of vertical lines without exposing the specimen to additional radiation. Because the pixel intervals overlap, the localization would be less accurate than that produced by simply increasing both the speed of the digitizing clock and the dose-rate by the factor of two. However, a small improvement ($\sim$30%) should still be possible as long as the two digitizing systems are well balanced; this should not be difficult if pulse-counting is used.

Pixel shape

Present commercial instruments in general use circular probes to elicit data which will eventually be displayed as square pixels. In the case of the laser scanning instruments, the situation is further complicated by the fact that the probing beam is continuously moving horizontally, and as a result, averaged over the digitizing time, the Airy disk is not even round but is effectively blurred in one direction. The limitations imposed by these approximations and the extent to which they can be ameliorated by the use of non-circular pinholes or improved digitizing techniques have yet to be fully determined. However, it is undoubtedly true that there are good reasons for using non-circular apertures for both illumination and detection when the pixel size is markedly larger than the diffraction limit of the objective lens. These matters are discussed at greater length in Chapters 4, 8 and 11.

Blind spots

When images are recorded on a "continuous" medium, there is no possibility that small but bright objects will be entirely missed. However, this is not true of sampling systems.

It is important to distinguish this problem from that of simply having an insufficiently small pixel size (referred to the specimen). The problem of blind spots refers to the fact that the system may be much less sensitive to signal emerging from some areas of the sample than that from others. In part, this can be attributed to mismatches between the diameter and shape of the probing beam and the distance between adjacent lines scanned on the specimen (undersampling), but the phenomenon of detector system dead-time is equally important. Unlike aliasing, blind spots are more likely to be a problem when the pixel size is much larger than the spot size.

Figure 6b illustrates the problem of deadtime. A series of identical pulses similar to single photon pulses from the PMT, has been fed to a digitizing system having significant dead time. The peak heights displayed in the figure are proportional to the values that the system has recorded for these pulses. The pulse arrival time is not synchronized with the digitizing clock so some pulses occur closer than others to the time at which the ADC cycles. Ideally all the pulses should be recorded as identical numbers from the ADC, but, as can be seen, the actual numbers vary by a factor of almost 20, depending on the match or mismatch between the arrival time of the pulse and the digitizing instant.

At best, such a system will add additional partition noise to the recorded signal (as detailed above). At worst, it may totally ignore small features that happen to be in the wrong place. In either case, digitization deadtime, as measured in this way, can unnecessarily limit the ultimate performance of a confocal imaging system (See Chapters 8 and 11 for a more complete analysis).

Practical Considerations Relating Resolution to Distortion

To obtain the theoretical spatial resolution of a confocal microscope, it is, of course, necessary to have a diffraction-limited optical system, but this is not sufficient. Leaving the practical aspects of alignment and optical quality for Chapters 7 through 11, I wish to discuss mechanical reliability and repeatability of the scanning system as it affects the performance of confocal microscopes because this allows me to highlight one of the most important differences between disk-scanning and laser-scanning instruments.

In disk-scanning instruments, the image is real and therefore cannot be distorted by the scanning system. If a solid-state sensor is used to detect it, geometrical distortion in the digitized image is extremely low and because of the inherent mechanical stability of the sensor, that distortion which remains can be corrected by digital image processing. The mechanical problems of this instrument are therefore confined to the effects of vibration and motion of the stage or lens.

In all confocal instruments, it is vital that relative motion between the objective and the specimen be kept to less than 10% of the resolution limit in X, Y, and Z. In the tandem instruments, both the rotating disk and the cooling system of the often-large illumination sources represent potential sources of vibration in addition to those normally present in the environment. They must all be maintained within tolerance levels or resolution will be degraded in a fairly straightforward manner.

Not so straightforward is the effect of vibration (and possibly stray electrical and magnetic fields acting either directly on the galvanometers or introducing spurious signals into the current amplifiers that control them) on the performance of the mirrors in the laser-scanning systems. In these instruments, accurate imaging depends on the mirrors causing the beam to scan over the sample in a precise pattern duplicating the mathematically perfect raster represented by the data locations in the image memory. Failure to duplicate this raster has the result that data will be displayed in the wrong pixel, producing distortion. On a system with a 1000-line raster and a 10:1 zooming ratio, keeping beam placement to within 1/10 of a pixel requires accuracy of one part in 10^5 (Fig. 10). No present systems preserve this level of performance even in the electrical signals used to drive their mirror-galvanometers, and the electro-mechanical properties of the galvanometers (mass, spring constant, frequency response, overshoot, resonant frequency, bearing tolerance, rigidity, etc.) can produce major additional errors. Image distor-

tions produced by these errors are often masked by the paucity of test samples having an accurately defined geometry and by the fact that, at high zoom, current instruments greatly oversample the image so the smallest, visible structural features are many pixels wide. (See also Chapter 17, Fig. 11)

This problem merits mention here because it is possible to measure the x, y, z position of the centroid of an object in a digital image to an accuracy of much smaller than the spatial resolution limit. Indeed, non-confocal light microscopy techniques have been used to measure motion on the order of 1 nm (Gelles et al, 1988). However, due to random imprecision in the systems used to position the mirrors, it is unlikely that measurements of similar reliability could be made on any present laser-scanning system. In this context, then, the accuracy and precision with which mirror position can be controlled is a fundamental limitation on the ability of laser-scanning confocal microscopes to determine position.

The presence of scan instability can be detected either by visually comparing sequential single-scan images of a diagonal knife-edge viewed at the highest possible magnification and contrast or, alternatively, by computing the apparent motion of the centroids of two fixed objects, each covering 100–200 pixels as they are recorded on a number of sequential scans. The variations measured by the second method should decrease rapidly with increasing illumination intensity because of improved statistical accuracy.

Another aspect of distortion becomes evident in Fig 11. In these images, the box in the low magnification image is centered on a feature. This feature is then scanned by applying the same voltages to the scanning mirrors that were present when the beam was being scanned over the box at low magnification. In

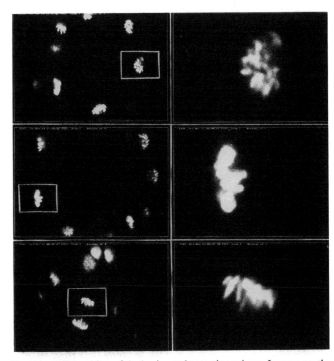

FIG. 11. Mistracking of the horizontal scanning mirror. Images on the left (a,c,e) show low magnification views with a superimposed box centered on features to the left, the right or centered. The right images were made by applying the voltages that were present while the low magnification image was scanning over the boxed area. The fact that the features are no longer centered in the field is a measure of the mistracking between the scan voltage from the computer and the actual position of the scan mirror.

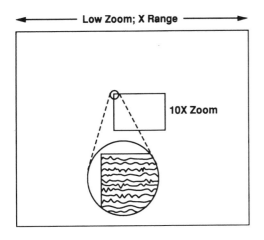

Low Zoom; X Range

10X Zoom

Jitter and distortion more important at (relatively) high NA / low mag

Mag	NA	# pixels / 20mm image field
10X	0.5	5000
100X	1.3	2000

FIG. 10. Effect of imperfections in the scanning system.

TABLE 1. LIMITATIONS OF CONFOCAL MICROSCOPY

Parameter	Theoretical		Practical
Resolution	Spatial:	Y $\lambda_1, \lambda_2, \alpha_1, \alpha_2$	Alignment, off axis aberrations
		X "	Alignment, off axis aberrations, bandwidth, ballistic scan
		Z " pinhole diam.	Alignment, off axis aberrations, Δ tube length
	Temporal:	Scan speed, signal decay times	Quantization of t
Position	Objective lens distortion Pixellation limitations Sampling time		Mirror accuracy, vibration
Quantitative measurement	Poisson statistics		Mirror and digitizing losses, detector DQE and noise, bleaching/photodamage, saturation, source brightness

the higher magnification images made away from the central vertical axis of the field, the position of the feature is no longer centered in the box, but is displaced in the direction away from the central vertical axis. This comes about because the horizontal galvanometer mirror is operating so close to its resonant frequency that its actual trajectory, while fairly linear, does not accurately track the theoretical sawtooth waveform assumed by the digitizing system. This is an important consideration when spot or vertical line illumination is to be used to monitor or bleach a specific area of the imaged specimen.

SUMMARY

I have attempted to highlight some aspects of confocal instrumentation that must be addressed in order to attain performance limited only by fundamental considerations (Table 1). Although I have addressed each of the constituent aspects of both photon efficiency and resolution separately, it has been evident that the effects of both of these factors overlap and interact in a fairly complex manner. To summarize, 1) All photons from the specimen should be counted as accurately as possible, 2) The system should work not only at a resolution limited by diffraction but also at larger spot sizes, 3) The effects of image quantization should not be ignored; if they are not at least somewhat evident, the image is probably over-sampled, 4) In laser-scanned instruments the relation between scanning precision and distortion can limit performance; and 5) Fluorescence saturation may place unexpected limits on the experiments that can be performed with the laser-scanning microscopes.

ACKNOWLEDGEMENTS

This chapter has benefitted greatly from my conversations with Sam Wells (Cornell) and Jon Art (Chicago) who also provided the images for Figs 7 and 10. Steve Paddock at the IMR was kind enough to help produce Fig 5b and Cheryle Hughes made the other drawings. This work was supported by salary funds from NIH Grant #00570–18 to the Madison Integrated Microscopy Resource.

REFERENCES

Crewe A.V. (1980) Theory of optical scanning in the STEM. Proc. EMSA 38:60–61.

Gelles J., Schnapp B.J., Steur E., & Scheetz M.P. (1988) Nanometer scale motion analysis of microtubule-based motor enzymes. Proc. EMSA 46:68–69.

Paddy M.R., Hiraoka Y., Chen H., Sedat J.W., & Agard D.A. (1988) A Structural overview of the nucleus as derived from CCD-based 3-D optical microscopy. Proc. EMSA 46:34–35.

Chapter 3

Quantitative Fluorescence Imaging with Laser Scanning Confocal Microscopy

K. Sam Wells, David R. Sandison, James Strickler and *Watt W. Webb

Developmental Resource for Biophysical Imaging and Opto-electronics, Applied and Engineering Physics, Cornell University, Ithaca, New York 14853

THE PROMISE OF SCANNING CONFOCAL FLUORESCENCE MICROSCOPY

Scanning confocal microscopy (SCM) offers a dramatic instrumental advantage for fluorescence microscopy through discrimination against out-of-focus background fluorescence, through inherent resolution perpendicular to the plane of focus and improved in-plane resolution. Quantitative measurements of fluorescence intensity in such images can provide precise image determinations of fluorescence marker distributions in three dimensions. This paper aims to define the realizable and ultimately limiting capabilities of SCM for quantitative fluorescence imaging.

The availability of selective, bright, fluorescent markers attached by monoclonal antibodies, specific ligand affinities or covalent bonds facilitates precise imaging of receptor concentrations with high specificity even in living cells. Bright, stable fluorophores provide high sensitivity. Fluorescent chemical indicators now provide measures of the chemical activity of Ca^{++}, H^+, Na^+, membrane potential, enzyme activity, and several additional species crucial in cellular activity. Spatial resolution at the diffraction limit in reconstructions of thick specimens should be obtainable by confocal fluorescence imaging. The dynamics of cellular chemistry should be observable in living cells using time series of fluorescence scanning confocal images.

These features, which promise significant improvement over conventional imaging methods, have yet to be realized with quantitative fluorescence SCM. The necessary criteria to achieve useful results are considered and the limitations and promise of scanning confocal fluorescence microscopy are appraised herein.

The crucial limitations of scanning confocal microscopy arise in essential features of photochemistry. A potential problem in fluorescence microscopy on living cells is photodamage by absorption of the radiation introduced to excite the fluorescence. To minimize this problem, the absorption of excitation radiation must generally be minimized. Confocal fluorescence microscopy alters the exposure chronology but does not inherently reduce the total exposure. However, fluorophore photochemistry becomes critical in SCM. Two fundamental features of fluorophore photodynamics—photobleaching of the fluorophore and saturation of the photoexcitation—impose strict limits on the method. The limitations these phenomena impose are all exacerbated by any inefficiency of fluorescence collection and detection including the inherent limitations of fluorescence microscopy and the additional fluorescence light losses incidental to the instrumentation for confocal scanning.

This paper presents preliminary analyses of these problems, presents some preliminary measurements of crucial parameters, reports the relevant properties of one typical commercial laser scanning confocal instrument (BioRad MRC-500) to illustrate the problems and, finally, offers some approaches to take maximum advantage of scanning confocal imaging for quantitative fluorescence image analysis.

Irreversible photobleaching limits the quantitation of fluorescence measurements. Usually, fluorescence emission even by the best fluorophore is limited to less than 10^5 photons per available fluorophore molecule. This is acceptable for recording individual two-dimensional qualitative images of specimens labeled with copious fluorescent stains. Measurements of specific selective stains for sparse species in living cells are more difficult. Compounding this problem is the low overall efficiency of collection and detection of fluorescence in the scanning confocal microscope. Even in the best conventional fluorescence microscopes less than 5% of the fluorescence emitted from within each resolution volume is detected. In laser scanning confocal microscopy (LSCM), we have found that this overall collection efficiency may easily be degraded to <0.1%. Therefore, the 10^5 photons emitted per molecule yield only about 100 total detected photons per fluorophore. For observation, imaging a 1 μm^2 area of a membrane stained with 100 fluorophores/μm^2 would provide ~1% measurement uncertainty in a single image which is usually quite satisfactory. However, SCM may be used to create a three-dimensional reconstruction of the fluorophore distribution of a translucent 3D specimen from a stack of 2D optical sections through a convoluted membrane structure. How the photobleaching accumulates in recording such a stack then becomes an important issue.

The illumination of a diffraction-limited spot in the object plane of a confocal microscope fills a converging cone as it passes through the specimen to reach the plane of focus and all, except the tiny fraction absorbed, passes out through a diverging cone. Thus, in the absence of intensity-dependent, nonlinear bleaching (see Chapter 16), the same amount of photobleaching occurs in all layers of the sample during the recording of each 2D section image. To assemble a 3D image of axial resolution r in a section of thickness R requires approximately $N = R/r$ sections, causing N times as much photobleaching as in a single 2D section. Therefore, the question of whether quantitative 3D fluorescence reconstruction will be improved by scanning confocal microscopy relative to conventional microscopy with optical transform methods will depend ultimately on

---

*To whom all correspondence should be addressed

the relative efficiencies of light collection and information utilization. The problem of fluorescence collection and detection efficiency thus becomes the major concern of this paper.

The stage-scanning confocal microscope (SSCM) offers strong optical advantages because all optical measurements are symmetric about the optic axis. Thus, the only extra optical element is a confocal aperture in an image plane (detector aperture). On the other hand, most of the full field of view of the optical system is utilized in LSCM. Compensating virtues of LSCM are that it allows much faster scan rates and the specimen remains stationary and accessible for manipulation. Because the greatest potential of quantitative fluorescence imaging is its application to the study of dynamic processes in living cells, it is appropriate to strive to retain the acquisition rate advantages of LSCM. An alternative instrumental approach employs disk-scanning confocal microscopy (DSCM). In that procedure, many dim illuminating beams serve in parallel. The analysis presented here will show results supporting the development of multi-beam alternatives.

The efficiency and accuracy of collection and detection of fluorescence radiation in quantitative scanning confocal microscopy is far more demanding of lens design than is scattering or refractive SCM. Chromatic aberration is the main problem. Confocality criteria must coincide for the exciting radiation wavelength and for the fluorescence wavelength; otherwise the confocal detector aperture excludes the fluorescence emitted from the conjugate confocal volume in the object plane that is most intensely illuminated by the diffraction-limited excitation beam. For stage-scanning microscopes, the problem is limited to repositioning the confocal detector aperture or refocusing to correct for chromatic aberration along the axis; for laser scanning instruments, the off-axis corrections may be more difficult. In LSCM, the off-axis curvature of field aberrations also introduce errors; they distort 3D image reconstruction, even in forming refractive images and the distortion disrupts measurements of planar objects as well.

The rate of fluorescence emission at low photoexcitation intensity is determined by the rate of absorption of excitation radiation times the quantum efficiency for fluorescence. At high enough excitation intensities, however, fluorophores will reside predominantly in the excited state and the fluorescence emission will be limited by the intrinsic rate of fluorescence emission, usually between 10^8–10^9 photons/s. For an effective dwell time of ~ 1 μs/pixel for formation of the scanning image, about 10^3 photons per fluorophore are emitted with less than one being detected per diffraction limited volume per scan. This raises the shot noise to the single quantum limit. Transitions to the metastable triplet excited state may further limit fluorescence emission. The effect of the saturation phenomena is to place a limit on the rate of fluorescence emission per molecule in SCM, which restricts the rate of useful image acquisition per confocal beam to rates less than those already obtainable by conventional fluorescence image acquisition methods. (See also Chapter 16.)

Diffraction limited excitation by more than a few mW of appropriate visible ion laser radiation saturates typical fluorophores. Therefore, far better fluorescence images have been obtained by integrating multiple scans at low excitation power than with 1 scan at full power (White et al. 1987). Saturation is the reason. This inherent limitation to image acquisition rate is lifted only by utilization of simultaneous confocal excitation beams as in DSCM or by very high fluorophore concentrations. Measurements of saturation effects on fluorescence are pre-

sented to demonstrate their ubiquitous presence under relevant operating conditions.

OPTICAL TRANSFER EFFICIENCY

The accuracy, sensitivity, precision and speed of measurement of the spatial distribution of fluorescent markers and indicators in LSCM depends in part on the efficiency of collection and the detection of fluorescence radiation from the image. Because laser-scanning confocal optics use most of the microscope field of view, the optical transfer efficiency both on-axis and off-axis is a crucial instrumental parameter. The total accessible information in the fluorescence image and its rate of acquisition depend on it. Photobleaching limits the number of photons and photosaturation limits the rate of emission of fluorescence photons. Therefore, the fraction of the emitted photons that are utilized must ordinarily be maximized in qualitative imaging experiments.

Fluorescence optical transfer efficiency in the laser scanning confocal microscope is subject to all of the losses of conventional microscopy and degraded further by losses in the scanning instrumentation and the slight losses specific to confocal optics. This section considers the factors affecting the optical transfer efficiency, reports new measurements of instrumental properties, describes some methods for measuring key parameters and identifies some problems that call for attention.

Measurements of Optical Transfer Efficiencies

We define the fluorescence Optical Transfer Efficiency (OTE) as the fraction of the fluorescence light emitted by fluorophores within the focal volume at the object plane that is detected by the photomultiplier tube. This efficiency usually varies with location in the field of view but the data here concentrate on the on-axis value. Later, the relative off-axis values will be considered. For an optical element, the OTE is simply the fractional transmission or fractional reflection.

A schematic diagram of the optical system of the BioRad MRC-500 LSCM is shown in Fig. 1 to identify the elements that are involved in determining the OTE. Since all optical elements function in series, the overall optical transfer efficiency for the system is the product of the OTE for each element. In conventional fluorescence microscopy, the elements determining the OTE are the collection efficiency and transmission of the objective lens, transmission of the eyepiece, any auxiliary lenses, filters, and the quantum efficiency of the photomultipliers. In the LSCM, there are additional losses associated with scanning and auxiliary mirrors. In addition, the confocal optical filtering may introduce losses due to chromatic aberration and curvature of field that might simply blur or distort images in conventional microscopy. This issue is considered more specifically in a subsequent section and in Chapter 7.

Table 1 shows the results of measurements of the transfer efficiency of each element of a commercial instrument, the BioRad MRC-500 LSCM. The overall fluorescence optical transfer efficiency of the instrument as measured with an efficient objective and fully open detector aperture is about 0.2% at best. That means that only 2 fluorescence photons are detected for 1000 emitted. (It is not ordinarily correct to attempt to record images with the detector aperture fully closed in this instrument where OTE $\sim 10^{-4}$.) In the corresponding conventional microscope the OTE is about 25 times larger at about 5%.

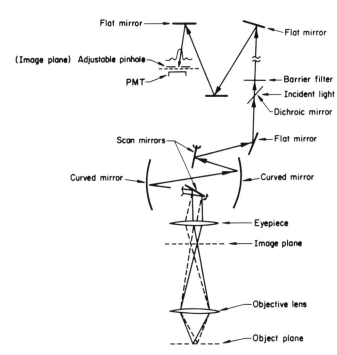

FIG. 1. Diagram of the optical path in the laser scanning confocal system (BioRad MRC-500). The optical surfaces where the light is collected and relayed are depicted, with their approximate relative orientations. The scan mirrors are located at conjugate aperture planes from which the path length to the detector aperture (field plane) is about 1.7 m. The curved mirrors allow the use of two orthogonal scan mirrors.

The principal losses in the Biorad MRC-500 laser scanning system are due to the low OTE of the flat relay mirrors and to the scanning duty cycle. In our instrument, the combined mirror OTE is about 0.32. Upgrade of the mirrors should produce an easy factor of three improvement in the light throughput of the laser scanning system. The duty cycle losses could be improved by blanking the laser during scan mirror deceleration and retrace. In both conventional and laser scanning confocal microscopy, the quantum efficiency of the photomultiplier tube can and should be improved substantially by appropriate photocathode optimization for the fluorescence wavelength. Improper electronic processing of the photomultiplier output may cause further losses particularly at low intensities where photon counting may become appropriate in some instruments. (See Chapter 12.) With sufficient intensity, a simple solution for avoiding electronic losses is to sample and digitize the photomultiplier current, after amplification and RC filtering, at a rate appropriate to match the scan rate and system resolution; about 1.6 μs/pixel for a 512×768 pixels/sec exposure. Photon counting may be appropriate in an apparatus designed for minimum dead time and having adequate dynamic range. With proper care, electronic losses can be negligible.

The photomultiplier is a source of inefficiency that can be only partially corrected. The tube in the BioRad MRC-500 that was tested contains a prismatic S-20 photocathode surface (model #9828B, Thorn EMI) which has a less than optimal quantum efficiency (QE) between 400 and 700 nm. The manufacturer specifies the QE to be ~0.13 to 0.03 for λ ~550 nm to 750 nm. These values should be improvable by a factor of about 2.

TABLE 1. OPTICAL TRANSFER EFFICIENCY (T.E.) FOR A LSCM SYSTEM

Optical Component	T.E.
*MRC-500 Mirrors	0.32
2 scan mirrors	
2 curved mirrors	
4 flat mirrors	
Nikon 8X Eyepiece	0.96
Objective Lens	0.5 to 0.95
Solid angle of collection	0.015 to 0.30
(NA = 0.25–1.4)	
Dichroic Mirror	0.75 to 0.9
(λ ~ 520 nm–700 nm)	
Barrier Filter	0.92
(λ ~ 540 nm–700 nm)	
S-20 PMT Quantum Efficiency	0.03 to 0.13
(λ ~ 550 nm–750 nm)	
Scanning Duty Cycle	~0.65
Dectector aperture Factor	0.05 to 1
(min.–max. diameter)	

Optimum overall fluorescence detection efficiency‡

Detector aperture max. diameter	0.002
Detector aperture min. diameter	0.0001

*MRC-600 mirrors have a combined T.E. of 0.7, increasing the total efficiency by 2.2.

‡ For λ emission = 600 nm, objective NA = 1.4, T = 0.65, PMT Q.E. = 0.06

The dominant unavoidable loss is the collection efficiency of the objective lens which varies as $[1 - \sqrt{1 - (NA/n)^2}]/2$, where NA is the numerical aperture and n is the refractive index of the immersion medium. With high magnification objectives now reaching NA = 1.4, nearly 1/3 of the fluorescence can be collected in suitable media. At sufficiently low excitation power, the rate of fluorescence photon emission per fluorophore molecule increases as $(NA)^2$ so the overall radiation detected per fluorophore molecule is proportional to $(NA)^2[1 - \sqrt{1 - (NA/n)^2}]/2$.

Methods of Measurement of Optical Transfer Efficiencies

The key to measurements of the optical transfer efficiencies reported in Table 1 is the use of a portable photodiode detector that can be inserted in the optical path of the LSCM to measure beam power at various points. With appropriate alignment and calibration, the ratio of beam power reaching the plane of the detector aperture to the incident power at the objective back aperture plane in the nosepiece, and various intermediate points could be measured without disassembly of the scanning mechanism. This LSCM system (Fig. 1) contains two orthogonal scanning mirrors, two curved mirrors, and four flats required to extend the optical path to the detector. The path to the detector is ~1.7 m in order to magnify the point spread of the object to a size, which can be accommodated with a conventional adjustable iris to serve as the detector aperture with a minimum diameter of ~1 mm and a maximum diameter of ~7mm. In our system the total magnification, with a 100× objective at zoom 1, is about 5500×.

The reflectivity of each mirrored surface was obtained by measuring the ratio of the reflected power to incident beam power with a large surface area photodiode (model #1723–06, Hammamatsu Corp.). The beam was obtained by steering the

LSCM laser through the bottom of the optical train to the scan mirror nearest the eyepiece plane (eyepiece removed). This allowed the laser beam to reflect off all of the mirrored surfaces simultaneously, in the absence of a filter pack.

The transmittance spectrum for a given objective lens is occasionally obtainable from the lens manufacturer; however, one can measure the objective transmittance directly by monitoring the exit and incident beam with a photodiode. Objectives were mounted on a spatial filter jig for access to the front and rear focal planes. The incident beam from a spectrofluorometer source was filtered for a single wavelength, collimated and passed through an aperture so that it just underfilled the objective back aperture (the incident light measured was not clipped at the aperture). Since photodiode responses are sensitive to incidence angle, the output of the objectives at the front focal plane were collected by a matched objective so the final output came out through the back aperture of the second objective as parallel radiation normal to the diode face. The only disadvantage of this method is the need for two identical objectives; however, once a good measurement or accurate manufacturer's value is obtained for one objective, the "calibrated" objective can be used to obtain calibrations for other objectives with nearly equivalent aperture dimensions and spectral characteristics. This can be done by ratioing the detector values for calibrated and uncalibrated objectives in the scanning microscope (see Chapter 2) without confocal optical filtering using a mirror or fluorescent dye for the sample.

Confocal Spatial Filtering for Depth of Field Compromises Optical Transfer Efficiency

In LSCM, the light approaching the detector surface is spatially filtered by the confocal detector aperture to select the depth of field. The ultimate theoretical confocal 3D imaging performance assumes a vanishingly small detector aperture (Wilson, 1988). The variable detector aperture provides the control of the depth of field and a small enhancement of lateral resolution. Resolution is gained at the expense of light collection efficiency by shrinking the aperture. Optimum overall performance can be achieved by judicious compromise of depth of field and associated background flare rejection to gain increased signal power for fluorescence applications. The following analysis of the dependence of depth of field, light collection efficiency and background flare rejection aims to show the trade-off amongst these parameters that is accessible by adjustment of the confocal detector aperture diameter (D_p).

Figure 2 shows the dependence of depth of field on D_p. Depth of field was measured as the full-width at half-maximum, $2\Delta Z_{1/2}$, of a point intensity profile along the optical axis by recording the light intensity collected from a small (<200 nm diameter) fluorescent bead with a Nikon planapo 60/1.4 oil-immersion objective as a function of object z-position along the optical axis for various values of D_p. The effect of the fluorescence Stokes shift on the depth of field is expected to be negligible compared with the other effects described here.

D_p can be expressed in dimensionless optical units (Born and Wolf 1983), $V_p = (2\pi/\lambda) (D_p/2)$ NA/M_t where λ is the wavelength of detected radiation, NA is the objective lens numerical aperture and M_t is the total magnification which is about 55 times the objective lens magnification in the BioRad MRC-500. The value NA/M_t is $\sim$ a/f, where a = the effective aperture plane radius and f = the effective distance to the image plane (detector aperture). These units, valid in the paraxial ap-

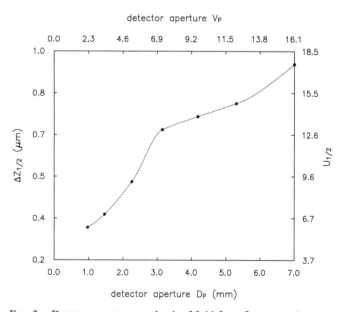

FIG. 2.   Detector aperture vs. depth of field for a fluorescent bead < 200 nm in diameter. The detector aperture diameter D_p is the measured quantity in mm and V_p is a dimensionless optical unit, which is proportional to the detector aperture radius. $\Delta Z_{1/2}$ is the measured half-width at half-maximum of the point intensity profile, measured along the optical axis (z), in microns. $U_{1/2}$ is a dimensionless optical unit which is proportional to $\Delta Z_{1/2}$. The depth of field is seen to decrease continuously with decreasing detector aperture size to a minimum of $\Delta Z_{1/2} \sim .35\ \mu m$, $U_{1/2} \sim 6.5$ at a detector aperture of $D_p \sim 1$ mm, $V_p \sim 2.2$. The inflection point near $D_p = 3$mm corresponds roughly to a detector aperture equal to the diameter of the Airy disk.

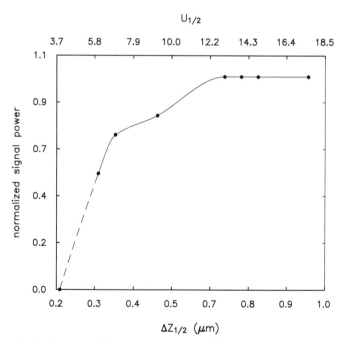

FIG. 3.   Integrated signal power vs. depth of field for a fluorescent bead <200 nm in diameter. The signal power was obtained by integrating inside the image area, for the x-y plane corresponding to the maximum signal in z, bounded by the half-maximum image intensity values and normalized to unity at the maximum signal obtained. $\Delta Z_{1/2}$ and $U_{1/2}$ are as described in Figure 2. The intensity is extrapolated to zero for a value of $V_p=0$, with the corresponding theoretical value of $\Delta Z_{1/2} = 0.22\ \mu m$, $U_{1/2} = 4$ for a point detector. An optimum detector aperture maximum, corresponding to $V_p \sim 7$, is suggested, leading to a depth of field of about twice the minimum obtainable, with little loss of power from a point source.

proximation, apply since the detector aperture resides in a paraxial region in our system. The data are plotted as the half depth-of-field ($\Delta Z_{1/2}$) in microns and dimensionless normalized optical units $\Delta U_{1/2} = \Delta Z_{1/2}(8\pi\eta/\lambda)\sin^2(\alpha/2)$, where $\lambda \sim 0.58$ μm for the emission wavelength, $\sin\alpha = NA/n = 0.93$, and $\eta = 1.33$ for the index of refraction of the medium surrounding the sample. It is necessary to use this high NA form for $\Delta U_{1/2}$ (Sheppard 1987,1988). In the image of a point source the theoretical lateral spacing between the first diffraction minimum and the peak corresponds to $V_p = 3.8$. V_p as plotted in our experimental data may be offset due to uncertainties in the optical dimensions of our system.

The trade-off of light collection efficiency for depth of field as the detector aperture size varies is depicted in Figure 3, where measurements of the signal power are plotted versus the half depth of field for a fluorescent point source measured at corresponding values of V_p. The measurements and units are as described above for Figure 2. The signal was measured at the axial position yielding a maximum signal by integrating (within the x-y plane) in the area of the image bounded by the half-maximum intensity values. Signal values were normalized to unity at the signal obtained with the maximum accessible V_p. Signal power $S = 0$ at $V_p = 0$ and the corresponding value of $U_{1/2} = 4$, $\Delta Z_{1/2} = 0.22$ μm are the theoretical results given by the value of the half-width at half-maximum of the function for depth of field in confocal microscopy $\{(\sin x)/x\}^4$ (Wilson 1984), where $x = 1 = U_{1/2}/4$. There appears to be an optimum value of V_p at a depth of field about twice the theoretical minimum with less than 25% incremental power loss from a point object. (See also Chapter 11.)

An important advantage of confocal microscopy is rejection of flare due to background fluorescence or scattering. The thin-

ner the depth of field achieved by confocal optics, the better the flare reduction. But again signal is sacrificed for flare reduction. Figure 4 plots the normalized signal collected from a fluorescent point (S), the signal collected for a large uniform scattering volume (B) to represent a background flare source, and their ratios (S/B) as a function of D_p and V_p. The integrated signal of the point source was measured as described above. The "background" signal from a uniform source is independent of x, y and z and its image field mean value B as a function of D_p provides a measure of background transmission through the confocal spatial filter. The ratio S/B of the point source fluorescence to the large volume scattering background provides a measure of the S/B improvement by confocal filtering as a function of D_p. The relative scale of the values of the fluorescence power from the point source and the extended source is arbitrary and the values are plotted relative to convenient maximum values.

OPTICAL ABERRATIONS IN FLUORESCENCE LSCM

The five primary monochromatic aberrations, described by the corresponding coefficients B,C,D,E, and F (Born and Wolf, 1983), are spherical, astigmatism, curvature of field, distortion and coma. Because stage scanning confocal microscopy (SSCM) requires only paraxial imaging, it escapes virtually all but the first of these aberrations. Although fluorescence SSCM is subject to the effects of longitudinal chromatic aberrations, they are easily correctable. Therefore, if slow image acquisition and limited specimen accessibility can be tolerated, stage scanning should be the method of choice to minimize aberration in image formation. For fast imaging, LSCM is indicated and off-axis aberrations must be considered and overcome. (See also Chapter 7.)

Electromechanical scanning and electronic image display can add further aberrations in SCM that are unique to scanning microscopy. If the nonlinearity of the scanning mechanism is not precisely compensated, additional image distortions appear. Any nonlinear scan must be compensated in both the scale of display and in the intensity calibration. Because nonlinearities appear at high excitation intensities due to photobleaching and photosaturation, intensity changes due to variable scan rates are not readily correctable and linear scanning is necessary for satisfactory intensity quantitation.

Video displays can introduce spatial asymmetry due to nonsymmetric pixel shape. In LSCM, the same effect can arise from improper calibration of the rotation of the scanning mirrors. Ordinarily, this effect is fully calibrated and compensated, but it remains a potential source of aberration associated with any video display or scanning system. Calibration of x, y and z scans as well as various optical and electromechanical aberrations that lead to planar image distortion are readily tested by measuring images of calibrated stage graticules in x and y (Inoué 1986). Calibration along the z-axis can be tested by viewing objects of known thickness with due regard for index of refraction.

Image fidelity in LSCM can suffer seriously from the effects of curvature of field. Plan objectives are carefully designed to minimize these effects and usually meet the needs of conventional microscopic imaging. However, LSCM can enhance curvature of field problems because confocal applications are designed to take advantage of the reduced depth of field. The LSCM provides a convenient tool for measurement of curvature of field as illustrated below. Figure 5 shows the axial displacement of the intensity maxima of light collected with confocal

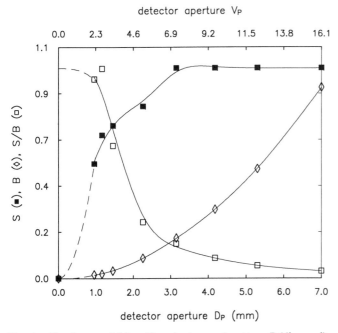

detector aperture V_P

FIG. 4. Signal power-S (■), uniform background scatterer-B (diamond), and signal to background ratio-S/B (□) versus detector aperture size. The signal was obtained from a fluorescent point <200 nm in diameter, as described in Figure 3. The signal, background and their ratios are arbitrarily normalized to unity at their respective maxima and extrapolated for $V_p = 0$. Detector aperture D_p and V_p are as described in Figure 2. This plot shows the relative effects of decreasing detector aperture size on "flare rejection" (B), point signal power and the trade-off in background rejection at the expense of object point power loss (S/B).

optics from a plane mirror in the object plane as a function of distance from the center of the field of view. The axial displacement is less than 0.7 μm across the field for a plan objective and is ~ 4.5 μm for a conventional objective. For comparison, the depths of field of these objectives are < 1 μm.

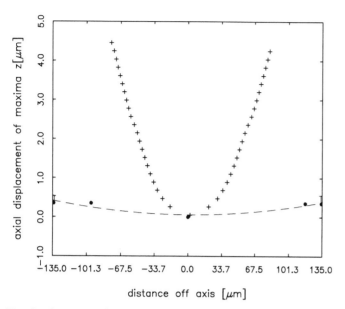

FIG. 5.   Curvature of field. The axial displacement, z, of the maxima of the signal detected from a plane mirror in a confocal geometry with minimum detector aperture is plotted vs. distance off axis in the object to display the curvature of field for two objectives [Nikon planapo 60/1.4 oil (·) and an objective not designed for flat field, a Zeiss 100/1.25 oil (+)]. These results are relatively insensitive to the size of the detector aperture. The data spans the full field of view for these objectives in the BioRad MRC-500; the curve for the plan lens is simply a guide to the eye.

The effect of the curvature of field on the intensity profile across the field of view is illustrated in Fig. 6. The bell-shaped curves show the intensity distributions across the field of view recorded by LSCM with minimum detector aperture using a plane mirror in the object plane. The distance off-axis is normalized to the full field of the objective lens. LSCM imaging of a plane mirror with a non-plan lens suffers a loss of the intensity to nearly zero over the outer half of the field of view. Imaging the same surface with a plan lens also reduces off-axis intensity as a result of inefficient collection of light reflected through large angles, but not as rapidly as the non-plan lens. Light scattered from an isotropic, uniform, deep sample should show neither curvature of field or the collection problems associated with reflected incident light. Indeed, the scattered light curves of constant intensity in Fig. 6 show uniform signal over the entire field of view for both types of objectives. This result also shows that spherical aberration, coma, and astigmatism do not introduce large intensity artifacts over the range of collected angles used here. The radially exaggerated loss of intensity in the non-plan lens is the result of imaging a flat surface with a curved field of view. This aberration distorts 3D reconstructions. Instead of reconstructing a 3D image out of thin slabs, the image is actually a compilation of thin dishes. Allowance for the departures from planarity of field can be incorporated in the image reconstruction procedure.

Chromatic Aberrations in Fluorescence LSCM Measurements

Chromatic aberration, to first order, refers to variation of focal length with wavelength. This variation leads to a dependence of magnification on wavelength. In conventional microscope images recorded with white light, the result is radial separation of colors that increases with distance off-axis in the image. In fluorescence LSCM, this dispersion separates the ac-

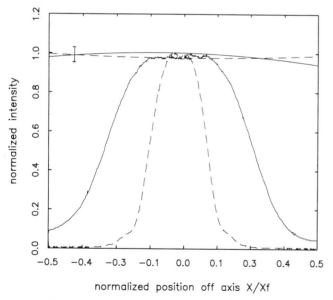

FIG. 6.   Effects of curvature of field on intensity in images of a flat reflecting object. The bell-shaped curves show normalized LSCM intensity profiles recorded with a plane mirror in the object plane and minimum detector aperture (_ _ _ Zeiss 100/1.25 oil, _____ Nikon planapo 60/1.4 oil). The distances off-axis, X, are normalized by the full field width, X_f, for each objective. The field widths are 160μm and 270μm respectively. The curves of constant intensity, corresponding to normalized signals from a thick, uniform layer of scatterers, show the uniformity of response from objects immune to curvature of field.

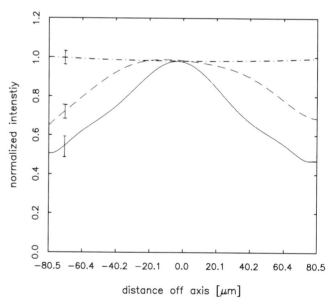

FIG. 7.   Losses in off-axis confocal collection efficiencies from a thick fluorescent sample due to chromatic aberration. Normalized fluorescence signals (_ _ _ maximum detector aperture, _____ minimum detector aperture) are plotted as a function of distance off-axis to show the reduction in collection efficiency even in a thick fluorescence source. The upper curve (_ . _ monochromatic scattering) shows the control signal, monochromatic scattering from a deep uniform back scatterer. Full field is 160μm.

tual fluorescence intermediate image from the scanning image of the exciting short-wavelength radiation. Confocal image filtering in the MRC-500 requires that both the incident and image forming radiation follow the same path through the optics. This condition is satisfied for monochrome images formed by scattered or refracted light. However, chromatic aberration separates the reciprocal pathway of the fluorescent radiation from the pathway of the excitation radiation and thereby attenuates or eliminates the off-axis areas of the LSCM fluorescence image because the detector aperture is not in conjugate apposition to the most brightly illuminated spot in the object. These effects are illustrated by the following experiments.

To demonstrate the effects of chromatic aberration on fluorescence measurements in the LSCM, a thick layer of dilute solution of rhodamine dye, which fluoresces at and above 600 nm, is illuminated with 514 nm laser light using a Zeiss 100× 1.25 N.A. oil-immersion objective and a Nikon 8× eyepiece. Many Zeiss objectives (including this one) are designed for use with a compensating eyepiece to correct for lateral chromatic aberration. The 8× Nikon eyepiece provided with the MRC-500 is not such an eyepiece. The LSCM is focused underneath the fluorophore surface and the absorption length in the dye solution is large compared to the depth of focus. To show that this geometry avoids curvature of field effects, the backscattering of the 514 nm laser light by the same chamber filled with homogenized milk was recorded. Figure 7 displays these results as normalized LSCM intensities plotted as a function of actual distance off-axis in the object field. The fluorescence signal recorded with a small detector aperture falls by a factor of 1/2 at the edge of the field. With the detector aperture full open, nearly half of the collection efficiency at the edge of the field is recovered.

To understand chromatic aberration effects in this microscope, notice that the fluorescence volume, which is conjugate with the detector aperture, should reside in the volume defined by the focus of the exciting light. Chromatic aberration separates the conjugate positions for different wavelengths. On the optical axis the displacement is perpendicular to the planes of focus leaving only longitudinal aberration; off axis there is also radial displacement. The local excitation intensity falls off rapidly with distance as the laser beam spreads out above and below the plane of focus in the object. The lower intensities illuminate the volumes above and below the object plane so that the volume that is conjugate with the confocal detector aperture in fluorescence radiation is weakly illuminated and a reduced signal is still received. If the detector aperture is opened, the fluorescence from a larger illuminated region above or below the plane of focus of the exciting illumination reaches the detector. The off-axis effects displayed in Fig. 7 may also include the results of higher order chromatic aberrations due to off-axis failure of the color correction. Note that the on-axis loss due to chromatic aberrations has been normalized out of this figure.

The full effect of chromatic aberration in fluorescence LSCM is only displayed by recording the fluorescence from a thin, planar fluorescent source. Figure 8 plots normalized intensity versus distance off-axis in the object for a 2-µm thick sample of concentrated rhodamine. The data were recorded at the maxima along z for each x coordinate to remove effects of curvature of field. Both curves for the thin fluorescent source fall off faster than those for the thick specimen of Fig. 7 since there is essentially no fluorophore present outside the plane of focus to be stimulated by the defocused excitation radiation. With a minimum detector aperture, the collected intensity at the edges of the field of view is 90% below that of a scattering sample and 80% below that of a thick specimen. In this case, the off-axis intensity decline is a measure of the loss of coincidence of conjugate points in the image planes for the excitation and fluorescence light. Slight misalignment is evident in one measurement.

With LSCM, only a minor degree of chromatic aberration is necessary to cause severe errors in fluorescence measurements. The objectives used for these experiments, a Zeiss 100× 1.25 N.A. oil immersion and a Nikon 60× 1.4 N.A. planapo oil immersion, showed qualitatively similar errors even for this visible dye. For UV and near UV excitation or near infrared emitters, the usual ranges of optimal color correction are likely to be far exceeded. Hence, the collected fluorescence light may be imaged far from the detector aperture, preventing the application of confocal spatial filtering. On the optic axis, these problems can be avoided by the insertion of an appropriate correcting lens in the light collection pathway or in the illumination pathway to bring the image plane for fluorescence and the detector aperture into appropriate superposition. There is no available information on the effectiveness of this approach, but the on-axis corrections by this method should be completely successful. Off-axis, this approach works only if the dispersive correction can be made before the scanning system.

PHOTODYNAMIC EFFECTS

Laser scanning confocal fluorescence microscopy invariably requires exposure of chromophores to very high light intensities sometimes exceeding 1 MW/cm². The rationale behind this is simple: the greater the power of incident irradiation, the greater the fluorescence emission rate and hence the shorter the period required to acquire a low noise image. If a dynamic cellular process is to be studied by time series imaging, low image acquisition time is essential. This section discusses the molecular

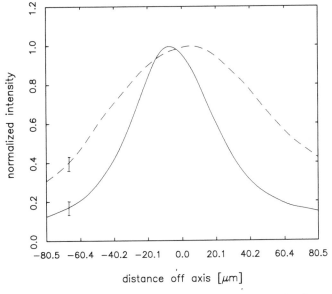

FIG. 8.   Reductions in off-axis confocal collection efficiencies from a thin fluorescent sample due to chromatic aberration. Normalized fluorescence signals (_ _ _ maximum detector aperture, _____ minimum detector aperture) are plotted as a function of distance off-axis to show the reduction in collection efficiency in a fluorescence source 2µm thick. The displacement of the center of the curves is due to very slight optical misalignments. (See also section on Lateral Chromatic Aberration in Chapter 7.)

photodynamic limitations to fluorescence emission rates and hence to the imaging speed of fluorescence LSCM. Specifically, it describes the effects of optical saturation, of intersystem crossing to a metastable triplet state, and of photobleaching. A brief theoretical treatment is given illustrating how populational dynamics are governed by the intensity of the exciting light along with transition rates between relevant electronic states. Experimental techniques used to measure these rate constants are described and a few results for two popular fluorophores are presented. (A slightly different treatment will be found in Chapter 16.)

Theory

The energy level system of a typical chromophore may be depicted in a Jablonski diagram as shown in Fig. 9a. The electronic singlet ground state, S0, is represented by a band of vi-

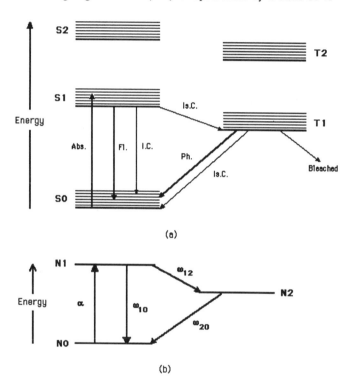

FIG. 9.   (a) Jablonski diagram for a generic organic chromophore. S0, S1, S2 represent singlet electronic energy levels, T1,T2 being the corresponding triplet states. Vibrational sublevels are shown as distinct lines while in fact these are blurred together by solvent interactions. Heavy lines denote radiative transitions while light lines show non-radiative interactions. Photon absorption excites molecules from S0 to S1 where they quickly relax to the lowest vibrational sublevel via radiationless internal conversion (not shown). From this level molecules relax to the ground state either by fluorescence (Fl.), or non-radiative internal conversion (I.C.). Molecules in S1 may also undergo intersystem crossing (Is.C.) to the triplet state T1, from whence they relax to the ground state S0 either by phosphorescence (Ph.) or by radiationless intersystem crossing. Bleaching of excited state chromophores may occur either from T1 as shown or from S1 (not shown).
(b) A simplified model of the energy level system depicted in (a). N0, N1, and N2 designate molecular populations of the S0, S1, and T1 energy levels of that diagram. α signifies the stimulated absorption rate between S0 and S1, and is equal to the product of illumination intensity, I, with the absorption cross section σ. ω_{10}, ω_{12}, and ω_{20} are rate constants for downward transitions between levels as shown. Note that ω_{10} and ω_{20} include both radiative and non-radiative rates, hence the fluorescence emission rate is given approximately by $\omega_{10}Q$ where Q is the quantum efficiency for fluorescence, and where $\omega_{10} \gg \omega_{12}$.

brational sublevels, the first excited singlet state is denoted by S1, the second by S2, etc. In addition to the singlet state manifold, the energy system has an adjacent "ladder" of triplet energy states T1, T2, etc., each of which has slightly lower energy than its corresponding singlet state. In the absence of radiation, these states will be populated according to Boltzmann statistics, the bulk of the molecular population residing in the ground state at room temperature. Upon absorption of a photon whose energy matches the difference between the ground state and some excited singlet state a chromophore will undergo an upward transition to the excited state. The frequency of this process of "stimulated absorption" is given by the product of the incident intensity I (photons/s.cm²) with the absorption cross section σ (cm²).

Absorption of a photon excites a chromophore typically into some vibrational state within the particular singlet band. The excited molecule will relax very quickly ($\tau \sim 10^{-12}$ s) to the lowest vibrational level of S1 by a radiationless process. This energy loss leads to the familiar Stokes shift between excitation and emission spectra of organic fluorophores. At this point there are several possible paths by which the molecule may give up energy. The most desirable from the point of view of the microscopist is that of fluorescence emission. Fluorescence, however, competes with other decay processes including intersystem crossing in which the excited electron undergoes a spin flip, thereby arriving in the T1 state. While this process is usually orders of magnitude less frequent than fluorescence emission, it may nonetheless have serious practical consequences to the fluorescence microscopist. Since de-excitation from T1 is relatively slow, usually not much less than 100 ns (J. P. Webb et al. 1970), molecules may become trapped in this state, thus reducing the effective concentration of fluorophore. Much has been written on this subject in the context of adverse effects on the dye lasing threshold (Schafer 1970). Relevant transition times are very sensitive to environmental quenching, and it is difficult to predict the consequences in LSCM without experimentation under the appropriate set of conditions.

An alternative non-radiative path for the excited dye molecules is photobleaching, an irreversible chemical change to non-fluorescent species. Photobleaching limits the total amount of fluorescence information thet may be extracted from a fluorescence labeled specimen. While photobleaching occurs from both singlet and triplet states (Linden 1988), we explicitly show only triplet bleaching on Fig. 9a, for simplicity.

Population Rate Equations

The dynamics of an optically-pumped dye system, as illustrated in Fig. 9a, may be predicted by population rate equations in which the rate of molecular transitions from a given state to another state is proportional to the population of the first state. The following system of equations models the simplified dye system depicted in Fig. 9b:

$$\frac{dN_0}{dt} = N_1\omega_{10} + N_2\omega_{20} - \alpha N_0 \tag{1a}$$

$$\frac{dN_1}{dt} = \alpha N_0 - N_1(\omega_{10} + \omega_{12}) \tag{1b}$$

$$\frac{dN_2}{dt} = N_1\omega_{12} - N_2\omega_{20} \tag{1c}$$

where N_0, N_1, and N_2 are populations of the ground state, first excited state, and corresponding triplet state; and α, ω_{10}, ω_{12}, ω_{20} are molecular transition rates for excitation ($S_0 \rightarrow S_1$), singlet relaxation ($S_1 \rightarrow S_0$), intersystem crossing ($S_1 \rightarrow T_1$), and triplet decay ($T_1 \rightarrow S_0$), respectively. The dye population is normalized to unity for convenience and is taken to be initially entirely in the ground state. This system incorporates enough detail to illustrate the essential features of real chromophore dynamics while still yielding an easily interpreted analytic solution. In the usual case where $\omega_{10} >> \omega_{12}$, ω_{20}, the general solution for the singlet excited state population may be written as follows:

$$N_1(t) = \frac{\alpha\beta}{\alpha + \beta\omega_{10}} - \left(\frac{\alpha}{\alpha + \omega_{10}}\right) e^{-(\alpha + \omega_{10})t} +$$
$$\left(\frac{\alpha}{\alpha + \omega_{10}}\right)\left(\frac{\alpha(1-\beta)}{\alpha + \beta\omega_{10}}\right) e^{-\left[\frac{\alpha(\omega_{12} + \omega_{20}) + \omega_{10}\omega_{20}}{\alpha + \omega_{10}}\right]t} \quad (2)$$

where $\beta \equiv \dfrac{\omega_{20}}{\omega_{20} + \omega_{12}}$

Since the fluorescence emission rate of this system is given by N_1/τ_f, where τ_f is the fluorescence lifetime, it is useful to examine the behavior of Eq. 2. In the saturated limit where $\alpha >> \omega_{10}$, the excited state population becomes:

$$N_1(t) = [\beta - e^{-(\alpha + \omega_{10})t} + (1 - \beta) e^{-(\omega_{12} + \omega_{20})t}] \quad (3)$$

such that for times $1/\omega_{10} < t < 1/(\omega_{12} + \omega_{20})$, $N_1 = 1$ and the fluorescence per molecule attains the maximum possible value $1/\tau_f$. This initial intensity at saturation decays to an equilibrium value β/τ_f with time constant $\tau_1 = 1/(\omega_{12} + \omega_{20})$, as molecules accumulate in the T_1 state. This reduction in fluorescence rate may be avoided in LSCM by scanning sufficiently fast that the dwell time of the exciting beam is short compared to $1/\omega_{12}$. This may be as short as 10^{-7} seconds (J. P. Webb et al. 1970), hence the scanning technology employed in an instrument is an important factor in determining its utility. It is quite possible that superior images may be obtained by summing many very rapid scans as opposed to scanning slowly for one frame.

A second interesting limit illustrates the case of photobleaching. If $\omega_{20} \rightarrow 0$, then any dye molecule which enters T_1 is effectively removed from the system since it cannot return to the ground state. The excited state population is given in this case by:

$$N_1(t) = \frac{\alpha}{\alpha + \omega_{10}} [e^{-\left(\frac{\alpha\omega_{12}}{\alpha + \omega_{10}}\right)t} - e^{-(\alpha + \omega_{10})t}] \quad (4)$$

Thus the fluorescence will decay with the characteristic time $(\alpha + \omega_{10})/\alpha\omega_{12}$, which in the saturated limit, $(\alpha >> \omega_{10})$, becomes simply $1/\omega_{12}$.

In the case that $1/\omega_{10} < t < 1/\omega_{12}$ we have:

$$N_1(t) \approx \frac{I\sigma}{I\sigma + \omega_{10}h\upsilon} \quad (5)$$

where we have explicitly written excitation rate, α, as the product of the incident intensity I with the absorption cross section σ and $h\upsilon$ accounts for the incident photon energy. The fluorescence per molecule may be written:

$$F \approx (1/\tau_f)\frac{I\sigma}{I\sigma + \omega_{10}h\upsilon} \quad (6)$$

Thus, fluorescence reaches half of its saturated value $F_{sat} = 1/\tau_f$ with a characteristic incident intensity $I_{sat} = h\upsilon\,\omega_{10}/\sigma$. I_{sat} may be calculated from fluorescence lifetimes and extinction coefficients taken from the literature as shown on Table 2.

Inverting expression (6) and inserting the above identities gives the following linear equation in $1/F$ and $1/I$:

$$\frac{1}{F} = \frac{1}{F_{sat}} + \frac{1}{F_{sat}}\left(\frac{I_{sat}}{I}\right) \quad (7)$$

Thus, I_{sat} may be determined by plotting $1/F$ vs $1/I$ and taking the $1/I$ intercept.

Experiment

Saturation parameters and fluorescence decay times have been measured for two dyes: 1,1'-dioctadecyl-3,3,3',3'-tetramethylindocarbocyanine perchlorate (DiI, Molecular Probes, Eugene, Oregon D-282), and laser grade Rhodamine B (Eastman Kodak, Rochester, New York).

Dye samples were dissolved in DMSO and pressed between slide and coverslip to create films of about 2.5 μm thickness. Dye concentration was chosen such that the films should be optically thin over the depth of field of the objective lens used here.

All measurements were made using a BioRad MRC-500 LSCM instrument in conjunction with a Nikon Optiphot microscope using a Nikon 60/1.4 NA plan apochromat oil-immersion objective lens. See Fig. 10 for a block diagram and description of the experimental apparatus.

Excitation was provided by a tunable argon ion laser (Coherent model CR-3). with a maximum output of ~450 mW for the 514 nm line. The beam intensity was regulated by an

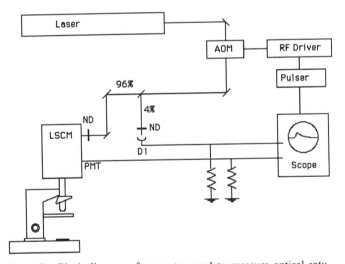

FIG. 10. Block diagram of apparatus used to measure optical saturation and fluorescence decay rates. CW light from a one Watt Ar+ ion laser is diffracted in an acousto-optic modulator (AOM) to produce a pulse train in the first order beam. Pulse width is varied between 1 μs and 100 μs, pulse amplitude is varied between ~.3mW and ~8 mW, and pulse frequency is kept below 20 Hz to allow bleached dye to be diffusionally refreshed between pulses. Pulse height is monitored by the pickoff photodiode (D1) after passing through neutral density filters (ND). The main beam enters the BioRad MRC-500 scanner head after passing through a switchable neutral density filter (ND). The pulse train is focused through a 1.4 N.A. objective lens into a thin film of dye dissolved in DMSO. The emitted fluorescence is collected with the confocal optics and measured on the photomultiplier tube (PMT) in the scanner head. Signals of both the pickoff diode and the PMT are measured on the oscilloscope, which is triggered by the pulse generator. Diode D1 is frequently calibrated against a second diode placed in the back focal plane of the objective such that, using the transmissivity of the objective lens, the total power incident on the sample may be determined from D1.

acousto-optic modulator system (Newport model N30085–3D), which in turn was controlled by a 20 MHz pulse generator (HAMEG HM 8035). Pulses of duration from one to one hundred microseconds were run at repetition rates of 2–20 Hz in order to diminish the effects of photobleaching. The diffusion coefficient of these dyes in DMSO was estimated to be $\sim 10^{-6}$ cm^2/s and the mean time for diffusion of the dye from the center to the edge of the focused spot was calculated to be ~ 0.6 ms for a beam waist diameter of $\sim 0.5 \mu m$.

Incident beam power was monitored continuously with a "pick-off" photodiode, which was periodically calibrated against the power incident on the sample. The incident beam waist was ~ 5 meters from the objective lens; thus the back focal plane of the objective was well overfilled.

Optical saturation was measured for the two fluorophores by recording the emitted fluorescence while varying the incident pulse power. Fluorescence signal power was measured at its peak which occurred atop the 200 ns rise of the signal. Data have not been corrected for the power dependent reduction in signal due to bleaching or intersystem crossing. This correction should be less than 10% of total signal amplitude, however, even at the peak incident power. Data are presented on Fig. 11 in raw form—F vs. I—and in reciprocal form—1/F vs 1/I—according to equation (7). The characteristic saturation intensities are 3.3 MW/cm^2 and 2.9 MW/cm^2 for DiI and RhB, respectively, both significantly higher than the 1.0 MW/cm^2 calculated on Table 2. The discrepancy may be partly due to effects of complex geometry which we have ignored by treating the 2.5-μm-thick illuminated layer of dye as a cylinder instead of using the true 3D transfer function of the objective lens.

Fluorescence decay records for Rhodamine B and DiI dissolved in DMSO are presented on Fig. 12 on both linear and semi-log plots. The curves may be roughly fit by a sum of three exponentials. It is likely that the initial fast decay, $\tau \sim 3–4 \mu s$, represents intersystem crossing to a metastable triplet state as described above.

The second decay time, $\tau \sim 30 \mu s$, represents destruction of fluorophore by photobleaching. Photobleaching limits the molecular fluorescence yield (MFY) to the value MFY $= \tau_b/\tau_f$ where τ_b is the bleaching time. Since image quality in fluorescence is often limited by shot noise as determined by the fluorescence yield, the MFY should be a useful parameter in determining the dye concentration required to achieve an acceptable image.

The third decay constant, $\tau \sim 0.2$ ms, probably represents depletion of the region surrounding the illuminated volume of viable fluorophore. As photobleaching progresses, the concentration of unbleached chromophore will decrease in the neighborhood of the illuminated volume, hence the photobleaching rate will not come to equilibrium with the rate at which fluorophore is refreshed. The exponential fit is, of course, very poor in this region since there is no reason to expect simple exponential behavior here.

The principal effect on fluorescence LSCM of saturation of the fluorophore excited state is to limit the useful excitation laser power to a few milliwatts in the diffraction limited focus of a high numerical aperture objective (Table 2). The resulting excitation intensity of around a megawatt/cm^2 excites typical good fluorophores to saturation where the fluorescence emission rate per molecule is around 10^9 photons/sec. Note that it may be necessary to scan fast enough to keep the dwell time below 10^{-7} sec. in order to avoid further fluorescence power

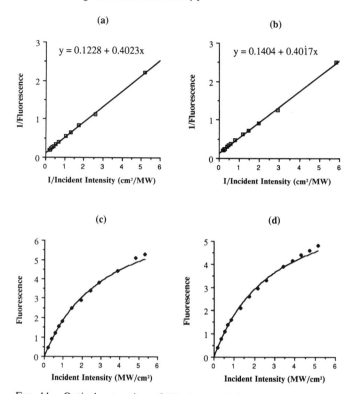

FIG. 11. Optical saturation of Rhodamine B (a,c) and DiI (b,d) in DMSO thin films. Figures a and b show linear fits to the inverse — inverse plots used to extract the saturation parameter I_{sat} according to equation (7) of the text. Figures c and d show the raw data with lines of best fit taken from a and b.

TABLE 2. PARAMETERS RELEVANT TO SATURATION

Parameters determining optical saturation. P_{sat} is the saturating beam power in mW equal to the effective saturation intensity, I_{sat}, times the focal spot area $\pi(w/2)^2$ where w = the beam waist diameter. The fluorophore extinction coefficient ϵ is expressed as absorption cross section σ.

Dye	ϵ (l/mole·cm)	σ (cm^2)	τ(ns)	$(\sigma\tau)^{-1}$	I_{sat} (W/cm^2)	P_{sat}(mW)
di-I	130,000[a]	$4.9 \cdot 10^{-16}$	.8[b]	$2.5 \cdot 10^{24}$	$9.8 \cdot 10^5$	1.5
Rh B	35,000[c]	$1.3 \cdot 10^{-16}$	3[c]	$2.6 \cdot 10^{24}$	$1.0 \cdot 10^6$	1.5

a. Haugland (1985); b. Packard and Wolf (1985); c. Berlman (1971).

reduction by pumping of slow decaying triplet states. Photobleaching probably saturates as does fluorescence, but it still limits the total number of fluorescence photons per fluorophore to about $\tau_f/\tau_b \sim 10^5$. Since the photobleaching rate τ_b^{-1} is strongly environment sensitive, it may be possible to design preparations to enhance substantially the total fluorescence yield. (See Chapter 16 for a discussion of conditions under which bleaching may not saturate.)

The problems associated with saturation of the fluorophore excited state and with photobleaching may be used to advantage in SCM through application of advanced techniques for imaging energy transfer (Jovin 1987, Jovin and Arndt-Jovin, 1989). The efficiency of fluorescence energy transfer between two spatially adjacent fluorophores with appropriately overlapping spectra and the efficiency of photobleaching from the singlet excited state can be saturation independent. Therefore, microscopic imaging of energy acceptor fluorescence or of photobleaching rates

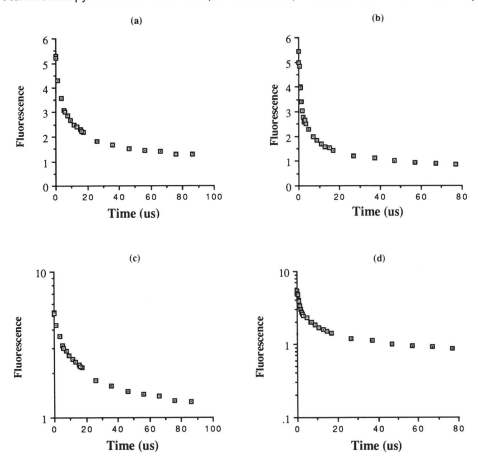

FIG. 12.   Linear and semi-log plots of fluorescence decay curves for Rhodamine B and DiI in DMSO thin films. Semi-log plots c and d show that the data are not fit by a single exponential; they are roughly fit by sums of three exponentials. The shortest decay time ~3–4 μs is believed to represent intersystem crossing, the intermediate time ~30 μs is attributed to photobleaching, and the longest decay time >150 μs is believed to result from depletion of fresh fluorophore from the diffusionally accessible volume surrounding the focal spot.

may be particularly useful in SCM. Jovin and colleagues have reported advantages of imaging with chromophores that optimized intersystem crossings to triplet excited states that decay by phosphorescence but that photobleach from the excited singlet state (Jovin and Arndt-Jovin, 1989; Tanke, 1989). A LSCM using an image dissector photomultiplier detector (Goldstein 1989) may provide useful technology for this elegant microspectrofluorometry approach because the scan geometry and dwell can be arbitrarily selected. Further opportunities to exploit fluorophore photodynamics in high intensity excitation are likely to appear as the high intensity photodynamics are studied more intensively with the motivation of SCM imaging applications.

FLUORESCENCE PHOTOBLEACHING RECOVERY WITH LSCM

Fluorescence Photobleaching Recovery (FPR) denotes a quantitative fluorescence optical technique which is used to measure diffusion, the dynamics of molecular mobility and the chemical change of fluorescent labeled molecular species. Measurements of molecular motion on the surfaces of living cells in

culture during the last two decades have become a ubiquitous biophysical procedure. These extended studies have shown that most cell surface proteins diffuse more slowly by several orders of magnitude than a simple fluid-mosaic model of the cell membrane would suggest. The origins of these constraints remain poorly understood and continue under study.

It is seldom appreciated that the most common FPR procedures utilize the best features of confocal optics. Therefore, adaptation of general-purpose fluorescence scanning confocal microscopes to FPR experiments appears to be appropriate. Although there is little experience to report at this time, the requirements of this promising method and some directions for future developments are briefly outlined.

In the simplest form of FPR, a dim beam of ion laser excitation light is focused to a diffraction limited spot on a fluorescence labeled cell surface and the fluorescence radiation power excited in that stationary spot is measured with a photomultiplier located behind a detector aperture just as in SCM. The spot is ordinarily not scanned, but instead, the excitation light is briefly pulsed to high intensity to photobleach most of the fluorophore within the illuminated spot. Then the dim beam is used to monitor the fluorescence of the remaining fluorophore in exactly the same spot and to record the time course of the recovery of the fluorescence as fresh fluorophore moves into the photobleached spot. For diffusion on a 2D surface such as a cell membrane, the time scale of the recovery $\tau_D \approx W^2/4D$ is determined by the diameter of the bleached spot W and the diffusion coefficient of the labeled molecules D. Typically, the recovery time might be many minutes for a cell surface protein and only seconds for a membrane lipid analog. A canonical quantitative procedure has been described fully by Axelrod et al. (1976). This technique can be accommodated readily in any SCM with a few milliwatts of laser power by the incorporation of a calibrated, reliable fast-attenuator in the exciting laser beam and appropriate time series recording of fluoresence power. The attenuator must not deflect or distort the beam. Insertion of filters with a fast solenoid to switch the intensity works if the filters are polished to perfectly parallel surfaces. Acousto-optical modulators can work if selected for tolerance of high beam power and function over sufficiently wide dynamic range. A factor of 10^4 dynamic range with a few millisecond risetime is useful. It is crucial to image the detector aperture at the focus of the beam on the specimen surface, and it is necessary to know and usually to measure precisely the effective beam size (Schneider 1981). Scanning confocal image inspection can assure focus, and a nanometer accuracy stage scan with a short range provides an easy means for beam diameter measurement that can also be used in other confocal applications.

An alternative geometry for FPR uses a linear pattern of parallel stripes as the bleaching pattern. Recovery can be monitored either by fluorescence excitation in the same pattern as the bleaching pattern or by analysis of the image excited by uniform or scanned illumination. Frequently, the bleaching pattern is formed by imaging a Ronchi ruling in the object plane, or better, by formation of the interference pattern of two slightly convergent laser beams within the object (Smith 1978, Davoust et al. 1982). Fluorescence SCM should be adaptable to pattern FPR experiments with an externally generated bleaching pattern with the LSCM used quite simply to monitor the pattern as it changes. A better alternative requires a suitably programmed scanning and beam intensity modulation system (using the programmed scanning system) to provide the photobleaching pattern. Then the recovery can be monitored with either attenuated repeats of the same pattern or overall with SCM. However, with this method the phase shift between the bleaching process and probe beam scans may have to be taken into account. This method appears easy for all but the fastest diffusion rates but has not been extensively tested.

The axial imaging resolution of the LSCM appears to allow easy applicability of pattern FPR to non-planar cells and to thick preparations. There can be an advantage, but it is essential to note that the geometry of the diffusion process is not simplified. The bleaching light does pass through the specimen above and below the plane of focus, leaving behind a more uniform bleach in those regions. The diffusion-mediated fluorescence recovery must therefore be calculated as a three dimensional diffusion problem for each geometry. It will be advantageous to utilize symmetric specimen geometry to facilitate the solution of these problems. Use of the axial resolution of the LSCM for FPR studies of non-planar cell membranes embedded in thick preparations may extend the applicabilities of the technique.

FPR experiments have long employed the photochemistry of photobleaching processes without much research or elucidation of the photobleaching process itself. Now the close approximation of the optical conditions of FPR to the conditions to be used in fast LSCM motivates more concerted and intensive studies of the photochemistry. It is expected that photobleaching is limited by saturation of the excited state just as is the fluorescence itself, but there have been few studies. Presumably bleaching can occur from either singlet or triplet excited states depending on the particular photochemical system, but information is sparse on the usual fluorophores. Oxygen interaction with an excited state is often implicated in photobleaching but it is not clear that this is the only possibility. Deoxidation of living biological tissues to minimize photobleaching can itself damage the tissue. Developments of protective procedures and selection of long wavelength radiation as established for erythrocytes (Bloom 1983, 1984) may become necessary. (See also Chapter 16.)

No fundamental limitations on the use of SCM instruments for FPR experiments have revealed themselves in this analysis. Therefore, it appears appropriate to recommend the development of software and hardware to implement FPR on LSCM. Successful development would make FPR measurements more readily accessible.

CONCLUSION

Quantitative fluorescence scanning confocal microscopy demands the highest possible efficiency of collection and detection of the fluorescence photons in order to maintain the sensitivity, speed and spatial resolution required for application to molecular cell dynamics. Efficiency as high as in conventional microscopy may be designed into the instrumentation for fluorescence scanning confocal microscopes. For some experiments, it may be necessary to trade off spatial x-y resolution against collection efficiency (see Chapter 11). It is always possible to improve signal-to-noise ratios at the cost of spatial resolution by local spatial averaging of acquired images during subsequent electronic processing.

The principal design components involved in optimization of fluorescence efficiency are the light collection efficiency of the objective, the transmission efficiencies of the scanning optical system and the quantum efficiency of the photodetector and its associated electronics. Because the product of these transmission efficiencies determines the overall instrumental efficiency, each one must be optimized. Problems can arise with the numerical aperture of the objective lens, coatings for high transmittance, reflectivity of scanning and beam steering mirrors, photodetector quantum efficiency and effective duty cycle of detection electronics. Nevertheless, for SSCM there is no fundamental reason why the overall efficiency cannot match conventional fluorescence microscopy. However, there are several limitations. Photodynamics places a fundamental limit on the fluorescence emission rate per molecule in SCM. In LSCM, chromatic aberrations of the objective lens appear to pose grave problems.

Chromatic aberration appears to limit the applicability of existing SCM to quantitative fluorescence imaging. However, for SSCM correction optics may adequately compensate for longitudinal chromatic aberrations in some circumstances, even with ultraviolet excited dyes. Stage scanning is optically preferable for those fluorescence SCM applications that can tolerate the relatively slow speeds and inaccessible specimens because the on-axis optical aberrations are much simpler to control. On the other hand, LSCM will be preferred for dynamical measurements and generally for most measurements on living cells. A combination of an imaging procedure using either conventional fluorescence imaging or fluorescence SCM in addition to selective small field (zoomed) scans for small area quantitation near the optical axis may provide a powerful tool for difficult cases.

Ultimately, the rate of data acquisition is limited by photodynamic saturation of the fluorophore excited state. Even with fluorophores of high absorbance, saturation occurs around 10^6 Watt/cm^2 which is generated at the focus of high NA objectives by about 1.5 mW of exciting laser power. Saturation limits may be further exacerbated by intersystem crossing to a slowly decaying triplet state. Evading this problem may limit the acceptable residence time of the exciting beam in a resolution volume and may demand very fast scan rates for dynamical experiments with ultimate sensitivity.

Photobleaching ultimately limits the total amount of information available per fluorophore to the order of 10^5 photons per molecule. The photobleaching process is environment (oxygen activity) sensitive, is frequently non-exponential, and is not yet sufficiently understood for satisfactory control. The applicability of convenient high intensity lasers and the motivation of fluorophore applications in LSCM and in dye lasers may lead to research that will lessen this problem.

Disk scanning microscopes avoid the photodynamic limitations of fluorescence LSCM but suffer from limitations of flexibility associated with the rotating disk and from limited experience in fluorescence quantitation. Because the exciting radiation is divided amongst many simultaneous exciting beams, the local intensities in each beam are small enough to avoid saturation although the overall data acquisition rates can be very high. The relatively low efficiency of utilization of the light source (usually about 1%) does not necessarily limit the rate of fluorescence acquisition. As in other SCM techniques, it is the efficiency of acquisition of the fluorescence signal that determines performance. The ultimate SCM for quantitative dynamical fluorescence may be a multi-beam LSCM with multiple electro-optical channels processed in parallel to assemble the image at high rates with intensities below saturation levels.

There is every indication that much of the early promise of SCM for quantitative dynamical fluorescence measurements is realizable. However, like any new technique, considerable developmental effort will be necessary to realize the full potential.

ACKNOWLEDGEMENTS

This work was supported primarily by an NIH grant (DHHS-P41-RR04224-0) for the Developmental Resource for Biophysical Imaging Optoelectronics at Cornell with additional support from the NSF (BBS-87-14069), the ONR (N00014-89-J-1656), and from the Cornell Biotechnology program which is sponsored by the New York State Science and Technology Foundation, a consortium of industries, the US Army Research Office and the NSF. D.S. and J.S. were predoctoral trainees in Molecular Biophysics and W.W.W. was a Scholar in Residence at the NIH Fogarty International Center during part of this work.

REFERENCES

Axelrod D, Koppel D E, Schlessinger J, Elson E, Webb, W W (1976): Mobility measurements by analysis of fluorescence photobleaching recovery kinetics. Biophys. J. 16, 1055.

Berlman I B (1971): Handbook of Fluorescence Spectra of Aromatic Molecules (2nd ed.). Academic Press, New York.

Bloom J A, Webb, W W (1983): "Lipid diffusibility of the intact erythrocyte membrane." Biophys. J. 42, 295.

Bloom J A, Webb W W (1984): "Photodamage to intact erythrocyte membranes at high laser intensities: Methods of assay and suppression." J. Histochem. Cytochem. 32, 608.

Born M, Wolf E (1983): Principles of Optics (6th ed.). A. Wheaton & Co., Great Britain.

Davoust J, Devaux P F, Leger L (1982): Fringe pattern photobleaching, a new method for the measurement of transport coefficients of biological macromolecules. EMBO J. 1, 1233–1238.

Goldstein S (1989): to be published in J. Microsc.

Haugland R P (1985): Handbook of fluorescent probes and research chemicals. Molecular Probes Inc., Eugene, OR.

Inoué S (1986): Video Microscopy. Plenum Press, New York.

Jovin T M, Jovin D A (1987): Microspectrofluorometry of single living cells. Edited by E. Kohen, J.S. Ploem and J.S. Hirschberg, Academic Press.

Jovin T M, Arndt-Jovin D J (1989): Luminescence Digital Imaging Microscopy, Ann. Rev. Biophys Biophys Chem. eds: Engelman D M et al 18, 271–308.

Linden S M, Neckers D C (1988): Bleaching studies of rose bengal onium salts. J. Am. Chem. Soc. 110, 1257–1260.

Packard B S, Wolf D E (1985): Fluorescence lifetimes of carbocyanine lipid analogues in phosopholipid bilayers. Biochemistry 24, 5176–5181.

Schafer F P (1977): Principles of dye laser operation, in Dye Lasers (2nd Ed.). Springer − Verlag, Berlin.

Schneider M B, Webb W W (1981): Measurement of submicron laser beam radii. Appl. Opt. 20, 1382–1388.

Sheppard C J R (1988): Depth of field in optical microscopy. J. Microsc. 149, 73–75.

Sheppard C J R, Matthews H J (1987): Imaging in high aperture optical systems. J. Opt. Soc. Am. /A 4, 1354–1360.

Smith B A, McConnell H M (1978): Determination of molecular motion in membranes using periodic pattern photobleaching. Proc. Natl. Acad. Sci. USA 75, 2759–2763.

Tanke H J (1989): Does Light Microscopy Have a Future? J. Micros 155, 405–418.

Webb J P, McColgin W C, Peterson O G, Stockman D L, and Eberly J H (1970): Intersystem crossing rate and triplet state lifetime for a lasing dye. J. Chem. Phys. 53, 4227–4229.

White J G, Amos W B, Fordham M (1987): An evaluation of confocal versus conventional imaging of biological structures by fluorescence light microscopy. J. Cell Biol. 105, 41–48.

Wilson T, Carlini A R (1988): Three-dimensional imaging in confocal imaging systems with finite sized detectors. J. Microsc. 149, 5l-66.

Wilson T, Sheppard C (1984): Theory and Practice of Scanning Optical Microscopy. Academic Press, London.

Chapter 4

The Pixelated Image

ROBERT H. WEBB AND C. KATHLEEN DOREY

Eye Research Institute of Retina Foundation*

INTRODUCTION

We think of images as smoothly continuous, but we frequently handle them in small pieces. This chapter is about the consequences of dividing the image space into small boxes called *pixels* and assigning each a number—the pixel value or *gray level*. We do not display *every* x position, but rather divide the x axis into perhaps 1000 parts and choose our x locations from those. Similarly, we don't display all the imaginable pixel values, but rather divide the intensity range into parts (gray levels) and choose our pixel values from those.

The ideal display would be one which shows all the information available for the image, but doesn't use more divisions in space or intensity than are needed. A microscope which can resolve only 100 separate points across the field of view doesn't need a 1000 pixel display. And a detector which can distinguish only 8 intensity steps doesn't need 256 gray levels. More often the reverse is true: the resolution in space or intensity is more than can be displayed economically, and we will discuss strategies for dealing with this. We will find that the image should be smoothed (the resolution spoiled!) to the point that the available number of pixels satisfies the Nyquist sampling criterion that there must be two samples for every resolvable point (in each direction). And we will see how best to match a limited number of gray levels to the range and resolution of the measured intensity. Throughout this chapter we are concerned with how best to *match* the choice of pixel characteristics to the optical detector and display characteristics.

All the images we perceive pass through a partitioning stage. The retina has discrete photoreceptors and there are only three color receptor varieties among them. In spite of this discrete sampling the world looks smooth to us, and we see an apparent continuum of color. To achieve this, the optics and computing apparatus of the human visual system are beautifully integrated with the photoreceptor matrix. For instance, the resolution element ("resel") of the eye spans roughly two photoreceptors. The microsaccadic motion of the eye "dithers" the image over the inter-receptor gaps. In the center of the visual field, the photoreceptor array is roughly hexagonal, so that packing is closest and special directions are not orthogonal. In the visual system, parts of the image are enhanced by a wide variety of selective amplifications and inhibitions of the neuronal signals that transfer the image to the brain. Each of the three color detectors measures intensity in its spectral region, and the differential signals are sufficient to distinguish millions of colors. Edges and motion (and possibly many other special features) are detected rapidly, and stable features are quickly de-emphasized. As a

final economy, only a small area is involved in high-resolution viewing, with the rest of the visual field contributing 'context' and special features (Cornsweet 1970, Alpern 1978).

Microscopes do not yet have the elegance of the human visual system, but microscopists must solve the same problems as best they can, and be satisfied to find that some of our cleverest solutions have been anticipated.

Pixelation

Pixelation is the process of partitioning the image, both in space and intensity, into discrete elements for storage and display. This process immediately comes to mind when images are to be stored in a digital computer. However, many other mechanisms may divide the image into discrete components, and such mechanisms tend to interact. We can often use 'pixel' to describe the results, without distinction as to mechanism, but here we will be more particular, in order to understand the interactions.

Optical Resolution: The Resel

Optical resolution is a topic well covered in other parts of this *Handbook*, so we will not discuss it in detail. Every microscope has an optical limit: somewhere on the scale between houses and atoms it becomes impossible to detect finer structures as resolved entities. In some cases the image is partitioned into pixels by the detector (CCD cameras, film, the human eye), and any resolution exceeding that of the detector is lost. In other cases of interest to us (scanning systems with a single detection channel like scanning laser microscopes) the partitioning occurs *after* detection and is performed by an explicit digitizer, often an analog-to-digital converter (A/D). In these cases pixel size is determined by the temporal resolution (bandwidth) of the transfer electronics in the digitizer.

Most typically, the apertures of the illumination system and of the observation system determine optical resolution. We will call the minimum optically resolvable entity on the object a *"resel"* (Dorey and Ebenstein). The resel familiar to most microscopists, shown in Figure 1, is defined by the Rayleigh limit—a circle whose radius is $r = 1.22 \lambda'/\sin \alpha$, where α is the angle subtended at the object by a radius of the exit pupil of the objective, and λ' is the wavelength of the measuring light in the medium of the object (Born 1959). The proper metric in microscopy is the wavelength, which is λ in vacuum. In a medium of refractive index n the wavelength gets shorter: $\lambda' = \lambda/n$. The only medium of interest for this measurement is that of the

---

*20 Staniford Street, Boston, Mass 02114, correspondence: RHW.

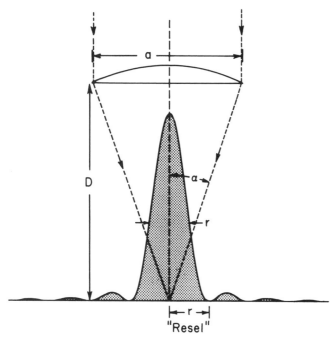

FIG. 1.   The geometry of the optics defining a resolution element (resel) for lenses, including microscope objectives. D is the distance from aperture to focal plane, a is the aperture diameter, and λ' the wavelength of the relevant light in the medium of the focus.

object itself (usually water in biology, n = 1.33). Resolution is often written in terms of Numerical Aperture: $r = 1.22\lambda/2NA$, and the factor 1.22 is generally dropped in acknowledgement of reality (Stone 1963).

So our *resel* is defined by the optics of the system. The confocal resel is slightly smaller than r, $r_c = 0.8\ \lambda'/2\sin\ \alpha$, and the axial resolution is $r_a = 1.4\ \lambda'/\sin^2\ \alpha$ (Sheppard 1978, Corle 1986). The *resel* is the smallest area of the *object* which can be discerned as different from its neighbors, regardless of detection and subsequent processing. In the three-dimensional world of confocal microscopy, we need a three-dimensional resolution element—sometimes called a *voxel*. As we are here reserving the word pixel for the display, we caution that both pixel and voxel are often used to mean both display partitionings *and* resolution elements at the object. As there is nothing inherently two-dimensional about a resel we will use this term for the resolution element at the object, imposed by the optics, whether in two or three dimensions.

Pixel

Now we go all the way to the other end of the microscope—the display. Typical display devices are film, TV monitors and computer memory readouts. Film has grains of some size, television has discrete horizontal lines and an electronic bandwidth, but computer memories are simplest. Suppose our image, like those returned from a spacecraft, is a string of numbers, each of which can be stored in some computer location. Each number is a pixel value. The indivisibility is obvious: if the 5th picture location has a value 27, there's no way to tell if the left half was 30 and the right half 24. So a *pixel* is the smallest area of the *image* which is presented as distinct from its neighbors. All pixels in the image should be of equal area and spacing.

Gray Level

The analogous division of the intensity range is the gray level. This may be displayed as the brightness of the (single dot) pixel on a TV monitor, the number of halftone dots in the pixel of a magazine picture, or the number of developed grains in the pixel of a photograph. In each case the value assigned to that pixel is chosen from a list of allowed numbers. In the computer image, a pixel value is a single number. If we are using 8 bit storage, the smallest number is 0 and the largest 255. So we must content ourselves with 256 gray levels. There's no way to tell if level 123 came from 123.2 or 122.6. Of course, we *can* store the number 123.2, but that requires more storage bits for every pixel, and the resolution of the detector may not justify such an expenditure.

If the display uses a fixed number of dots—all either black or white—we might use each as a pixel in a line drawing, or we could make up a half-tone print by using groups of dots to indicate a pixel's intensity. As such pixels grow in size, we will notice their 'graininess' if we are too close. So we need to balance pixel size against the need to render intensity. Video displays, of course can use one dot per pixel and vary each dot's brightness, but hard copy taken from such a display may be disappointing. A good display should have enough dots to appear smooth. With 20/20 vision, we can distinguish dots 1 arc-second apart (that's 200 μm at 1 meter), so dots on billboards can be bigger than those on a page (Cornsweet 1970). As a rule of thumb, 300 dots/inch on a page at normal reading distance looks pretty smooth. A parsimonious display shows all its information at its expected viewing distance, and rewards further magnification with mere graininess. Pictures in handbooks are generally parsimonious. Photographs have grain sizes of about 10 μm, and about 64 gray levels (8×8 grain pixels: 400/inch) (Jones 1961).

In Between

Between the optical front end, which is responsible for resolution, and the display, which partitions the image into pixels, there may be one or more stages which also partition the image in some way. Typical of this is a fiber optic face-plate on a video tube, or a half-tone mask on a published picture. We will refrain from naming this image element, but we will remember its existence, particularly as we discuss *aliasing*, where the interaction among the various partitionings may result in a visual artifact.

MATCHING IMAGE SPATIAL CHARACTERISTICS

The Nyquist Theorem

All of this chapter might well be summed up by saying "Don't ignore the Nyquist Theorem". So before going on with images we will state this important conclusion of sampling theory. Nyquist asked what is the minimum number of times that we can sample a sine wave of (temporal) frequency f in order to reproduce it faithfully. By sampling he meant taking an instantaneous reading and then waiting a while and taking another. His conclusion is that the *sampling* frequency must be at least 2f. That means that we must read the meter at least twice during each cycle of the wave (Oppenheim 1983, pg 519). (The reality that ideal low-pass reconstruction filters are unavailable suggests 2.3f as a minimum sampling frequency, and this is a safer course.)

The frequencies of interest in imaging are likely to be spatial ones, but the theorem holds for them as well. Images (signals) are seldom made of pure sine waves, but they can always be separated into components which are sine waves of various frequencies—each with an associated intensity and phase (if a sine wave isn't present, its intensity is zero). This is the ubiquitous technique of Fourier analysis, a very important concept to keep in mind. If we want the image to look like the object, we must not ignore any of the object's spatial frequencies.

What we should note here is that most objects have sharp edges, small spots, or other features which contribute very high frequency components. The typical gaussian or sin^2x/x^2 blur of our optical system will truncate these components, so that the edges are only sharp up to the optical resolution limit. Once that truncation has taken place, we don't need the capacity to record higher frequencies, because they carry no information. But below that limit, failure to record all the frequency components can lead to *mis*information.

It is important to keep in mind exactly what is being resolved. If the goal is to distinguish two particles lying close together, then the required frequency will be 2.3/D, where D is the space separating the particles. On the other hand, if it is necessary to decide whether the particles are circles or hexagons, the frequency satisfying the Nyquist theorem will be much higher: the information sought requires resolution of very small differences at the *edge* of a particle, and there are higher frequencies present in the edge. Similarly, to reproduce properly the small changes of position of a moving particle, we must sample at a high enough frequency to describe its edge. We can think of this situation as trying to resolve the edge in two sequential frames—if we superimposed them. Then the slower the particle moves, the closer we must sample.

Having said this, why do we recommend sampling at a little more than twice the highest frequency? This is because the image isn't formed until the sampled information is *reconstructed*. Reconstruction always takes place through some filter, which limits the *image* to lower frequencies. This is necessary in order to remove the sampling artifacts and make the image look like a continuous entity. Typical filters are: the eye, smoothing half-tone dots into a continuous tone picture; an integrator (capacitor-resistor pair), smoothing the sharp changes from the A/D as the voltage stream goes through a D/A to the monitor. When such a filter is not used—as in the blocky images of a "zoomed" computer display or in a close view of Byzantine mosaics, the extraneous information (about the sampling) actually detracts from the display. We solve that by stepping back until the divisions are below the resolution of the eye.

We leave details here to the references.

Sampling at 3 times the highest frequency present (f_H) is unnecessary. Why does it sometimes seem to work? Because we have misjudged f_H ! After all, the only way to find what frequencies are present is to look with ever higher resolving power. For practical purposes, f_H is determined by the optics: $f_H = 1/resolution$. When sampling can't keep up with this, such as a low zoom setting on a high NA, low magnification lens we can get aliasing. When sampling is significantly higher than $2.3f_H$, it is wasted for purposes of image reconstruction.

We say f_H is the optical *bandpass* of the system. More precise work on determining these frequencies uses the Modulation Transfer Function (MTF) to define what we are calling the optical bandpass (Inoué 1986, pg 123). For our purposes the simpler approach is adequate.

Scanning devices convert spatial frequencies to temporal ones, so the temporal bandpass of the electronics will have the same function of limiting the frequencies present in the image (along the fast-scan direction). That is why we say that the electronic bandpass can determine the image resolution.

So what does the Nyquist theorem tell us? A true rendering of the image should use a sampling frequency matched to the optical and electronic resolution: sample at over twice the highest frequency in the image. Since this is not always possible, much of the rest of this chapter deals with the consequences and trade-offs of sampling at a non-ideal rate.

Hyper-resolution: Oversampling

Sometimes it makes sense to sample at frequencies far above the Nyquist limit. This is variously referred to as super-resolution, hyper-resolution and sub-pixel resolution. In our terminology, sub-pixel resolution would be an oxymoron, but the intent would be *sub-resel* measurement. (Super-resolution is also used for a number of other effects.) By these names we mean a situation in which it is useful to locate the position of an unresolved object to a fraction of the resolution of the microscope. That sounds contradictory, but it isn't: to *locate* an object, we don't need to resolve it. Consider a true point object—a delta function entity. Our microscope will turn this into a blur which we have decreed to be one resel across. If we sample this blur 20 times as we scan across it, we can never describe whether it is a true point or a resel-sized thing. But if it isn't imaging we're after, we can gain some useful information from the oversampling: we can tell *where* the entity is. Astronomers run into this problem often: their stars appear as blurs of a size determined by the aperture of the telescope, but two stars which are resolved can be located to a fraction of a "blur". The size of the fraction involves not only the number of samples but also the noise in the signal—the centroid of a bright blur (resel) is more surely measured than that of a dim one. This is beyond the scope of our treatment here (Morgan 1989), but we may consider its implications for scanning microscopy.

Let us suppose that our microscope is properly set up with electronic and optical bandwidths matched, and no artifacts. To reconstruct an image of the object, we will need to sample at the Nyquist limit. But suppose we want to watch the motion of tiny entities well below the system's resolution. For imaging, it would be a waste to use more than a pair of pixels in any direction in which the entity is not resolved. But if we sample Z times across the resel (usually by 'zooming' the display), we can image the diffraction pattern of the microscope aperture itself. If the motion is 1 resel in T seconds, and we would like to see its new position every second, we will need 2T samples per resel. Eventually, neighboring pixels look alike (plus or minus the noise), so further oversampling doesn't help. We will discuss this in the section on Matching Image Intensity Characteristics, but it should be apparent that if we need to collect 10 photons in each of 2 samples to declare that the entity is there (for imaging), we will need 10 photons in each of our 2Z samples to locate it to 1 Zth of a resel. That's Z times as long, at the same light level. By which time it may have moved a full resel! This is the principle of conservation of difficulty, and it suggests that hyper-resolution is of use only in special cases.

A more familiar use of hyper-resolution is in the smoothing of diagonal edges or lines. A line at a shallow angle to the rasterization shows up the pixelation steps—it looks jagged. We think of this as due to diagonal drop-out (below): the sampling perpendicular to the line is too slow, and a higher sampling rate would aleviate this. But we can also think of the benefit of a higher sampling rate as due to hyper-resolution: although the line may be unresolved, we can *locate* it very exactly by over-sampling, and display that location on an image of much finer pixelation. The resulting smooth line has thus benefited from sampling at a frequency far above that specified by Nyquist for the optical resolution of the instrument. Note that this is a problem solely *due* to pixelation of the image.

The resel/pixel ratio

Our pixels, then, are generated by sampling, while our resels come from the optics. The Nyquist theorem states that we need 2.3 samples for each point in a resolved pair: 2.3 pixels per resel (remember how the retina is organized?)[2]. It can be easily understood that if the microscope resolves two bright points it is because there is a perceptible dark space between them. To keep them resolved in the image, we need two bright pixels separated by a dark one.

We know that we should make a two-to-one match of the pixels to the resels. But that is along a *line*. Our images are two dimensional, so we need *four* pixels per resel. In the scanning system, where the resel is scanned over the object, that means that we would undersample unless the horizontal scan lines overlap! Not only should we have no dark gaps between our *measuring* raster lines, the odd ones should "touch" each other and the even ones fall squarely on the join. The the TV raster lines, or the computer pixels, can then be made to "touch"—thus giving the required two pixels per resel vertically as well as horizontally.

Confocal microscopy complicates things further: we are interested in axial resolution too! That's right—*eight* pixels per resel. The three-dimensional resel will not be spherical, so successive image planes need not be as close as the lateral pixelation, but for faithful reproduction in a digitized image we need to record in two image planes per axial resolution element. This is appalling, but true:

8 pixels/resel in three dimensions.

The standard digitized field in computer imaging is 512×512 pixels—roughly that imposed by television technology. But the standard field in microscopy is about 1000 resels across, which needs 2000×2000 pixels for proper display in two dimensions. CRTs which are not limited to TV format can display many more pixels than TV monitors. The penalty in scan time, cost and image handling is severe, but in some circumstances this is an appropriate technique. But as soon as we want to *measure* our image data, we are likely to present it on a monitor or in computer memory.

Confocal microscopes are capable of aggravating the problem of too few pixels: a scanned stage confocal microscope can have 10,000 resels per field diameter and as many axial sections as time allows. The *computer* is (in principle) perfectly capable of storing four hundred billion pixels. To perceive such an "image" we might view it at low resolution, then zoom in on interesting parts, or we could make a "tour" around it, always at higher resolution but never seeing the whole. However, we quickly arrive at another limitation: it is only *in principle* that computers easily store $20,000 \times 20,000$ pixels *per image*. This is at least 400 MBytes, and we might want to look at a *series* of images, moving axially through the sample, or sequentially in time. This is not simply a question of buying more memory. Rather, it takes time—both computer access time and experimenter interaction time—to use such a quantity of data. This problem is generally handled by indexing. Although library techniques are improving, they are not yet really adequate to this problem. Rather, remembering the retina, we might store and view images at low resolution, only keeping at high resolution those parts deemed interesting while the record was being made. Whatever our strategy, we are unlikely to *display* pixel fields of more than a few million.

The usual TV screen has about a 4:3 aspect ratio. Its horizontal resolution is determined by the electronic bandwidth (some few MHz), while its vertical resolution is a true pixelation—there are a discrete number of (horizontal) lines spread vertically down the screen. Resolution on TV monitors is specified in terms of "TV lines". In the vertical direction this means just what it seems to. In the horizontal direction the electron beam forms a continuously moving spot which turns on and off as rapidly as the electronic bandpass allows. A 5 MHz bandpass implies 200 nsec from crest to crest of the fastest possible modulation. The horizontal line takes 53 μsec, so there are 265 such crest-to-crest variations, or 265 line pairs. That's 530 pixels. This is high for most common monitors, and it will be true only in the center of the picture. Edges are worse, and corners are hopeless.

The familiar US standard TV has 525 lines vertically, of which as many as 10% are blanked or off the screen, and manufacturers claim 500 to 600 "TV lines" horizontal resolution. This latter allows an electronic bandpass of 4.5MHz—imposed by broadcast considerations. For computer displays the broadcast standards aren't involved, but the business community defines the needs—mostly for text and graphs. Consequently, image handling software expects to send 512 x 480, or at most 640 by 512 pixels to the monitor, which may not display the edges. Resolution of monitors is often given with "per picture height" implied, though it is the (higher) horizontal resolution which is quoted. There are all sorts of ways to rectify this, but the simplest is to specify the actual number of lines displayed. This is not the "resolution" anyway, as we have seen. One hears of monitors with "square pixels"—that usually has nothing to do with the pixel shape but rather means that a circle on the object plane looks round on the monitor. The round dots making up the pixels are spread vertically and horizontally until this desirable match is achieved. A complete and reliable reference for television matters, specialized to microscopy, is Inoué's book (Inoué 1986).

The message here is that quality images need quality monitors. The image-handling software must be capable of dealing with the more flexible non-standard monitors, *or* we may even adopt strategies to display parts of the image at high resolution.

Diagonal Dropout

Pixel arrays interact with image features in strange ways. One of these is illustrated in Figure 2. Here the pixel frequency is 2/image line both horizontally and vertically, but on the 45° diagonal, the spacing is 1.4/line, and at a shallower angle it is

a

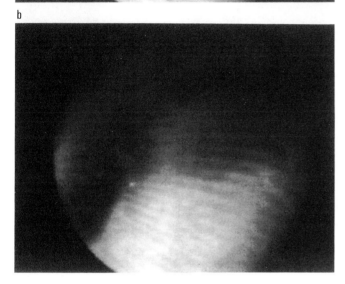

b

FIG. 2. TSM image of *Stentor Coeruleus*. As the organism rotates, stripes appear in the lower right of the image (a). These false features are due to an aliassing between vidicon target pixellations and an unresolved regular structure in the *stentor*. In the next video frame (b) the rotation has eliminated the aliasing again. These are from a video tape kindly supplied by V.K-H. Chen (Chen, 1989).

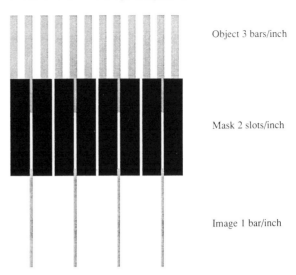

Object 3 bars/inch

Mask 2 slots/inch

Image 1 bar/inch

FIG. 3. Aliasing of a 3 cycle/inch structure. The sampling mask can only pass 2 cycles/inch, but instead of ignoring the higher frequency structure, it presents it as a 1 cycle/inch image, when no such structure is present in the original at all. Smoothing after sampling would turn this into a 1 cycle sine wave, but only low-pass filtering (to less than 2 cycles) before sampling would eliminate it.

spot taller than it is wide (by allowing astigmatism in the electron gun, for instance), or by moving the spot's vertical position a little bit (and very fast)—"dithering". While the image appearance is improved by this, it is not quite a true representation. The same is true of the use of Ronchi gratings—a technique for doubling each line and adding it to the dark spaces above and below (Inoué 1981). Some of the hardcopy systems now available use a diffusion process to achieve horizontal line blurring. Only spatial filtering at a Fourier plane truly smooths without loss, as shown by Ellis (Inoué 1986 appendix 1). Most probably, the ideal is to display on the best monitor the project can afford, and to produce hard copy—photographs or similar material—with the same attention to preservation of the stored information.

Aliasing

The various partitioning mechanisms in the image formation process—optical resolution, detector characteristics, and display pixelation—can be mismatched. One result of this is a type of moiré pattern called aliasing, in which features appear in the image which are not present in the object (Oppenheim 1983 pg 527). The name arises because the features in the object which give rise to these artifacts are really quite different—they show up "under an assumed name". The phenomenon responsible is the mismatch of sampling and resolution: high frequencies present in the object have not been excluded from the image data before sampling took place at a lower frequency. A simple example is to sample a 300 Hz wave 200 times per second (Figure 3). The sampling misses whole cycles, but "measures" a 100 Hz wave—which isn't really there. The 300 Hz wave thus masquerades as a 100 Hz one. Unfortunately, the only way to avoid the possibility of recording a spurious signal is to increase the sampling rate.

If there is no chance of using enough pixels for proper representation of the object, we should spoil the resolution before pixelation. Otherwise those higher frequencies will appear un-

below 1/line and the structure is no longer resolved. It might pay to rotate the sample and look again, but a more likely strategy is to oversample, as suggested above under hyper-resolution.

Pixel shape distortion

For presentation reasons, the pixels may be made unround. As usual, we need to distinguish between the aspect ratio imposed by the display (the pixel's aspect ratio) and that which may have been imposed by the detector (or even the optics). We will concern ourselves here only with the shape of the pixel in the display. The usual reason for unround pixels is to bridge the dark gaps between the horizontal raster scan lines in the display. Remember that in a laser scanning microscope these gaps may be real, in the sense that, at certain low zoom settings, the path of the scanning beam may not overlap properly. It is possible to blur the gaps between TV scan lines by making the

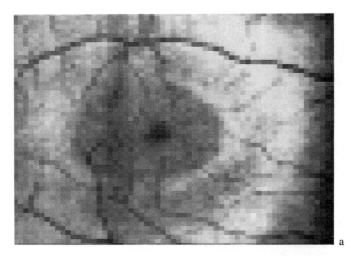

a

b

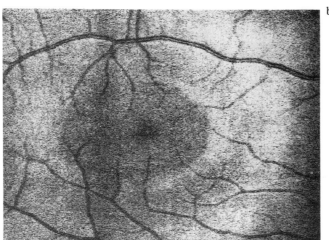

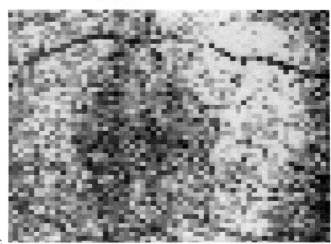

c

FIG. 4. Averaging before and after sampling. The "original", 4a, has been stored in a computer and plays the role of an "object", with each stored pixel a "resel". In 4b the resolution has been spoiled before sampling by averaging. The "resels" are taken in groups of 4 (2 × 2) and averaged, so that one of the new large pixels of 4b is an average of the group of resels of 4a. In 4c sampling is done without resolution spoiling. Each 2 × 2 group of 4 pixels was assigned the value of the upper left "resel": the resulting pixelation did not match the resolution.

der a different name—aliased into some lower frequency. Spoiling the resolution in order to get better images is treated below.

THE MECHANICS OF PIXELATION

Pixelation occurs in a number of ways. Let's assume the optical resolution is adequate, and that we have an analog image reaching the digitizer/partitioner. Typical are signals from: a CCD [RCA 1974] array camera, or a PMT [RCA 1970] producing an analog voltage stream.* These result in two very different partitioning processes. The CCD has a discrete spatial partition, which will be the pixel. This camera accumulates charge as photons fall on it during the TV frame period (1/30 sec in US standard). Thus it integrates both temporally during the frame and spatially over the pixel. If we have correctly ar-

ranged a resel to be sampled by 2.3 detector elements, it is not possible to violate the Nyquist theorem. The single detector, on the other hand, can violate sampling procedure with ease: the instantaneous voltage represents the light returned from the resel at that instant. A *pixel* is derived by an analog-to-digital converter (A/D) which samples this voltage stream (Chapter 12 of this handbook; Analog Devices 1986; Gates 1989). The flash A/D works as follows: when the pixel clock says "NOW", it samples the analog voltage at *that* instant, taking perhaps 1% of the available time to do the reading. For the rest of the sample period, the sampled-and-held voltage is being transferred to the storage. So the pixel value as read is not an average over the time between clock pulses, but a sample *at* the pulse. Any frequencies in the voltage stream above the Nyquist frequency are going to contribute misinformation to the image. Therefore all

---

*Other common detectors fall in the second category: solid state detectors such as avalanche photodiodes [Brown 1987] are obvious analogs of PMTs, and are probably more appropriate for scanning laser microscopes. Vidicon cameras [RCA 1974] may be a common detector for tandem scanning microscopes. These resemble the CCD array in storing the image in a nominally discrete diode array on a target— usually made of silicon. But the read-out resembles a raster-scanned

laser microscope: an electron beam moves continuously over the target in a raster pattern and discharges each target cell onto a single wire, where the voltage stream is more like the continuous output of a PMT than the discrete "bucket brigade" of a CCD. The pixelation here comes about at the A/D, not at the target. The best vidicons have targets with cells much smaller than the subsequent pixels will be, but it is a good idea to check that they are not of comparable size, lest various moiré patterns appear.

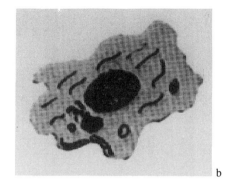

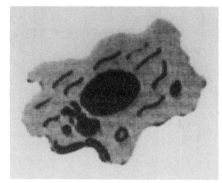

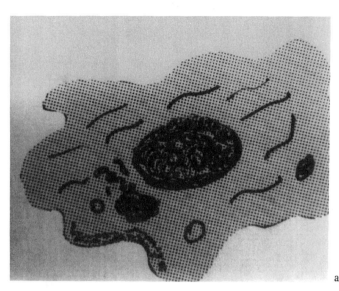

FIG. 5 (a-c).   Spoiling the resolution by defocussing. The "cell" here has been recorded by a vidicon camera. At high magnification, internal structure is visible (a). At half the magnification this structure isn't resolved, but aliases with the vidicon's target matrix to exhibit a non-existent coarser structure (b). When the camera is slightly defocussed, this aliasing pattern goes away, without loss of any real structure that is resolvable at this magnification (c).

frequencies higher than the Nyquist frequency should be suppressed before sampling.

An analogy is the following: suppose you want to measure the pattern of rainfall on your yard. You can put out test-tubes on a one foot grid, and measure the levels of their collection. That is fine as long as there are no significant differences in rainfall over distances shorter than a foot. You might, of course, miss the drip line from your roof and the rainshadow of a branch on your prize pansy. This sampling partition can be turned into an integrating partition by equipping each test tube with a one foot square funnel. Details of spacings shorter than a foot will not be shown here, but they will at least be integrated into the picture, rather than distorting it. "Pixels" which include the roof drip will be wetter and the one including the pansy will be dryer.

If you *must* use the sampling method, (and with scanned laser confocal microscopes you must), then to avoid the artifacts of sampling below the Nyquist limit, *spoil the resolution*. That sounds frightful to a microscopist, but do it. In the analogy, either use bigger raindrops or install funnels. In a microscope, the best thing is to match your resolution to the pixelation: use a low enough power and a sufficiently small field to be sure you are sampling twice per resel. In the case of a CCD camera, do the same thing. There is no benefit to using a resolution higher than the camera is imposing, so avoid it. Again, with the PMT system, resolution can (and should) be spoiled electronically as well. To do this put in an appropriate integrator (most simply a capacitor) before the A/D in order to limit the bandwidth so it will be less than one half of the sampling frequency. Then the voltage signal will be sampled by the A/D converter at a frequency twice the video bandwidth of the electronics. The

voltage cannot vary faster than half the sampling rate. This process, like the optical resolution spoiling, is an integrating one, so that all the energy in the higher frequencies gets used—signal from the drip line in the rain pattern gets included in the average over the square foot in which it falls.

Figure 4 shows the impact of this procedure on a real image. The "original" is an image from a scanning laser ophthalmoscope of the macular area of a human retina. It has been stored in a computer and here plays the role of an "object", with each stored pixel a "resel". The other two pictures show the results of rendering this with new, larger pixels—in obvious violation of our favorite theorem. In 4b this is done by an averaging procedure, spoiling the resolution. The "resels" are taken in groups of 4 (2 × 2) and averaged, so that one of the new large pixels of 4b is an average of a group of resels from 4a. Resolution is lower, but that is all, since we have brought the system into conformance with the Nyquist requirement.

In 4c sampling is done without resolution spoiling. Each of the large pixels corresponds to the upper left "resel" from the 2 × 2 groups in 4a. When the group spans a large feature, this is much like averaging, but for the smaller features—small retinal veins and arteries—the sampling is an inadequate method and the information content of the image is substantially impaired. Nothing subtle like aliasing is going on here—we're simply not matching the resolution to the pixelation. It should be clear that if we had lowered the resolution first and then sampled, we would get the same picture as in 4b. Averaging in a computer is, of course, artificial compared to proper resolution matching − use of a lower resolution objective or (and) bandpass limiting in the electronics.

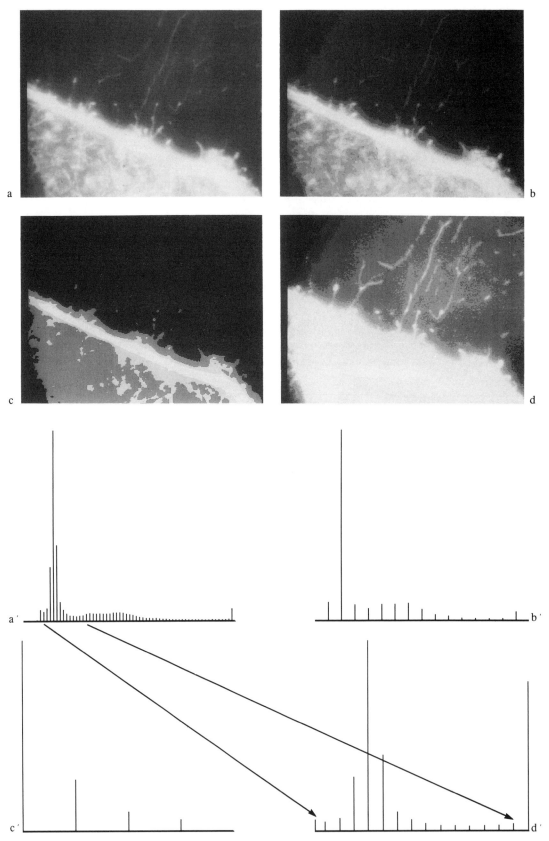

FIG. 6 (a–d). The cells in this videomicrograph were recorded over 64 levels of intensity, and are so shown in (a). These intensities are counted and displayed in the histogram of (a'). If we had to display them with only 16 levels, we could show the whole range as in (b) and (b'), where every pixel of value 9, 10, 11, or 12 has been assigned to level 3. If we have only 4 levels, the situation is as shown in c and c'. In (d) and (d') we have "zoomed" the intensity scale and show only the pixels with values from 33 to 48, assigning them values 1 for 33, 2 for 34, up to 16 for 48. This preserves the intensity resolution at the expense of the overall picture—exactly the same case as spatial zoom. With color coding, we could render the range 0–20 as blue(say), 21–42 as green, and the rest as red, thereby retaining the resolution *and* the overall picture—using false color to multiplex the three ranges.

RESOLUTION CAN BE SPOILED EITHER BY LIMIT-
ING THE BANDWIDTH OF THE ELECTRONICS OR BY
USING A LOWER RESOLUTION OPTICAL SYSTEM (eg A
LOWER MAG OBJECTIVE). IN FACT, PROPER MATCH-
ING THROUGHOUT IS ACHIEVED IF BOTH PROCE-
DURES ARE FOLLOWED. The electronic matching depends
on the A/D sampling rate, so it need not change with optical
changes like magnification. If the resel/pixel ratio is determined
by the optics, it must be chosen at each magnification and field,
and attention should be paid here constantly. The electronic
bandwidth affects only the fast-scan direction (horizontal), so
problems with vertical pixelation can be avoided only by optical
spoiling as shown in Figure 5. The "cell" here has been recorded
by a vidicon camera. At high magnification, internal structure
is visible (a). At half the magnification this structure isn't resolved, but aliases with the vidicon's target matrix to exhibit a
non-existant coarser structure (b). When the camera is slightly
defocused, this aliasing pattern goes away, without loss of any
real structure that is resolvable at this magnification (c).

MATCHING IMAGE INTENSITY CHARACTERISTICS

Gray scale

Gray scale refers to the number of distinct intensity levels
in the displayed pixel. Here again, we may find confusion between measurement and display.

This is a very similar situation to that of the spatial partitioning which gives us resels and pixels. An intrinsic resolution
in intensity is given by the measurement's signal-to-noise ratio,
and we want to map this properly onto the available digital
steps provided by our digitizer. We would also like to *present*
these steps in a way that is felicitous to the human visual system
which will view them, but that comes last.

Detection

The analog of the resel in intensity terms is determined as
follows: a pixel value is the result of a measurement of N photons. The uncertainty (noise) associated with this measurement
is $\sqrt{N}$ or $\sqrt{N_{dark}}$, whichever is bigger, where N_{dark} represents
instrument noise--dark current, amplifier noise or whatever,
translated into "equivalent dark photons". N_{dark} is the noise still
present with no light reaching the detector. Let us assume that
the instrument is "ideal" ($N_{dark} = O$), so that it is quantum
noise which controls the brighter pixels. A measurement of N
photons is significantly different from one of $N \pm \sqrt{N}$ photons.
So the next distinguishable level of intensity is $N \pm \sqrt{N}$, and
$\sqrt{N}$ must be the intensity analog of our spatial resel. Any "sampling" involved has been taken into account by the statistical
analysis which produced this step size, so we need just one
display step to represent the intensity resolution step. But, of
course, this is a step size that varies with intensity. How many
steps do we need?

The brightest pixel comes from N_b photons. The dimmest
worth measuring must come from N_{dark}. So the *dynamic range*
is $N_b - N_{dark}$, and there are $\sqrt{N_b} - \sqrt{N_{dark}}$ meaningful levels associated with it. For example, if our dark current is equivalent to
10 photons, and our brightest measurement during a pixel is
10,000 photons, the dynamic range is 9,990 and there are 97
meaningful levels. The problem here is that these levels are not
equally spaced: the lowest one is $\sqrt{10}\,(=3)$ photons wide, while
the highest is 100 photons. Completeness demands that we

make the Least Significant Bit (LSB) in our digitizer equal to
3 photons (meaning the current or voltage produced by 3 photons). If the digitization is linear, we need $10,000/3 = 3,333$
steps to cover this dynamic range. The nearest power of 2 is 2^{12}
$= 4048$, so we would need a 12 bit digitizer, with 4048 levels
to represent faithfully the 97 actually meaningful levels.

This works out to give us the required number of bits:

$$B = \log_2 \{(N_b - N_{dark})/\sqrt{N_{dark}}\},$$

or

$$= \log_2 (N_b - N_{dark}) - .5 \log_2 N_{dark}.$$

with the number of meaningful levels being:

$$L = \sqrt{N_b} - \sqrt{N_{dark}}\,.$$

Now fortunately (!) we seldom get such good signal-to-noise
ratios. We generally scan fast enough so that a peak signal of
100 photons per pixel would be brightest, with its S/N of 10.
But suppose we have a peak of 1000 photons, with S/N = 32.
Good detectors should allow a dynamic range of 1000 ($N_{dark} =$
1). This would require 10 bits. If the detector is not as good,
say $N_{dark} = 4$, we could use a 9 bit converter for our 31 useful
levels.

What can the common 8 bit converter do? $2^8 = 256$, so we
know our dynamic range can only be as big as 256, and then
only if dark noise is insignificant. This is a situation in which
photon counting often makes sense—if you're scanning slowly
enough. There are only 16 meaningful levels in this range, appalling as that seems.

Frame grabbers (Mize 1985, Data Translation 1986), which
are organized around fast A/D converters, usually provide 8
bits per pixel. If the dynamic range requires more, some
compression before "grabbing" may be more useful than the
expense in money and memory of a 12 bit A/D. For instance,
if we were to derive the square root of the current from an
analog processor and then digitize that, 32 useful levels could
be encoded by a 5 bit A/D. This is a compression scheme, so
data must be decompressed (squared) in order to be manipulated arithmetically (averaged, summed, etc). Its advantage is
that it is a parsimmonious compression without information
loss.

Display

Now let us turn to the question of displaying the data. Figure
6 shows an image using various levels of gray. Photographic
prints generally are capable of rendering 16 levels, transpar-
encies 128, and TV monitors possibly 64. These are levels whose
intensity can be measured as distinct by a photometer. The
human eye's Just Noticeable Difference (JND) is about 0.03 log
units (Graham 1965, pg 210)—a *factor* of 1.07. In a single scene
we can manage a brightness range of 3 log units—a factor of
1000. (Incidentally, the total dynamic range of the eye is 11 log
units -10^{11}, but not all in one scene). So we would like to present
an image with 100 levels meaningful to the eye, each representing a factor of 1.07. We will need 10 bits to *write* a range
of 1000 to the display, and most of the 1024 values that represents will not be distinguishable by the viewer. Notice the
similarity to the detection situation above—the eye is a detector
obeying the same laws of physics as any other.

Since the detectors used in confocal microscopes are capable
of wide dynamic range, images can be presented in other ways.
One such is to spread the intensity range of local interest over

the available grayscale and black out everything else—a technique called intensity windowing (Zimmerman 1988, Pratt 1978), and equivalent to zooming in the spatial domain. Figure 6 shows the mapping used to display one intensity range of the image shown over the full range of the display device's grayscale.

Most scientists are now familiar with *false color* coding, which assigns an arbitrary color chosen from a palette. Although the number of useful shades is a lot less than that claimed by computer sales people, we can stretch the pixel intensity range by color coding steps which might be below the JND (less than 0.01 log unit) for visual inspection. False color presentation is also a very valuable way of encoding another data dimension in the image—such as time or axial depth. Keep in mind, however, that only the (properly sampled) original information is there. No process can ever *add* information to an image after it is recorded.

IMAGE PROCESSING REMOVES DISTRACTING UNWANTED INFORMATION. IT NEVER ADDS NEW INFORMATION.

Color displays

Color is rendered in the display very much as intensity is. The color separation at detection depends on the detector(s), and, in general, three numbers are associated with each pixel location (RGB). We can treat these as three separate displays, each having the same pixelation problems as a monochrome image. Color *monitors* introduce some new problems by having generally lower bandwidths—hence less TV resolution—and by having yet another level of pixelation for the color overlay: each TV pixel is now composed of three adjacent dots, so the actual pixel for a pure red image uses one third of the pixel real estate for that location. A white pixel uses all three colors, but the sub-pixel structure may be apparent, and may alias with image features. This is particularly true when the color alignment is not perfect—the usual situation. In general, the best presentation is on a black and white monitor.

For laser microscopy, it is not possible to display the true color. This is because pure spectral sources like lasers lie on the edge of the CIE color space—they are perfectly saturated. But TV monitors and color film use a more limited color space defined by a triangle whose corners are the phosphor or separation layer coordinates in CIE space (Conrac 1985, appendix III). The rendering is fairly true—good enough for most work, but not really what the data have found.

In fluorescence, the source has lots of spectral width, and most of the color can, in principal, be rendered truly by the common media. Moreover, the data here may be the spectral values themselves, so that a false color rendition may present them more usefully.

CAVEATS

Spectral variation of detectors

Many applications in confocal microscopy utilize the measured value of the pixel to assess absorbance or fluorescence of a particular probe. The color property of the probe may change, reflecting the biological property to be measured, and this is reflected in the pixel value. Data distortions are introduced by the spectral sensitivity of the detector, and digitization simply reads these into a permanent record. *All* of the detectors used in confocal microscopy should be treated as suspect—they all have different sensitivities at different wavelengths, and these are seldom adequately corrected in the software. In every application involving real color detection and display, a standard should be measured and corrections applied appropriately.

Automatic Gain Control

Television cameras, such as those sometimes used to record confocal images from disk-scanning microscopes, often have built into them a dynamic range stretching device (i.e. an automatic gain control) which increases the gain (the ratio of photons to output voltage) when the light level is low. That is very helpful for home movies, but fatal to quantification of data. We do not record number of photons, we record a voltage. If these two quantities are not linearly related, our pixel values will not represent light output, and N_{dark} will be unmeasurable. It is, in principle, possible to assess the changing transfer function, but discretion suggests we disable the AGC.

Even with the AGC off, most system electronics are AC coupled. This results in a residual AGC-like behavior, as pictured in (Spomer 1988). Similarly destructive to the quantitative accuracy of the stored and displayed intensity signal are non-linear amplifiers installed before the digitizers of some commercial instruments such as the Bio Rad MRC-600.

STRATEGY FOR MAGNIFICATION AND RESOLUTION

How should we choose magnification and resolution? First, of course, always use as much light as your specimen can endure. Then, for imaging, match the sampling rate to the resolution—adjusting whichever is free to the constrained entity. For sub-resel measurement, oversample by Z, where Z is the number of distinguishable gray levels.

Example: The display is 500 pixels (square). Microscope resolution is 0.2 μm. Zoom until the field is 250×0.2 μm = 0.5 mm. (If the task calls for a bigger field, use a lower NA objective). Now scan slowly enough to display the features of interest—this can only be done with the object itself as a test, since contrast and reflectivity (or fluorescence) will vary. As long as there are no non-linear processes like heating or fluorescence saturation, one scan of T seconds is identical to M scans of T/M seconds each (it's the total number of photons per pixel that matters). If some features are unresolved, but stand out by 20 gray levels above (or below) their neighbors, then their spacing or relative positions can be measured to 0.01 μm. To do this, increase the zoom (decrease the field size) by 20.

ACKNOWLEDGEMENTS

Our thanks to Michail Pankratov, Tom Clune, George Hughes and Eli Peli, who have all been most helpful in understanding and explaining these matters.

REFERENCES

Alpern, M. (1978) *The Eyes and Vision*, in *Handbook of Optics*, Driscoll, W. G. and Vaughan, W. eds., McGraw-Hill.
Analog Devices (1986) *Analog-Digital Conversion Handbook* 3rd ed.

Analog Devices, Inc. PO Box 796, Norwood, Mass 02062.

Brown, R.G.W., Jones, R., Rarity, J.G. and Ridley, K.D. *Characterization of silicon avalanche photodiodes for photon correlation measurements* Appl Optics **25** 4122–4126 (1986) and Appl Optics **26** 2383–2389 (1987).

Born, M. and Wolf, E. (1983) *Principles of Optics,* 6th ed. Pergamon Press.

Castleman, K. R. (1979) *Digital Image Processing,* Prentice-Hall. Chapter 12 is a fine description of sampled data.

Chen, V.H-K, and P.C. Cheng (1989) Real-time confocal imaging of STENTOR COERULEUS in epi-reflective mode by using a Tracor Northern Tandem Scanning Microscope Proc EMSA 47 138–139.

Conrac Corporation (1985) *Raster Graphics Handbook* Van Nostrand Reinhold Co.

Corle T.R., Chou C.-H. and Kino G.S. (1986) *Depth response of confocal optical microscopes.* Opt. Lett. **11,** 770–772.

Cornsweet, T. N. (1970) *Visual Perception,* Academic Press.

Data Translation (1986) *Applications Handbook* Data Translation, Inc. 100 Locke Drive, Marlboro, Mass 01752–1192.

Dorey, C.K. and Ebenstein, D.B. (1988) Quantitative multispectral analysis of discrete subcellular particles by digital imaging fluorescence microscopy (DIFM). Visual Communications and Image Processing '88 SPIE 1001, 282–288.

Gates, S.C. (1989) *Analog To Digital Converters in the Laboratory* Scientific Computing and Automation 49–56. Gordon Publications, Morris Plains, NJ 07950–0650.

Graham,C.H. (1965) *Vision and Visual Perception* John Wiley & Sons.

Inoué, S. (1986) *Video Microscopy* Plenum Press. A fine general reference on many of these topics.

Inoué, S. (1981) *Video image processing greatly enhances contrast . . .* J Cell Biol **89** 346–356.

Jones, R.C. (1961) *Information Capacity of Photographic Films,* Jour Opt Soc Am **51** 1159–1171.

Mize, R.R. (1985) *The Microcomputer in Cell and Biology Research* Elsevier.

Morgan, J.S., Slater, D.C., Timothy, J.G. and Jenkins, E.B. (1989) *Centroid position measurements and subpixel sensitivity variations with the MAMA detector* Appl Optics **28,** 1178–1192.

Oppenheim, A.V., Willsky, A.S. and Young, I.T. (1983) *Signals and Systems,* Prentice-Hall. Chapter 8 describes sampling theory very well.

Pratt, W.K. (1978) *Digital Image Processing* John Wiley & Sons pg 309ff.

RCA *Electro-Optics Handbook* EOH-11 RCA Solid State Div, Electro-Optics and Devices, Lancaster, PA (1974).

RCA *Photomultiplier Manual* PT-61 RCA Electronics Components, Harrison, NJ (1970).

Sheppard C.J.R. and Wilson T. (1978) *Depth of field in the scanning microscope.* Optics Letters **3,** 115–117.

Spomer, L A and Smith, M A L (1988) *Image Analysis for Biological Research: Camera Influence of Measurement Accuracy* Intelligent Instruments & Computers **6,** 201–216

Stone, J. M. (1963) *Radiation and Optics,* McGraw-Hill pg 182.

Zimmerman, J.B. et. al. (1988) *An Evaluation of the Effectiveness of Adaptive Histogram Equalization for Contrast Enhancement* IEEE Trans Med Imaging **7** 304–312.

Chapter 5

Laser Sources for Confocal Microscopy

ENRICO GRATTON AND MARTIN J. VANDEVEN

University of Illinois at Urbana-Champaign, Department of Physics, Laboratory for Fluorescence Dynamics
1110 W. Green St., Urbana, IL 61801

INTRODUCTION

In this chapter we will describe the characteristic properties of a number of lasers commonly used in fluorescence microscopy. We will concentrate on the characteristics of lasers in relation to their use as an illumination source. Lasers have a number of unique properties compared to other sources emitting electro-magnetic radiation, such as arc lamps, which make them an almost ideal light source for use in confocal microscopy. These properties are:

- high degree of monochromaticity
- small divergence
- high brightness
- high degree of spatial and temporal coherence
- plane polarized emission (for many types)
- a Gaussian beam profile (can be obtained by special optics)

Over the last 30 years, since the realization of the first experimental laser, a wide and still expanding variety of lasers has been developed. Available laser systems cover an extremely wide range, differing from each other in physical size, principle of operation, optical, temporal and mechanical properties, such as beam divergence, output power, polarization properties, duty cycle, stability of the beam, and vibration sensitivity related to the mechanical design, emission wavelengths and tunability, ease of operation, maintenance costs, reliability, and safety aspects. This chapter will introduce the microscopist to the operation of the laser, the most important laser parameters, and their influence on the quality of the confocal image.

LASER POWER REQUIREMENTS

First, we introduce an estimation of the order of magnitude of emission intensity that can be obtained in fluorescence microscopy using a given illumination power. The amount of laser power needed depends crucially on the quantum efficiency of the contrast medium being studied. The most common factors are sample fluorescence and backscatter.

It is convenient to express our quantities in terms of photons per second per pixel per mW of incident light at a given wavelength, since, for modern detectors, it is better to compare the number of photons per second detected with the intrinsic dark noise of the detector. Also, expressing the flux per pixel, provides a quantity which is independent of the illuminated area. The useful relationships are the following:

$$\text{Energy of one photon} = h\lambda = hc/\lambda = 4 \times 10^{-19}\text{J}$$
$$\text{at } \lambda = 500 \text{ nm}$$

1 mW of light intensity at 500 nm represents
$2 \times 10^{+15}$ photons/second
Assume that an image of 1000×1000 pixels, 1 mW of incident light, uniformly distributed, is equivalent to

$$\text{flux per pixel} = 2 \times 10^9 \text{ photons/(sec.pixel.mW) at 500 nm.}$$

There are two considerations. First, how many photons will be emitted per pixel? Second, how many photons can be tolerated per pixel before saturation of the fluorescent molecules occurs?

Let us analyze the first question. Using fluorescein, one of the most common probes, the molar extinction coefficient is about 100,000 per cm of optical path. Assuming an effective optical path of about 1 μm (the depth of field) the molar extinction is about ten. The local concentration of fluorescein can vary, depending on the spatial location and the degree of labeling. Let us assume that a concentration of 10^{-5} M is reasonable, then the O.D. of one micron pathlength is about 10^{-4}. The number of photons absorbed is then

$$\text{photons absorbed} = 2 \times 10^5 /\text{(sec.pixel.mW) at 500 nm.}$$

Assuming a quantum yield of 0.8 and a collection efficiency of 1/10, we should have at the detector

$$\text{photons at the detector} = 2 \times 10^4/\text{(sec.pixel.mW of incident light).}$$

Given the quantum efficiency of good detectors (0.1 at 500 nm), the final detected photon flux should be about

$$\text{flux detected} = 2000 \text{ photons/(sec.pixel.mW of light).}$$

This flux should be compared with the dark noise of most detectors, which can vary between 10 and 1000 photons equivalent per second per pixel. In our estimation, the only quantities that can vary over a wide range are the power of the laser and the effective concentration of the probe. Lasers can have up to watts of power and the concentration of the probe can be larger than we have assumed. The efficiency of detection can be smaller than we estimate and the noise can be larger. The purpose of our calculation is to give an idea of the kind of power that the laser must furnish to be usable for fluorescence microscopy.

Our conclusion is that 1 mW of incident power is close to the detection limit of a microscope system, if that power is spread on 10^6 pixels. Tsien and Waggoner (see Chapter 11) find an optimal power with the best S/N with respect to autofluorescence and elastic and inelastic scattering of 76 μW at 488 nm and 590 μW, when triplet formation is neglected. Our calculation gives some overestimation of the required power. Therefore, a laser power of 1–2 mW should be sufficient for most applications. This depends on the efficiency of the light path optics.

With regard to the saturation problem, we must take into account two different types of effects. One is related to the number of molecules that can absorb light in a given area with respect to the amount of incident light. In a given pixel, assuming a volume of 1 μm^3, the volume is 10^{-15} liter. At a molar concentration of 10^{-5}, we should have approximately $6 \cdot 10^{+3}$ molecules per pixel. Since the number of photons absorbed per mW of incident light is about $2.5 \cdot 10^{+5}$/sec on a single pixel, each molecule is excited about 40 times per second. From the photophysical point of view, the decay of fluorescein (and in general all of the single state decays) is very fast ($4 \cdot 10^{-9}$ sec), so that the ground state should be repopulated very rapidly. However, there are many possible photochemical processes which are either irreversible or have a cycle of several milliseconds to seconds. In this latter case, even if the quantum yield for these effects is below 1/1000, and the exposure times on the order of several seconds, they will pose severe limitations on the overall intensity that can be used without large linearity distortions. Of course, for quantitative microscopy this is the most important limitation.

Having discussed the power requirements, we continue with a concise description of the basic elements of a laser, its principle of operation and other important aspects, such as heat removal and mechanical and optical stability.

THE BASIC LASER

The acronym laser stands for *Light Amplification by Stimulated Emission of Radiation*. Laser action, i.e., the emission of coherent radiation, has been observed for a large number of different media, but all lasers have several features in common, see Figure 1a.

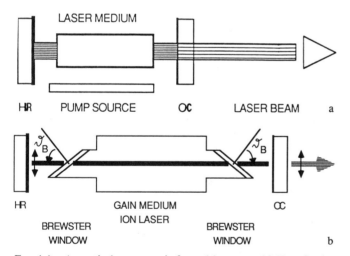

FIG. 1a). An optical resonator is formed between a highly reflective mirror (high reflector, R = 99.99%), HR, and a mirror with a reflectivity of e.g., 80%, the output coupler (OC). Within this resonator we find the active lasing medium (a crystal, semiconductor, liquid or gas) and its energy supply: the pump source, an arc lamp or flash lamp, another laser, etc. 1b). Emission of linearly polarised laser light from an ion laser equipped with Brewster angle plasma-tube windows. Only vertically polarised light is amplified. It experiences no reflection losses at the Brewster angle: theta Brewster = $\tan^{-1} n$, with n the refractive index of the pure crystalline quartz window. Horizontally polarised light suffers reflection losses and stays below the lasing threshold. Windows normal to the optical axis of the laser would introduce reflection losses and could prevent the laser from operating at all or introduce a set of reduced length resonator cavities.

Active laser medium: atoms, molecules, and atomic ions in pure or mixed gases, vapors, liquids, or solids.

Excitation source: An external source of energy used to pump the laser medium. This can be another laser, arc lamp or flash lamp, electron beam, proton beam, electrical discharge and radio frequency (rf) excitation, electrical current, etc. The choice of pump source is determined by the optical, thermal, and mechanical properties of the active medium and the wavelength region of interest.

Optical resonator: The laser medium is enclosed between two parallel mirrors which form a Fabry-Perot interferometer. The mirrors are placed at each end of the laser medium. One mirror, the high reflector (HR), totally reflects, the other mirror, the output coupler (OC), only partially reflects.

Principle of Operation

Upon excitation a particle absorbs energy and goes to an excited level. It returns to the lower level by emission of radiation. Under normal conditions, a Boltzmann equilibrium exists for the population of the energy levels. When an excited, metastable level with a long lifetime exists in the laser medium upon excitation, energy will accumulate in this level. An inversion of the Boltzmann distribution normally present will occur if the excitation source is intense enough, then photons emitted from this energy level will interact with the population of the metastable level, forcing energy to be released back to the lower level. This process is called stimulated emission of radiation. The stimulated emitted light is coherent, i.e., a certain phase relationship exists between the photons because the excited level is stimulated to emit by a traveling electromagnetic wave in the laser medium. Every laser works via this process of stimulated emission of electro magnetic radiation. The radiation will have a high degree of monochromaticity or spectral purity, since emission occurs from a well-defined transition. Also, the emitted radiation will have excellent spatial and temporal coherence.

A convenient way to couple the laser medium with the electromagnetic radiation is a resonant cavity. At optical wavelengths this is achieved by a Fabry-Perot type interferometer. Two plane parallel mirrors, one highly reflective, the other semi transparent, are separated by a distance of an integral multiple of half the lasing wavelength. This resonant cavity increases the probability of stimulating de-excitation because the electromagnetic radiation stays in contact with the laser medium longer. It also provides the necessary feedback to let the emission grow coherently.

So far we have only discussed a three-level laser, i.e., ground-state, upper excited-state, and lower excited-state. In a four-level laser, the population inversion is more easily obtained (Arecchi, 1972). Other improvements relate to the replacement of the Fabry-Perot mirrors by corner cube reflectors or crossed roof prisms for increased stability. An interesting approach is the use of optical fibers in a laser cavity. (For further information see Arecchi, 1972; Bass and Stitch, 1985; Bertolotti, 1983; Stitch, 1979.)

Laser Modes: Longitudinal and Transversal

The two plane-parallel mirrors of the Fabry-Perot interferometer cavity form an optical resonator. A standing wave pattern of an integer multiple, m, of half wavelengths, $\lambda/2$, exists in this optical cavity of length L: $m = L/(\lambda/2)$. The frequency, ν, for the mth vibration along the long axis of the laser (an axial or longitudinal mode) is, therefore, $\nu = mc/2L$, with c the speed of light in the laser cavity. The frequency spacing between adjacent longitudinal modes is $c/2L$, and it is the inverse of the round trip time. A very large number of longitudinal modes exist in the laser cavity unless bandwidth limiting devices such as Fabry-Perot etalons are installed in the cavity.

Transverse modes, vibrating perpendicular to the long axis of the laser, also exist. These modes are known as transverse electro-magnetic modes, TEM_{mn}, with m and n integers describing the nodal points in the two directions perpendicular to the laser axis. For each transverse mode many longitudinal modes can exist. (For an indepth derivation, see laser handbooks, e.g., by Arecchi, 1972; Bass and Stitch, 1985; Demtröder, 1982; Hecht and Zajac, 1977; Stitch, 1979.)

For light microscopy, the TEM_{00} is desired for most experiments. It has a Gaussian beam profile with no phase shifts across the beam. The maximum intensity is in the center of the beam, it has complete spatial coherence with the smallest beam divergence, and it can be focused to the smallest spot size. Donut-shaped transverse modes TEM_{01}^* (TEM_{10} in overlap with TEM_{01}), such as obtained from some He-Cd lasers operating at 325 nm, are not desirable, since they possess no intensity in the center of the beam. In this case spatial filtering is necessary. (See later section)

Polarization

The output of many lasers is linearly polarized with the polarization vector vertical.

A convenient and inexpensive way to minimize reflection losses and to generate linearly polarized light is the installation of a Brewster surface in the resonator. Horizontally polarized light incident on such a plane parallel plate, (which is tilted so that the normal of the plane and the incoming beam form a specific angle, theta Brewster), will be completely reflected. Vertically polarized light will be completely transmitted without any reflection losses (Fig 1b). In laser resonators, this plate is usually a quartz or a fused silica plate. In solid state lasers, the rod is sometimes cut at the Brewster angle to minimize reflection losses. In gas lasers, the exit windows are usually placed at the Brewster angle to obtain vertically polarized light. When the Brewster windows are pointing upward they are the most likely spot for dust to collect, damaging the coating. Therefore, they must be kept absolutely clean using a dust cover and a slightly positive pressure in the laser head. In the jet-stream dye laser the jet is placed at Brewster angle in order to minimize losses due to reflection of the pumping beam, thereby maximizing the pumping efficiency. For the same reason, the tuning element of the dye laser, is also placed at Brewster angle. Brewster surfaces are usually the origin of very dangerous reflections. Eye protection should be worn.

Lasers built without Brewster windows will still show some polarized output due to birefringence within optical components. However, the plane of polarization may change with time even though the total intensity stays constant. After passing this light through a polarizer, large intensity fluctuations may be observed.

Randomly polarized beams contain two orthogonal components but the phase and ratio of the two components vary rapidly in time: polarization noise. Dichroic mirrors, and, in fact, any mirror or lens surface, not at right angles with the incoming radiation will reflect vertically and horizontally polarized light differently (directions are taken with respect to the plane of incidence formed by the reflected and transmitted beams). A convenient way to depolarize the laser emission is to install a polarizer or polarizing beamsplitter and a 1/4 waveplate (See Chapters 1 and 6 for methods of phase randomizing.) This waveplate converts linearly polarized light into circularly polarized light when placed at an angle of 45° with respect to the incoming linear polarization. These waveplates usually are designed for a specific wavelength. Achromatic retarders, e.g., Fresnel rhombs, are sometimes preferred, but are quite expensive (Hecht and Zajac, 1977; Driscoll and Vaughan, 1978). Another advantage of this arrangement in optical microscopy is preventing reflected or backscattered light from reaching the detector.

Coherent Properties of Laser Light

Temporal coherence. The coherence time is the time interval for which two points in space maintain a phase difference less than π.

Coherence length. The path travelled by the wave during the coherence time is called the coherence length, $L_c \sim c/\Delta\omega$, with $\Delta\omega$ the spectral width of the laser. For a typical gas laser, the bandwidth is a few GHz with L_c a few centimeters. In single mode operation with $\Delta\nu \sim 1 MHz$, L_c is 50 m. Dye lasers equipped with tuning elements, diode, and other lasers usually have bandwidths on the order of tens of GHz with L_c a few millimeters or less. Depending on the type of line narrowing element installed, L_c can increase by a factor 10^3 to 10^6.

Spatial coherence. Spatial coherence occurs when a constant, time independent, phase difference exists for the optical field amplitude at two different points in space.

Coherence surface. The coherence surface defined as the region of space for which the absolute phase difference of the optical field is less than π.

Coherence volume. The coherence volume is the product of coherence length and coherence surface. Interference between superimposed coherent waves will only be visible within the volume.

The long coherence length of lasers will cause laser speckles (i.e. interference effects) and scatter from out of focus particles to interfere with the image. Normally this light is removed by the dichroic mirror but a polarizing beamsplitter and 1/4 waveplate can be equally effective for removal of backscattered light (see Chapter 7).

Pumping Power Requirements

In order to sustain laser action, the gain of the optical resonator needs to be larger than the losses due to resonator walls and other optical elements. The minimum pumping power P necessary is proportional to ν^3. This means that going from the infrared (IR) through the visible (VIS) towards the ultra violet

(UV) an ever increasing amount of energy is needed to obtain laser action. This puts limitations on the possible pumping mechanisms.

Heat removal. A substantial amount of excitation energy is converted into heat, which must be removed to prevent destruction of the active laser medium. Small laser systems can use convective air cooling, but larger laser systems need forced-air or water cooling. Especially for the largest systems, fans and turbulent water-flows will introduce vibrations in the system (microphonics). These unwanted mechanical vibrations are inevitably coupled to the mirror mounts of the resonator cavity, causing a noise increase of the optical output. Pumps that recycle liquid laser media are a well known source for vibration. In this case, the vibration is transferred via hoses to the active medium in the resonator. To minimize these effects, the hoses should be clamped or fastened as close as possible to the laser head. The generated heat will also put thermal stress on the mechanical parts of the resonator. Laser systems with a less than ideal design will, therefore, quickly loose their proper alignment or may need an unacceptably long warm-up time. The installation of a laser system in a room with large daily or annual temperature fluctuations or a ceiling fan continuously blowing cold, dusty, air directly onto a laser will also hamper operation and cause performance to deteriorate.

Other Installation Requirements

Manufacturers usually describe the electrical power requirements and flow rates for cooling water (Gibson, 1988, 1989; Rapp, 1988). Before installation of a laser system, sufficient room temperature control and air conditioning should be available, an exhaust for noxious fumes should exist and systems should be established which prevent calamities such as power outages and coolant flow interruption. Mechanical vibrations due to nearby traffic can be eliminated by installing the system on commercially available vibration-free laser tables.

TYPES OF LASERS

The earliest lasers available were solid state lasers, using ruby as the active laser medium (Bertolotti, 1983). Subsequently, a wide variety of lasers were developed (Arecchi, 1972; Bass and Stitch, 1985; Brown, 1981; Eden, 1988, Weast and Tuve, 1971). Essentially, all continuous wave (CW) gas lasers (Bloom, 1968) and some solid state lasers, with emission in the visible part of the electro magnetic spectrum, satisfy the minimum intensity requirements estimated above for fluorescence microscopy. As we already mentioned, one of the essential characteristics of a laser to be used in fluorescence microscopy is the wavelength of emission. Some other important parameters are the output power at each wavelength, efficiency, and stability. Table I lists the major options for CW lasers. Table II lists the major options for pulsed laser systems.

CONTINUOUS WAVE (CW) LASERS

Continuous Wave (CW) lasers can be divided into several classes:

- gas lasers
- dye lasers
- solid state lasers

TABLE 1.   CW GAS LASERS: HIGH POWER

Argon ion, water cooled

25W multiline, cost \$\$\$\$\$*. (Specification for Innova-200-25/5 (Coherent) typical high power argon laser.)

Emission (nm)	Power (mW)	
multiline visible	25000	
528.7	1800	
514.5	10000	
501.7	1800	
496.5	3000	
488.0	8000	
476.5	3000	
472.7	1300	
465.8	800	
457.9	1500	
454.5	800	
333.6–363.8	5000	(multiline)
274.4–305.5	600	(multiline)

Krypton ion, water cooled

Cost \$\$\$\$\$* (Specification for Innova 200-K3, (Coherent) typical high power krypton laser.)

Emission (nm)	Power (mW)	
multiline IR	1600	
multiline red	4600	
multiline green/yellow	3300	
multiline blue/green	3500	
multiline violet	3000	
multiline UV	2000	
799.3–793.1	300	
752.5	1200	
676.4	900	
647.1	3500	
568.2	1100	
530.9	1500	
520.8	700	
482.5	400	
476.2	400	
468.0	500	
415.4	280	
413.1	800	
406.7	900	
337.5–356.4	2000	(multiline)

Stability of high power ion lasers

Example of most powerful ion laser, model Innova 200 (Coherent Inc, Laser Products Division, Palo Alto, Ca (800)-367-7890). Long term stability over 30 minutes after 2 hour warm-up. Values given for 514.5 nm (Ar) and 647.1 nm (Kr).

Laser type: model:	Argon ion Innova 200–25/5	Krypton ion Innova 200–K3
Light regulation	0.5%	0.5%
Current regulation	3.0%	3.0%
Current regulation w/Power Track	1.0%	1.0%
Optical noise (rms)		
Light regulation	0.3%	0.3%
Current regulation	0.4%	0.5%
Current regulation w/Power Track	0.3%	0.3%
Beam parameters		
Diameter (mm)	1.9	2.0
Divergence (mrad)full angle	0.4	0.5
Mode	TEM$_{00}$	TEM$_{00}$
Polarization	V	V

Advantages
- sturdy design, 2 inch invar bar.
- possibility to pump UV absorbing dyes.
- good beam pointing stability with hands off operation and active stabilization via Power Track system.

Disadvantages
- expensive, large system

CW GAS LASERS: MEDIUM POWER

Argon ion, water cooled

100 mW multiline, model 75-.1, Lexel, cost $$* (typical low power)

Emission (nm)	Multimode version Power (mW)	(200 mW multiline)
528.7	5	10
514.5	50	75
501.7	5	10
496.5	10	20
488.0	50	75
476.5	10	20
457.9	5	10

Example of typical low power Ar and Kr ion laser, models 75-.1 (Lexel Laser, Inc Fremont, Ca. (415)-770-0800)

model:	75-.1 (Ar)	75-.1 (Kr)
Long term stability		
Light control	0.2%	0.2%
Current control	2.0%	2.0%
Optical noise (rms)		
Light control	0.5%	0.5%
Current control	1.5%	1.5%
Beam parameters		
Diameter (mm)	0.9	1.0
Divergence (mrad) full angle	0.8	1.2
Mode	TEM_{00}	TEM_{00}
Polarization	V	V

Advantages
- small, portable, rugged invar bar resonator construction
- similar systems are available with air cooling
- Berillium-oxide plasma tubes long tube lifetime, years.

Disadvantages
- no UV or violet laser lines

Many manufacturers make models with similar specifications.

Helium-Cadmium, air cooled

Cost $* (Omnichrome, high power laser)

Emission (nm)	Power (mW)	
441.6	150	(model 4112×M) multimode
325.0	40	(model 3112×M)

White Light, Helium-Cadmium laser based on hollow cathode design. Nikon Dempa Kogyo Co. ltd, Sayama Factory, Japan, ph 0429(52)7211, FAX 0429(54)3968.

Emission (nm)	Power (mW)
887.8	
865.2	
853.1	
806.7	
728.4	
723.7	
636.0	
645.5	
537.8	25 total
533.7	
441.6	
325.0	

Example of Helium-Cadmium laser, most powerful models 3112×, 3112×M, 4112× and 4112×M (Omnichrome, Chino, CA, 800-525-6664)

Laser model	3112X	3112XM	4112X	4112XM
Wavelength (nm)	325	325	442	442
Average power (mW)				
CW specified	10		50	
typical (new)	12	40	75	150
Stability (over 2 hours)		5%		5%
Beam parameters				
Diameter (mm)	0.64		1.13	
Divergence (mrad)	0.65		0.5	
Mode	DONUT	multi-mode	TEM_{00}	multi-mode
RMS noise				
resonance region (240–300khz)	<4%		<4%	
10 hz–10 Mhz	<2%		<2%	

Advantages
- rigid and rugged
- no optics cleaning or adjustment
- 6000 hour expected tube life
- portable
- extra low noise sytems available upon request
- low power consumption 580 W under operating conditions after warmup (650 W from 0–5 min)

Disadvantages
- plane polarized output available for less powerful models
- forced air cooling may cause some vibration
- DONUT, TEM_{01}^* (overlapping TEM01 and TEM10) mode gives increased power, but like other multimode units may require a spatial filter to clean the laser beam.

Other manufacturers provide similar systems. Liconix (Sunnyvale, CA, 408-734-4331), makes many systems with plane polarized (V) output and with passive, convective air cooling.

Helium-Neon, air cooled

Multiline, model ML500, Spindler and Hoyer, Inc., Milford, MA, 508–478-6200, cost $*

Emission (nm)	Power (mW)
1523.1	0.5
1206.6	0.1
1198.5	0.3
1176.7	0.4
1161.4	0.4
1152.6	15
1140.9	0.2
1084.4	0.7
1079.8	0.4
632.8	50
629.4	0.6
611.8	1
604.5	1
594.5	1
543.0	0.75

Advantages
- rugged, long-lived, portable.

Disadvantages
- relatively low power

CW SOLID-STATE LASERS

High power

Neodymium-Yttrium Aluminum Garnet (Nd-YAG) and Neodymium-Yttrium Lithium Fluoride (Nd-YLF) system, (Coherent) cost $$$$$$*
Example of recently developed Nd-YAG, Nd-YLF laser system (Coherent, Laser Products Division, Palo Alto, Ca (800)-367-7890)

Laser model	Antares Nd-YAG			Antares Nd-YLF		
Wavelength (nm)	1064	532	355	1053	527	351
Average power (W)						
CW	24			22		
Modelocked (76 22)	2	0.55	18	2	0.55	
		or 3	or 1		or 3	or 1
Pulse width (ps)	100	70	70	50	35	35
Peak/Peak stability						
light loop off	<4%	<8%	<12%	<1.5%	<3%	<4.5%
light loop on	<1%	<2%	<3%	<0.75%	<1.5%	<2.5%
Beam parameters						
Diameter (mm)	1.3	1.3	0.7	0.5	1.5	0.7
Divergence (mrad)	1	0.5	0.6	3	0.5	0.6
Mode	TEM_{00}			TEM_{00}		
Polarization	V	V or H	V	V	V or H	V

Advantages
 • Easy to operate
 • reliable, stable system not sensitive to vibration, warms quickly up, system uses two krypton arc pumping lamps for homogeneous thermal load on laserrod.
 • microprocessor controlled console
 • automatic Q-switch protection for frequency doubling crystal
 • good manuals
 • operating costs low, replacement of pumping krypton lamps every 400 to 800 hours dependent on pumping power.
 • system can be Q-switched at up to 20 khz with 120–130 ns pulsewidth and mode-locked and Q-switched at the same time at up to 1.2 khz with a pulsewidth of 200–300 ns.
 • possibility to pump dyes that absorb 355 nm: extended spectral region

Disadvantages
 • large system takes up a lot of space
 • expensive
 • requires 30 kW electrical power and 2–8 gallons of cooling water per minute

Low power

Diode pumped Nd-YAG, model DPY 115 C, AB Lasers, Acton, MA, 508–635–9100, cost $$*

Emission (nm)	Power (mW)
1064	40
532	5

Advantages
 • compact and rugged
 • no high voltage
 • very high efficiency

Diode lasers, cost very low

Emission (nm)		Power (mW)
830	GaAlAs	25
810	"	4
790	"	3
780	GaAlAs	16
750	GaAlAs	15
670	InGaAlP	14

Semi-conductor or diode laser

Model DC25B Spindler & Hoyer, Milford, MA, 508–478–6200.

Wavelength (nm)	670 ± 20
Output power (mW)	0.5–2.0 adjustable
Long term stability	5%
Beam parameters	
Diameter (mm)	3×7 elliptical
Divergence (mrad) full angle	1.5
Mode at 2 mW	Single transverse, single longitudinal
Polarization power dependent	V

Advantages
 • compact size and rugged
 • tunable
 • low maintenance
 • no cooling water required

Examples

Titanium sapphire, CW tunable, model 3900, Spectra Physics, Mountain View, CA, 800–227–8054, cost $$$$*

　　　670–1000nm,　　　　3500mW @ 800nm

Another manufacturer is Schwartz Electro-Optics, Inc., (SEO), Orlando, FL, 305–298–1802. Pumping with a 5W, all line argon ion laser, 500 mW at 800 nm is obtained.

*$ = $10,000; $$ = $20,000 etc.

1. Gas lasers

Three major types of CW gas lasers are available (Bloom, 1968):

■ Argon Ion, Krypton Ion, and a mixture of Argon and Krypton
■ Helium-Neon
■ Helium-Cadmium

The CO and CO_2 lasers emit around 5 μm and at 10.6 μm and are not discussed here. In general krypton, and helium-neon lasers are not used, except if red excitation is necessary. Argon-krypton mixed gas ion lasers often form a cheaper alternative for the purchase of both an argon and a krypton system with additional power requirements and beam-steering optics.

Argon-ion

By far the most common laser in microscopy is the argon ion laser. Its stability is better, compared to that of a krypton laser, with less gas slushing. Commercial systems provide a large variety of emission wavelengths and output power, Figure 2. Recently quartz plasma-tubes have been changed to versions with metal-ceramic (Berillium oxide) tube envelopes with tungsten disks, crystalline-quartz, coated windows and quartz-metal

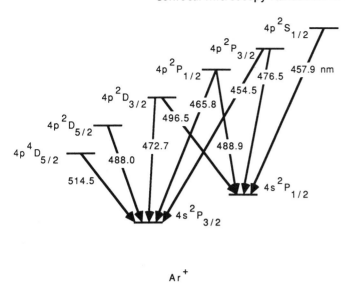

FIG. 2. Schematic energy diagram for Argon ion laser.

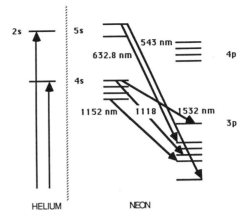

FIG. 3. Schematic energy diagram for Helium-neon laser.

seals, thereby increasing their reliability. The graphite and tungsten disks have a central bore, which passes the laser beam. The discharge pumps ions to the cathode end of the tube. This causes a pressure gradient between the anode and cathode. Return holes around the outer edge of the disks form an internal gas return path, which maintains a uniform gas pressure along the length of the plasma tube. Current systems have an operational lifetime from 3000–5000 hours. The stability of these lasers, especially the small- and medium-sized models, is good because they can be cooled by convective or forced air and their power requirements are modest. Some models are portable and easy to use, especially with the newly introduced features like Power Track (Coherent) or a new resonator design Stabilite (Spectra Physics).

The largest models are not so stable, and the heat they generate must be removed with a large amount of cooling water. The turbulent flow causes some vibration in the systems and insufficient water flow will cause the cooling water to boil and may lead to the destruction of the plasma tube. The large amount of heat generated also puts more strain on the resonator cavity. Longer warm-up times are necessary. The operational lifetime of these systems is on the order of 2000 hours. However, if the experiment requires reliable use of deep UV radiation at elevated power levels, these systems form a more stable alternative with respect to the solid-state UV generating lasers which require more steps to generate UV light.

Commercially available argon lasers have emission wavelengths extending from 275 to 528 nm. The emission is not continuously variable, but occurs at discrete wavelengths. Wavelength selection is obtained by installation of an angle tuned quartz prism or other appropriate optical elements. Starting in the UV, some of these lasers can generate hundreds of mW of power in the region were proteins absorb; however, microscopes with quartz optics are necessary.

A more accessible region of laser emission occurs between 334 and 364 nm. Lasers with powers of several watts are available and they are used to pump a dye laser which can cover a continuous spectral region from 390 nm extending well into the infrared. The output power of these pumped-dye lasers reaches several hundreds of mW.

The most common spectral region for lasers in microscopy is between 488 and 514 nm, although argon ion laser emission can be obtained from 454 to 528 nm. Both multiline or single line lasers are available from different manufacturers with powers ranging from a few mW for the small air cooled systems, to 10–20 W for the large frame, water cooled systems. The air cooled lasers are most commonly used in fluorescence microscopy. They are relatively stable and have tube lifetimes ranging from 5000 to 10000 hours. Partly, this is due to the fact that these units often are sealed. The optics provided by the manufacturer selects a single wavelength or the lasers may emit several wavelengths simultaneously. In the latter case, the user can externally select the proper wavelength by installation of interference filters, a prism monochromator, etc.

Krypton

When strong red emission is necessary, a krypton laser is the system of choice. Its stability, however, is slightly less than that of a comparably sized argon ion system. Also the gas retention in the graphite disks is slightly larger.

Helium-Neon

The use of these lasers in microscopy has been severely limited, essentially due to two major factors: the relatively low intensity and the red emission. With respect to emission wavelength, several manufacturers have recently introduced He-Ne lasers with emission at 534, 594, 612, 632 nm and lines in the infrared, Figure 3. However, the power of the multiline systems is relatively low, 1 to 2 mW, due to the introduction of wavelength-selecting elements in the resonator.

Helium-Cadmium

Helium-Cadmium (He-Cd) lasers have found several applications in microscopy. Essentially, they have two emission wavelengths at 325 and 442 nm, Figure 4. The lower wavelength requires special optics and is very rarely used in fluorescence microscopy. The emission at 442 nm is ideal for excitation of flavins and other fluorescent molecules with absorption in that spectral region. The power available at 325 nm is generally on the order of a few mW, while at 442 nm lasers with up to 150 mW are now available. The stability of these lasers is substan-

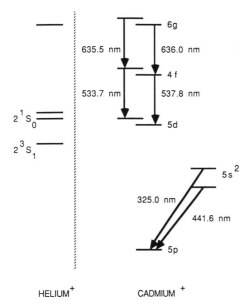

FIG. 4.   Schematic energy diagram for Helium-cadmium laser.

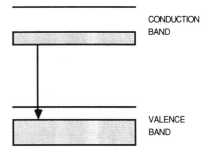

FIG. 5.   Schematic energy diagram for semiconductor laser.

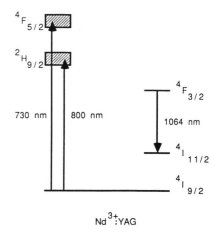

FIG. 6.   Schematic energy diagram for Neodymium-Yttrium-Aluminum Garnet (Nd-YAG) laser.

tially less than that of the argon ion lasers. In the 325 nm region, intensity fluctuations of 10 to 20% are not uncommon. The He-Cd laser tends to be more stable at the 442 nm emission. Some manufacturers provide special accessories to improve the intensity stability. These devices are based on external modulators with a fast feedback system. This method, of course, reduces the total power of the laser. In principle, these external modulators can be used to stabilize the output power of any CW laser. Most systems have an operational life of a 1 to 1.5 years, equivalent to 1000 to 2000 hours. The smaller lasers, operating at 325 nm, have a limited life-span. Some manufacturers require six weeks or more for tube replacements. Recently the so called "white light" He-Cd laser source has been introduced. It uses the negative glow region of a hollow cathode He-Cd laser (Nihon Dempa Kogyo Co., see Table I), and the powers for several lines have been balanced to produce a white light output. In addition to the 325 and 442 nm lines, wavelengths in the green at 533.7 and 537.8 nm, and in the red at 635.5 and 636.0 nm, are available with more lines in the near infrared from 723.7 to 887.8 nm. The manufacturer states a stability of 2% after a 10 minute warm-up.

2. Dye lasers

All dye lasers are optically pumped with powerful lasers. For continuous operation, the dye is circulated to prevent heating and bleaching of the dye, to reduce the competing triplet population, and to remove aggregates. Tuning of the laser is accomplished by a prism, a diffraction grating, and a stack of birefringent plates placed under Brewster angle or by etalons (Mollenauer and White, 1987; Demtröder, 1981). The laser medium is easy to handle, inexpensive, and consists of an organic dye dissolved in a solvent. Upon excitation, the dye emits radiation at longer wavelengths: fluorescence. Because of so-called "forbidden transitions," the molecules tend to pile up in the first excited triplet state. Rapid pumping, or the use of a jet stream, will prevent this triplet state from being populated. In order to keep the quantum yield high, i.e., the ratio of emitted photons versus the number of absorbed photons, the dye is

usually cooled. In this way, competing processes, like collisional and vibrational deexcitation, are minimized. High optical efficiencies (20 to 30%) can be obtained. The dye lasers have an extremely broad tuning range. Cuvettes with laser dye have to be cleaned regularly because the pumping beam cooks the dye molecules at the optical surfaces.

3. Solid state lasers

Semiconductor or diode injection lasers

Charge carriers in the semi-conductor material can be pumped optically, or by an electron beam but the most common method simply uses an externally-applied current in the forward-biased direction. Figure 5. Most of the devices still operate in the near infrared. The trend in recent years has been the development of diode lasers with output in the red. Present development of this type of laser towards wavelengths from the infrared to the red and their increased power will make this type of laser a formidable threat to the He-Ne lasers. When selecting a drive current source, it is important to select one with a low noise current, good stability and having a controllable temperature, because the diode lasers can choose their emission wavelength by varying their drive current and junction temperature.

Diode-pumped lasers

A different class of laser, based on solid state technology, has recently appeared (Kaminskii, 1981); i.e., Neodymium-Yttrium Aluminum Garnet (Nd-YAG) (Figure 6) and Yttrium

Lithium Fluoride (Nd-YLF) pumped by a diode laser. The advantages of diode lasers over conventional pump sources such as lamps, are reduced cooling requirements, higher efficiencies due to a collimated and focused output, and enhanced frequency stability (Baer, 1986). A typical improvement in electrical-optical conversion efficiency from 0.5% (TEM_{00} mode) to 6% can be obtained. The infrared output at 1064 (YAG) or 1054 nm (YLF) is frequency doubled to provide radiation at 532 and 527 nm, respectively. These lasers are extremely compact, efficient, and have an output power up to 15 mW. This new technology is expanding and the output power will increase in the near future. The stability of these lasers is quite good and the emission wavelength is ideal for excitation of rhodamine dyes.

Tunable solid state laser

One of the exciting new developments is the recent release of the CW Titanium-Sapphire laser (Hammerling, et al., 1985). These lasers can be pumped by a CW Nd-YAG or an ion laser. Their tuning range extends from 700–1000 nm. Power output is 3.5 W at 790 nm when pumped with a 20 W all line argon ion laser. This laser is bound to replace the IR dye lasers; it is much easier to operate, no dyes have to be changed, the stability is better than 3%, and the rms noise between 10 Hz and 1 MHz is less than 1%.

PULSED LASERS

Nitrogen lasers

The use of pulsed lasers in fluorescence microscopy has been limited. In principle a pulsed laser, after intensity integration, can provide performance similar to a CW laser. Pulsed lasers are characterized by large power per pulse (see Table II), which is very useful for a pumping a dye laser. Among the most common pulsed lasers are nitrogen lasers. Generally nitrogen lasers are not used directly, but in conjunction with a dye laser. Nitrogen lasers can provide intensities between 10^{-5} J to 10^{-3} J per pulse with repetition rates on the order of 20 to 100 pulses/sec. The average power is between 1 mW to 1 W, and the wavelength emission is at 337 nm. Due to the high instantaneous power, relatively large dye laser pumping efficiencies (30%) can be obtained. These lasers can provide easy tunability in the region from about 360 nm to the extreme red, depending on the dye used. The pulse width of these lasers varies between a fraction of a microsecond to subnanosecond. However, the time characteristic of laser emission has not yet been exploited in fluorescence microscopy.

Excimer Lasers

Over the past ten years excimer lasers have increasingly been used as light sources in the VUV and UV. They combine a high power with tunability (Figure 7). Although it is a well known fact that the rare gases in the ground state are chemically inert, it was found that in the excited electronic state, stable excited molecules were formed. Molecules with these properties are called excimers (excited-state dimers). Pumping of these lasers can be carried out with an intense beam of very high speed (relativistic) electrons. Since electron beams are not widely available, so far the only pumping technique is the avalanche electric discharge. Typical gases used in the excimer laser are the rare gases, Xe_2, Ar_2, and the rare-gas halides, KrF, XeCl, XeF, ArF, and N_2.

Excimer Lasers generally provide much more power than nitrogen lasers and higher repetition rates. Powers as high as 1–2 J are possible at repetition rates up to 500 Hz (Mollenauer and White, 1987; Rhodes, 1983). Their characteristic emission wavelengths are reported in Table II.

Metal vapor lasers

Metal vapor lasers (Lewis et al., 1988) are also extremely powerful and can be operated at much higher repetition rates. The average power can exceed 100 W and the repetition rate can be as high as 20–50 KHz. Their characteristic emission wavelengths are also reported in Table II.

A logical classification for pulsed laser systems is according to their temporal pulse behavior.

Normal mode, free running—When observed with a fast diode and oscilloscope, solid-state lasers can generate a continuous train of random spikes with varying intensity caused by the interaction of the various modes. This type of operation is not very useful.

Q-switched lasers

The term Q-switched is derived from the radio and microwave terminology, and this type of operation relates to a forced change in the quality factor, Q, of the resonant cavity. A low Q would indicate a resonator which hardly supports laser action. A simple implementation of a Q-switching device is the installation of an optical shutter in the resonator. The sudden opening of the switch releases all the stored energy in one giant pulse.

Active mode-locked—In a resonant cavity, many simultaneously oscillating, optical modes are present at the same time (Arecchi, 1972; Mollenauer and White, 1987). Usually these modes interact with each other in a random way. No phase relationship exists between the various modes. The output power fluctuates randomly according to the time dependent interaction between the various modes. Installation of an intracavity modulator with a resonance frequency exactly matching the round trip time in the laser resonator will lock all modes to that resonance frequency through gain modulation at exactly the frequency c/2L of the spacing of the cavity modes. This will generate many sidebands with the same frequency spacing of c/2L. The side bands provide for the required mutual phase locking of the modes. A certain phase relationship is maintained. This in turn causes the laser to generate a train of narrow optical pulses.

In dye lasers, one can obtain a train of optical pulses by pumping with an optical pulse train from another mode-locked laser (Herrmann and Wilhelmi, 1987; Muckenheim et al., 1988). A requirement is that the cavity length of the dye laser must exactly match that of the pump laser, i.e., a synchronously pumped laser.

TABLE 2. PULSED LASER SYSTEMS

Dye Laser

Examples of dye lasers pumped with various commonly used excitation sources.

Pump source:	Flashlamp	Ar/Kr ion	Copper vapor	Excimer	Nd-YAG	Nitrogen
See note:	a	b	c	d	e	f
Wavelength range (nm)	390–950	380–950	600–950	320–970	410–880	380–1000
Average power	50 W	5/100 W/mW	5 W	14 W	2 W	200 mW
Repetition rate	10 Hz	cw/80 MHz	12 KHz	25–500 Hz	10–40 Hz	300 Hz
Energy/pulse	5 J	1 nJ	0.5 mJ	40–120 mJ	20–120 mJ	700 μJ
Pulse width (FWHM)	2.2 μs	<10 ps	30 ns	7–25 ns	5–10 ns	6 ns
Amplitude jitter (%)	3					
Beam parameters						
Diameter (mm)	10	2.5				
Divergence (mrad)	1.2		0.5			

a: model LFDL-20 dye laser pumped with 2 60 cm long flash lamps, Candela Laser Corp., Wayland, Ma (617)-356-7637
b: mode-locked synchronously-pumped dye laser. Values depend slightly on dye laser configuration, Lambda Physik data.
c: model DL20 dye laser, shorter pulse widths can be obtained. Oxford laser,
d: model FL 3002 dye laser, Lambda Physik, Acton, Ma (617)-263-1100
e: Lambda Physik data
f: model ALCR 1 dye laser, Sopra, Bois-Colombes, France, 331-424-20447

Excimer lasers

Excimer pump lasers combine the high repetition rate of the Nitrogen pump laser with the high pumping power of the Nd-YAG. They still require elaborate maintenance (gas handling).

Excimer, max. 500 pps, EMG 200 MSC series excimer laser, Lambda Physik, Acton, MA, 617-263-1100, cost $$$$*.

	Emission (nm)	Power (mW)	(Energy/Pulse (mJ)
Fluor, F2	157	50	6
Argon Fluoride	193	60000	300
Krypton Chloride	222	10000	150
Krypton Fluoride	248	120000	500
Xenon Chloride	308	100000	400
Nitrogen (N2)	337	600	8
Xenon Fluoride	351	60000	300

Metal vapor, air cooled

Cost $$$$$*

	Emission (nm)	Power (mW)	(Energy/Pulse (mJ)
Copper vapor	578.2	5000	2.75
	510.6	10000	
Gold vapor	627.8	1500	0.15

Examples of several typical metal vapor lasers, Gold and Copper vapor lasers, models AU2 and CU10 are air cooled, medium power system. Models AU10 and CU60 are water-cooled, high power systems. Oxford lasers, Acton, Ma (508)-264-9110

Laser model	AU2	CU10	AU10	CU60
Laser medium	gold	copper	gold	copper
Wavelength (nm)	627.8	510/578.2	627.8	510/578.2
Average power (W)	1.5	10	9	60
Pulse energy (mJ)	0.2	2	1.5	10
Pulse width (ns)	20–40	10–40	15–60	15–6
Repetition rate (KHz) standard	9–11	8–14	6–8	5.5–7.5
Beam parameters				
Diameter (mm)	20	25	42	42
Divergence (mrad) full angle, standard cavity	3	4	6	6
Run time on one load of Au/Cu (hours)	>300	>300	>300	>300

Neodynium-YAG

Neodymium-Yttrium Aluminum Garnet (Nd-YAG), 10 pps, cost $$$$$$$$* (ultra high power)

Emission (nm)	(Energy/Pulse (mJ)
1064	800
532	350
355	170
266	100

Neodynium-YLF

Q-Switched system for very high pump power. Neodymium-Yttrium Lithium Fluoride (Nd-YLF), 10000 pps, diode pumped

Emission (nm)	Energy/Pulse (mJ)
1047	20 μJ
523	5

(See Table I for mode-locked, Nd-YAG and Nd-YLF systems.)

Nitrogen

Nitrogen, max. 100 pps, cost $$*

Emission (nm)	Power (mW)	Energy/Pulse (mJ)
337	330	9000
428		

Examples of a low and high power Nitrogen laser, models LN103 and model UV22, Laser Photonics, Orlando, FL, 306–281–4103.

Laser model	LN103	UV22
Wavelength (nm)	337.1	
Average power (mW)	4.2	330
Pulse energy (uJ)	70	6000
Pulse width (ns)	0.3	10
Repetition rate (Hz)	60	100
Beam parameters		
Diameter (mm) VxH	2×3	6×32
Divergence (mrad) VxH	3×7	1×7

*$ = $10,000; $$ = $20,000 etc.

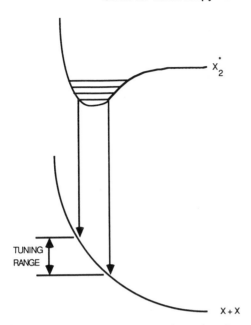

FIG. 7. Schematic energy diagram for excimer laser.

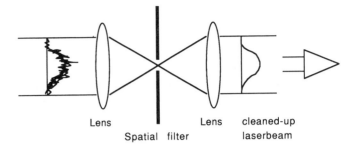

FIG. 8. Diagram of a spatial filter.

Trends in time-resolved spectroscopy applied to microscopy

The study of the time-resolved properties of fluorescence and phosphorescence emission from biological samples has advanced rapidly over the last couple of years due to the availability of several experimental techniques: time-correlated single photon counting (TC-SPC) and multifrequency cross-correlation phase and modulation fluorimetry (MCC-PMF). These developments have been aided by a rapid development in reliable, easy to operate laser and synchrotron light sources which generate stable nano- and picosecond optical pulse trains. Furthermore, by the availability of fast, 2-dimensional photodetectors like multi-anode microchannelplate photomultipliers (see e.g. Knutson, 1988) for parallel multiwavelength detection and the application of digital techniques, e.g. Jovin et. al. (1989). Extensive literature exists both for TC-SPC and MCC-PMF, which describes the status of state-of-the-art equipment in detail. The interested reader is referred to a number of review articles. For TC-SPC: O'Connor and Philips (1984), Cundall and Dale (1983). For MCC-PMF to Alcala et. al. (1985), Lakowicz (1983), Cundall and Dale (1983). A compilation of TC-SPC, MCC-PMF and similar time-resolved techniques, e.g. Wilson et. al. (1985) who describe a laser mode-beat frequency-domain method, is also given in Anal. Instrum. Vol. 14 (1985). Schemes to increase the data acquisition speed for MCC-PMF have recently been developed, see e.g. Birmingham and Garland (1988), Feddersen et. al. (1989a,b). Results of time-resolved spectroscopy on microscopic samples with a laser lightsource coupled to a microscope have been reported by e.g. Borst et. al. (1987), Kinosita et. al. (1988), Kusumi et al. (1988), Keating et. al. (1989).

WAVELENGTH EXPANSION THROUGH NON-LINEAR TECHNIQUES

Many gaps in the spectral region have existed in the past. Although dye lasers cover an extended portion of the spectrum, most dyes rapidly bleach. An alternative was found in the generation of non-linear optical (NLO) effects in certain classes of optically anisotropic crystals (Lin and Chen, 1987; Tebo, 1988). Focusing intense laser light into these crystals generates radiation at half the wavelength or double the frequency. This process, therefore, is known as "frequency doubling" or "second harmonic generation" (e.g., Huth and Kuizenga, 1987). The intensity of the frequency doubled light is proportional to the square of the incoming light intensity. When the incoming beam is very intense even third, fourth, or fifth harmonics can be generated. However, this usually only occurs for giant pulse lasers. The efficiency of the harmonic generation decreases at higher orders. Most doubling crystals can be angle or temperature tuned. Presently it is possible to combine even less powerful tunable dye lasers, semiconductor lasers etc., to continuously cover the wavelength range from 170 nm to 18 μm.

Another technique of generating different wavelengths from the basic laser wavelengths is sum or difference mixing. When two laser beams of high and low intensity and of frequency ω_1 and ω_2 respectively are simultaneously focused into a non-linear optical crystal, a sum signal is generated. The intensity of the sum signal, I $(\omega_1 + \omega_2)$ is proportional to the product I $(\omega_1)\cdot$I (ω_2). The higher-intensity, ω_1 laser helps in generating enhanced UV output I $(\omega_1 + \omega_2)$ with an extended tuning range. In a similar way, difference mixing, I $(\omega_1 - \omega_2)$ leads to a tuneable IR laser. (For examples, see Adhav, 1986; 1987; Demtröder, 1981, Dunning, 1978, Herrmann and Wilhelmi, 1987; Kaiser, 1988).

SPATIAL BEAM CHARACTERISTICS

Although lasers provide excellent beam divergence, the uniformity of the intensity in the beam cross section is relatively poor. Fortunately, this is generally not a problem, since the uniformity of illumination can be easily improved by spatial filtering. Filtering is very efficient when there is good spatial coherence of the beam. Several devices are available for spatial filtering; the most common is the gaussian spatial filter, which consists of a focusing lens that converges the beam toward a very small pinhole. After this pinhole, a second lens, one focal length away, is used to generate a parallel beam. This configuration is also used to expand or decrease the beam diameter. Spatial filtering takes place because diffraction effects at the pinhole produce an out-going wavefront which is the Fourier transform of the pinhole and is not effected by the spatial properties of the light impinging on the pinhole (Fig 8). It should be noted that dust particles moving in the vicinity of the pinhole can modulate the transmitted intensity, so great care must be taken to ensure that this does not occur.

INTENSITY FLUCTUATIONS OF CW LASERS

Several factors can be identified that produce high-frequency (noise) and slow variations (drift) in beam power, e.g., power supply variations, thermal drift of the cavity and mode competition. Noise and drift in dye lasers are caused by air bubbles and dye inhomogeneity. Gas lasers have plasma noise and instabilities caused by the optical pump (see Figure 9). Water cooled systems suffer from mechanical resonances and turbulence of the coolant. Nontheless, CW lasers can easily be intensity stabilized using either tube current stabilization or the external modulation of the light intensity (Miller and Hoyt, 1986). External modulators use a Pockels' cell between two crossed polarizers. An electrical signal is applied to the cell which causes a rotation of the plane of polarization. Depending on the voltage applied, more or less light can pass through the modulator. A photocell measures the transmitted light intensity and an electronic feedback system changes the Pockels' cell voltage to maintain the same transmitted intensity. Intensity fluctuations of up to 50% of the maximum power can be corrected in this way with a reduction of 50% in the total available power. The bandwidth of this intensity stabilizer is very good, generally on the order of 200 KHz. This modulator can effectively stabilize the intensity to more than 0.05% of the average intensity. Unfortunately, the modulator cannot work with low repetition rate pulsed lasers.

Another way to stabilize a gas laser is active stabilization (Peuse, 1988). Active stabilization corrects for misalignment of the resonator with a feedback mechanism. The advantages are that the resonator structure becomes independent of changes in the environment, e.g., temperature, and as a result provides an extremely rapid warm up time (seconds). This enables hands-off operation. Optical alignment occurs completely automatically and the system can run unattended for extended periods.

MAINTENANCE

After initial installation, a laser system usually performs well above the guaranteed specifications given by the manufacturer. The consumable parts (i.e., laser tubes) cannot be covered by any extended warranty. Depending on the type of laser used these costs can be substantial.

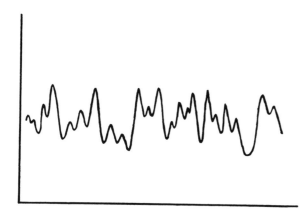

FIG. 9.   Typical high frequency noise spectrum of a gas laser measured with a HP8590A spectrum analyzer. Hor. axis: Displayed frequency range 0–100 KHz. Vert. axis: Intensity (arb. units).

A factor usually forgotten at the time of an initial laser purchase is the acquisition of peripheral equipment necessary for proper maintenance of the system. Extra dyes, filters, power meters, sampling oscilloscopes and sampling units, fast diodes, infrared viewers, spectrum analyzers, beam dumps, radiation shields, covers, laser goggles, explosion and fire proof cabinets for solvent storage and hazardous waste disposal, etc., are often not included.

Maintenance of active laser media

Laser tubes

Ion lasers need new plasma tubes due to sagging of the cathode or a deterioration of the bore of the graphite disks. Cracks may form in cooling tubes, usually leading to an immediate failure of the tube. Introduction of Berillium-Oxide tubes has significantly reduced the complexity of these laser systems and increased their reliability. Medium power systems last for about 3000 to 5000 hours (see Tables I and II) and high power systems for 2000 hours. Lasers systems presently come with warranties of 18 months. Some self-contained sealed systems carry a warranty for up to 5 years. Technology has significantly improved over the last couple of years so that the deposition of graphite disk material and other contaminants on the inner surface of the Brewster windows has been eliminated. As a standard, a getter, to improve the quality of the gas, is installed in the laser system. For Helium-Cadmium lasers, regular tube replacements are necessary at least once a year.

Gases

Excimer lasers need regular gas changes. Ion lasers refill their gas from a ballast tank via a micro computer controlled valve system. This has reduced the risk of overfilling the plasma tube and deteriorating the performance, or losing laser power altogether. To keep dust out of laser systems, the laser should be connected to a permanent supply of clean, dry, room temperature, oil free air or nitrogen gas. A slight over-pressure helps to prevent dust from entering the laser head. Commercial air filters used in these systems should not introduce additional dry powders into the laser system. Synchronously pumped systems perform markedly better and the intensity stability improves when dust is kept out.

Dyes

Dye lasers can pose a source of hidden costs. Rhodamine 6G is one of the least expensive dyes, and is the most stable: with a total of 2000 WH (i.e., the output power of the dye is reduced to 50% when it is pumped for 1000 H at 2 W or 400 H when pumped at 5 W). Dye aggregates are filtered. Evaporation of the solvents necessitates refilling. When the dye pump inadvertently starts to suck in air, air bubbles are generated and cause an immediate contamination of the optical mirror surfaces. This problem can be prevented by careful dye laser startup. Any weak, sharp clicks at the nozzle position indicate air bubbles. Operating the dye laser with the wrong solvent, e.g., viscosity not correct, may cause dye foam, which will quickly clog the system. In order to reduce downtime and contamination of dyes, it is recommended that every dye is run with its own pump module. It is more expensive, but results in a much faster hookup. Used dye and leftover solvent should be discarded in a manner which does not pose a threat to the environment. Dye nozzles should be cleaned regularly in a sonicator, especially when the system has not been used for a while. A non-laminar flow from the jet nozzle is an indication of nozzle problems.

Laser rods

Solid-state media, at least for CW lasers, are quite reliable. Pulsed systems, however, need a very good Gaussian beam quality, otherwise the rod coating will get damaged. Often one can hear this as sharp clicks indicating that the laser needs immediate attention. In the worst case, continued operation may damage the bulk of the laser rod (Soileau, 1987). Degradation of the surface layers of the medium, caused by the intense illumination of the pumping system and referred to as solarization, is less of a problem.

Maintenance of pumping media

For CW or pulsed lasers which are pumped by arc lamps, the lamp must be replaced when the output power of the laser decreases. On the inside of the arc lamp, dark deposits can be seen, which, over time, may cause a reduction in heat conduction and a catastrophic failure. Defective lamps usually fail within the first 10 to 20 hours after start-up (Smith, 1986; Littlechild and Mossler, 1988).

Maintenance of the optical resonator

Dust is one of the major enemies of the laser. Smoke should be absolutely prohibited in a laser laboratory. At all times dust covers should be kept in place and any dust on optical surfaces should be removed, e.g., on wavelength tuning prisms, or birefringent plates, mode locker or Pockels' cell surfaces, or mirrors. Using the wrong solvent to clean optics can destroy the optical coating, therefore, use only ultra-pure solvents recommended by the manufacturer and follow the proper procedure. Most laser manuals describe in detail the proper cleaning methods. Never use the same side of a cleaning wipe twice. A patterned movement should be used when cleaning optical surfaces. The optical coatings on laser cavity mirrors and external mirrors or fibers, especially in the UV, cannot withstand prolonged exposure to UV radiation. Colored rings will appear on the coating surfaces or they may look hazy or foggy. The formation of color centers, and thereby increased absorption, occurs in fused quartz materials: lenses, optical fibers, etc.. At high power, too tight, or self-focusing, conditions can produce mechanical damage. Damaged parts must be replaced immediately to prevent damage by a deteriorated beam on other components. This is especially true for pulsed systems. Frequency doubling elements should be inspected regularly or when laser intensity fluctuations occur. A microscope may be necessary to see damage to the coating. Heating of some crystals (e.g. KTP) seems to reduce these effects.

Maintenance of other system components

Cooling water

A gradual decrease in laser power can be caused by the growth of algae in the cooling water. A small addition of Sodium Azide (NaN_3) prevents a reoccurrence of the growth. An annual check of the rubber rings in the cooling hoses is recommended. The use of tap water for cooling should be limited as much as possible. Internal cooling circuits connected to a refrigerated bath are preferred. For proper operation of the laser, the resistivity of the cooling water should follow the recommended range given by the manufacturer. When the resistivity is too low, the lamps will not start. If the resistivity is too high, the plating on the inside of the elliptical resonator will dissolve and cause a decrease in laser power. Water filters and deionizing filters should be replaced regularly as demanded by the performance of the laser.

External optics

All optical surfaces should be kept as clean as possible. Mirror surfaces exposed to UV radiation will have to be replaced regularly, depending on the impinging power density. Apertures in spatial filters should be inspected and replaced when damage (burn) occurs.

SAFETY PRECAUTIONS

All lasers are generally divided into 4 classes:

- Class 1. Lasers and laser systems
- Class 2. Low power visible lasers and laser systems
- Class 3. Medium power lasers and laser systems
- Class 4. High power lasers and laser systems

General safety precautions, more stringent with increasing classification, must be followed when operating a laser. See ANSI-Z-136 classification. Every laboratory should have a "Laser Safety Officer" (LSO) who should be consulted when necessary. This person should be responsible for proper training of users of laser-assisted equipment. Lately laser companies (e.g., Coherent) are making a laudable effort in supplying users with a video cassette explaining the safety procedures to be followed.

Outside the laser laboratory, a "laser in use" warning sign must be posted and a red warning light should be positioned at the entrance to the laser room.

Inside the laser laboratory many safety precautions are necessary.

Curtains

Curtains should be made of a non-combustible material, preferably black in color. If a visual control is necessary from outside the room, a radiation-absorbing plastic window should be mounted in the door or wall. Tape should not be used to hold curtains together, since this could help to contain poisonous gases. An often disregarded possible source of trouble is clothing, famous are the stories of halved neckties.

Screens

Where possible, anodized, flat black aluminum pipes should be used to enclose the laser beams.

Beam stops.

Beam stops should be made out of anodized, flat black metal in such a way that no radiation is reflected back into the room. Stray reflections must be prevented; powerful IR or visible beams may easily start a fire on electrical cables, rubber parts, or other areas.

Each laser system must be equipped with the proper warning signs and interlocks. The listed references (Winburn, 1985; Sliney and Wolbarsht, 1980; Rockwell, 1983; 1986) describe in detail electrical hazards, e.g., reflections from rings, watches, etc., Biological effects are also extensively covered, i.e., thermal and photochemical effects upon exposure to CW and pulsed laser radiation, and the maximum permissible exposure to eyes and skin. Chemical hazards may be caused by laser dyes, such as mutagenic effects. Dye solvents and laser gases must be properly handled. Some protective measures recommended are laser goggles (Burgin, 1988), cleanliness, and proper handling of chemicals.

ACKNOWLEDGEMENT

This work was supported by National Institutes of Health Grant PHS-1P41-RR03155. The authors gratefully acknowledge Julie Butzow for her assistance in typing this manuscript.

REFERENCES

Adhav R.S., January, 1986. Data sheet 714. Sum frequency mixing and second harmonic generation. Quantum Technology, Inc., Lake Mary, FL (407–323–7750).

Alcala, J. R., E. Gratton, and D. M. Jameson. A multifrequency phase fluorometer using the harmonic content of a mode-locked laser. Anal. Instrum. 14, 225–250 (1985).

Arecchi, F.T., and Schultz-Dubois, E. O., 1972. Laser Handbook, Vol. 1, North-Holland Publishing Co., Amsterdam.

Baer, T. M., June 1986. Diode Laser Pumping of Solid State Lasers. Laser Focus/Electro Optics. 82–92

Bass, M. and Stitch, M. L., 1985. Laser Handbook, Vol. 5, North-Holland Publishing Co., Amsterdam.

Bertolotti, M., 1983. Masers and Lasers. An historical Approach. Adam Hilger Ltd., Bristol.

Birmingham, J. J., and P. B. Garland. Laser spectroscopic measurements of triplet-state lifetimes in both time and frequency domains. SPIE 909, 370–376 in Time-resolved laser spectroscopy in biochemistry, SPIE, Los Angeles (1988).

Bloom A. L., 1968. Gas lasers. John Wiley and Sons, New York.

Borst, W. L., S. Gangopadhyay, and M. W. Pleil. Fast analog technique for determining fluorescence lifetimes of multicomponent materials by pulsed laser. SPIE 743, 15–23 in Fluorescence detection, SPIE, Los Angeles (1987).

Brown, D. C., 1981. High-Peak-Power Nd-Glass Laser Systems, Vol. 25, in *Springer Series in Optical Sciences,* Springer-Verlag Berlin.

Burgin, C. D., 1988. A guide for eyewear for protection from laser light. LLL-TB-87, LLNL, P.O. Box 808, Livermore, CA.

Cundall, R. B., and R. E. Dale. Time-resolved fluorescence spectroscopy in biochemistry and biology. NATO ASI Series A: Life sciences, Vol. 69, Plenum Press, New York, (1983).

Demtröder, W., 1982. Laser spectroscopy. Basic concepts and instrumentation. Vol. 5, in *Springer Series in Chemical Physics*, Springer-Verlag, Berlin.

Dunning, F.B., May 1978. Tunable-untraviolet generation by sum-frequency mixing. Laser Focus Magazine, 72–76.

Driscoll W. G., and Vaughan W., 1977. Handbook of Optics. McGraw-Hill Book Co., New York.

Eden J. G., April 1988. UV and VUV lasers: Prospects and Applications. *Optics News*, 14–27.

Feddersen, B. M. vandeVen, and E. Gratton. Parallel wavelength ac-

quisition of fluorescence decay with picosecond resolution using an optical multichannel analyzer. Biophys. J. 55, 190a, (1989a).

Feddersen, B., D. W. Piston, and E. Gratton. Digital parallel acquisition in frequency domain fluorimetry. Rev. Sci. Instrum. 60, 2929–2936 (1989b).

Gibson J., November 1988. Laser Cooling Water. The key to Improved Reliability, Photonics Spectra, 117–124.

Gibson, J., April 1989. Laser water cooling loops deserve attention. Laser Focus World, 123–129.

Hammerling, P., Budgor, A. B. and Pinto, A. 1985. Tunable Solid-State Lasers, in *Proceedings of the First International Conference*, La Jolla, Ca, June 13–15, 1984. Springer-Verlag, Berlin.

Hecht, E. and Zajac A., 1977. Optics, 2nd Ed., Addison-Wesley Publishing Co., Reading, PA.

Herrmann J. and Wilhelmi, B. 1987. Lasers for Ultrashort Light Pulses. North-Holland Amsterdam.

Huth B. G. and Kuizenga D., October 1987. Green light from doubled Nd-YAG lasers. Lasers & Optronics, 59–61.

Jovin, T. M., D. J. Arndt-Jovin, M. Robert-Nicoud, T. Schormann, G. Marriott, and R. M. Clegg. Luminescence digital imaging microscopy. Biophys. J. 55, 432a (1989).

Kaiser, W., 1988. Ultrashort laser pulses and applications, Vol. 60, in Topics in Applied Physics, Springer-Verlag, Berlin.

Kaminskii, A. A., 1981. Laser Crystals Their Physics and Properties, (translation) ed. Ivey H.F. Vol. 14, in *Springer Series in Optical Sciences*, Springer-Verlag Berlin.

Keating, S. M., T. G. Wensell, T. Meyer, and L. Stryer. Nanosecond fluorescence and emission anisotropy kinetics of fura-2 in single cells. Biophys. J. 55, 518a (1989).

Kinosita, K., I. Ashikawa, M. Hibino, M. Shigemori, H. Yoshimura, H. Itoh, K. Nagayama, and A. Ikegami. Submicrosecond imaging under a pulsed-laser fluorescence microscope. SPIE 909, 271–277 in Time-resolved laser spectroscopy in biochemistry, SPIE, Los Angeles (1988).

Knutson, J. R. Fluorescence detection: schemes to combine speed, sensitivity and spatial resolution. SPIE 909, 51–60 in Time-resolved laser spectroscopy in biochemistry, SPIE, Los Angeles (1988).

Kusumi, A., A. Tsuji, M. Murata, Y. Sako, A. C. Yoshizawa, T. Hayakawa, and S-I Ohnishi. Development of a time-resolved microfluorimeter with a synchroscan streak camera and its application to studies of cell membranes. SPIE 909, 350–351 in Time-resolved laser spectroscopy in biochemistry, SPIE, Los Angeles (1988).

Lakowicz, J. R. Principles of fluorescence spectroscopy (1983). Plenum Press, New York (1983).

Lewis R. R., Naylor G. A., and Kearsley A. J., April 1988. Copper Vapor Lasers Reach High Power. Laser Focus/Electro Optics, 92–96.

Lin J. T. and Chen C., November 1987. Choosing a Non-linear Crystal. Lasers & Optronics, 59–63.

Littlechild J. and Mossler D., November 1988. Knowledge od Arc-Lamp Aging and Lifetime Effects Can Help to Avoid Unpleasant Surprises. Laser Focus/Electro Optics, 67–76.

Miller P. and Hoyt C., June 1986. Turning Down Laser Noise with Power Stabilizers. Photonics Spectra, 129–134.

Mollenauer L.F. and White J. C., 1987. Tunable Lasers, Vol. 59, in *Topics in Applied Physics,* Springer-Verlag, Berlin.

Muckenheim W., Austin L. and Basting D., June 1988. The pulsed dye Laser: Today's Technology, Today's Uses. Photonics Spectra, 79–84.

O'Connor, D. V., and D. Phillips. Time-correlated single photon counting. Academic Press, New York, (1984).

Peuse B., November 1988. Active Stabilization Of Ion Laser Resonators. Active Stabilization offers Advantages in Several Areas. Lasers & Optronics, 61–65

Rapp E. W., September 1988. Design Your Cooling System For Good Laser Performance, Laser Focus/Electro Optics, 65–70.

Rhodes Ch. K., 1983. Excimer Lasers, 2nd ed., Vol. 30, in *Topics in Applied Physics,* Springer-Verlag, Berlin.

Rockwell Associates Inc., Cincinnati, Ohio 1983. Laser Safety Training Manual, Sixth edition.

Rockwell, R. J. Jr., May 1986. An introduction to exposure hazards and the evaluation of nominal hazard zones. Lasers & Applications, 97–103.

Sliney D. H. April 1986. Laser Safety. The newest face on an old standard. Photonics Spectra, 83–96.

Sliney, D. and Wolbarsht, M., 1980. Safety with lasers and other optical sources. A comprehensive handbook. Plenum Press, New York.

Smith B., September 1986. Lamps for Pumping Solid-state Lasers: Performance and Optimization. Laser Focus/Electro Optics, 58–73.

Soileau, M. J., November 1987. Laser-Induced Damage, Photonics Spectra, 109–114.

Stitch, M. L., 1979. Laser Handbook, Vol. 3, North-Holland Publishing Co., Amsterdam.

Tebo, A. R., August 1988. Scientists develop Useful Optical Materials.

Laser Focus/Electro Optics, 103–110.

Weast, R.C., and Tuve, G.L., 1971. Handbook of lasers with selected data on optical technology, CRC Press. The Chemical Rubber Co., Cleveland, Ohio.

Wilson, D. A., G. H. Vickers, and G. M. Hieftje. Novel techniques for the determination of fluorescence lifetimes. Anal. Instrum. 14, 483–502 (1985).

Winburn, D.C., 1985. Practical laser safety. Marcel Dekker Inc., New York.

Chapter 6

Non-laser Illumination for Confocal Microscopy

Victor Chen

K.H.C. Associates, P.O. Box 21, Amherst, New York 14226

INTRODUCTION

Why use non-laser sources?

Non-laser light does not catch our imagination in the way that laser light does, but besides being practical and available, non-laser light sources have attractive practical and technical features for illuminating confocal microscopes, especially those that use disk-scanning methods (see Chapter 10).

First among the practical features is the fact that non-laser light sources are familiar to most light microscope users. Many microscopists feel that there are enough new aspects of confocal microscopy to be concerned about (such as those discussed in other chapters in this book) without having to learn about lasers as well. Common non-laser light sources, such as tungsten-ribbon lamp, quartz-halogen lamp, and xenon, mercury, carbon and zirconium arc lamps, are already part of conventional microscopes and are thus familiar to microscopists.

In addition, these sources are readily available as parts of conventional light microscopes. They can easily be transferred for trial use on a confocal microscope from conventional instruments already in the laboratory. As several of the commercial confocal microscopes are built around conventional light microscopes, incompatibility is not a major problem.

Finally, the care, alignment and replacement of these non-laser sources are familiar to microscopists, as are the associated purchase and maintenance costs. For example, users of conventional microscopes know when to rotate a darkening arc-lamp. They know when and how to center it, order a replacement, or replace a bulb. Users readily spot and replace fittings on the lamp housings which have been aged by prolonged exposure to heat and ultraviolet (UV) light. In contrast, most microscopists are unfamiliar with lasers. Besides the greater cost of purchasing and using a laser light source, more expensive optical elements are required to direct and shape laser light for use in a microscope. Furthermore, maintenance for laser light sources is more complex because of the requirements for special cooling, safety and power systems.

Aside from cost, familiarity and availability, there are several technical reasons which make non-laser sources important and desirable for confocal microscopes. This is especially true of disk-scanning instruments which utilize many confocal points within the field of view and so do not usually require the high brightness of a laser. The other advantages of non-laser light sources have to do with wavelength flexibility and coherence.

WAVELENGTH

The most desirable wavelengths for bright-field (436 nm, 546 nm, 579 nm) or for fluorescence (365 nm, 405 nm) are all avail-able as arc emissions lines (Fig. 1). Objectives are designed to give optimal correction at several of these specific spectral lines. Where more intensity is needed, mercury and carbon arcs lamps provide these wavelengths for conventional microscopical techniques. The super-pressure xenon arc provides intense illumination (without prominent spectral lines in the UV and visible) at wavelengths between the intense spectral lines of the mercury (Fig. 2). A modulated (Hg-I) arc lamp made by LTM Corp. has a useful spectrum (Fig. 3) and goes on and off at 120 hz amercury halide producing 110 lumens per watt, compared to the 30 lumens per watt of xenon arcs. The deep modulation greatly reduces the heat produced, allowing the housing to be compact. The high output suggests that it could be of use in confocal microscopy.

The sun, which has a similar spectrum but a higher brightness was used for confocal microscopy by Petran with a helostat. The difficulties in using the sun are the dependence on season, cloudiness and time of day for brightness and availability. The broad continuous spectra of the sun easily allows selection of the desired wavelengths for microscopy. Although the sun is considered an incoherent source, under high-resolution optical conditions a definite degree of coherence becomes apparent.

Second, several desirable wavelengths are available from each of the different types of arc and a particular wavelength band to can be selected with filters or gratings without changing lamps. The intensity provided by tungsten ribbon and quartz-halogen lamps is more than sufficient for disk-scanning confocal microscopy of highly reflective specimens. Quartz-halogen lamps provide very high stability over a broad range of wavelengths but at lower intensities than the arc lamps. Dichroic mirrors can be used to remove undesirable wavelengths, including heat, from the illumination path.

Finally, because of the historical selection of fluorochromes, arc lamps provide the most desirable wavelengths for fluorescence microscopy (Fig 1). The fluorochromes most used in microscopy today such as fluorescein and rhodamine were selected because they were easily excited at wavelengths available from non-laser sources. The widely used DNA label, DAPI is easy to excite using wavelengths from arc lamps but difficult to excite using wavelengths commonly available from lasers (see Chapter 16). The broadened spectral lines from high pressure arc lamps actually excite the fluorochromes more efficiently than an intense, narrow laser-emission line unless the latter is actually on an absorption maximum. The availability of broadened spectral lines in superpressure arc sources allow the simultaneously activation of several fluorochromes with differing emission wavelengths in conventional fluorescence microscopy (De Biasio et al, 1987) and this should certainly be possible in confocal microscopy with an efficiently configured arc source.

In biological science the current trend towards observing functioning cellular processes requires limiting the intensity of light reaching the specimen plane to well below that which just alters the processes being studied. This limit is already uncomfortably close for the quartz-halogen or arc sources used in conventional microscopy. This is exemplified by the action of intense light altering microtubule assembly and may also be true for more efficiently used arc sources in confocal microscopy as well.

The wavelengths used for illumination also need to be carefully chosen to be non-interfering with the process under study, and this is another advantage of having a light source with several wavelengths available. This is especially true for the case of a fluorochromes attached to functioning macromolecules in a living cell. Specimens living under the microscope should be illuminated only when data are actually being gathered. The trend in studying functioning cellular processed requires a decrease in light exposure of the specimen though decreased illumination levels while improving both the light-gathering efficiency and the detection sensitivity (see Chapters 3 and 12).

COHERENCE

Non-laser light is distinguished from laser light by its much lower degree of coherence. Both incoherent light and coherent light are theoretical concepts. They permit one to write the equations of image formation for the microscope under these two extreme conditions (see Chapter 11), but neither condition can be totally realized as a real source for practical microscopy. In microscopical practice, we have not paid much attention to the degree of coherence of the light used in illumination except when considering diffraction and interference effects. Roughly speaking, we consider light to be incoherent when we do not get such interference effects and to be coherent when we do. Actually several coherence properties of the light from a source are important in microscope image formation. These include spatial coherence (from the angle of the source subtended) and temporal coherence (from the wavelength band width of the source). In most practical microscopical image formation situations, we have a mixture of incoherent and coherent light. In the two extreme cases,

$$\text{Incoherent } I = \sum_i |\Psi_i|^2$$
$$\text{Coherent } I = |\sum_i \Psi_i|^2$$

where Ψ_i is the wave function added to give the resultant image intensities (Reynolds et al, 1989). The two forms of wave addition are very different. Even in imaging situations well described by incoherent phenomena, coherent effects may be detected if the results are examined with sufficient optical resolution. (Reynolds et al, 1989). In general, for microscopy, light with a low degree of coherence is needed for bright-field and reflection modes while high coherence is required for phase and interference modes. The process of fluorescence emission has so many steps that a high degree of coherence in the illuminating light may be important only in special situations.

If the coherence of the light is too high, it gives rise to interference fringes by interacting with the many optical surfaces of lenses and mirrors relaying the light from the source to the specimen. Even dust or minor surface defects will generate interference patterns, and when these become sufficiently complex we observe speckle in the image, making small details of the image uninterpretable. As a result, aside from a few special situations, low-coherence illumination of the specimen is desired in microscopy and this is available from non-laser sources. On the other hand, by reducing the spatial extent of the effective source emitting surface, non-laser sources can be arranged to deliver a high degree of spatial coherence.

WHICH TYPES OF CONFOCAL MICROSCOPE CAN USE NON-LASER SOURCES?

As many commercial confocal microscopes using beam-scanning (Biorad: MRC 500–600, Heidelberg Inst., Leitz, Sarastro, Zeiss) or stage-scanning (Biorad: SOM 100, Meridian Inst.) use only laser illumination, there is a popular notion that confocal microscopes must use laser illumination. The spectacular fluorescence micrographs of chromosomes and cytoskeletons made with laser-illuminated confocal microscopes have reinforced this idea. This impression is strengthened by the fact that these microscopes make no provision for the user to adapt a non-laser light source for use in the confocal mode.

In spite of this widely held belief, confocal microscopy does not require laser light. Minsky used a zirconium arc illuminator in the functional prototype stage-scanning confocal microscope he built in the 1950's (Minsky, 1988). Current commercial disk-scanning confocal microscopes include those made by Technical Instruments (see Chapter 10: single-sided optical system, glass Nipkow disk), Cambridge Technologies (Petran double-sided optical system, circular aperture copper Nipkow disk) and Tracor Northern (double-sided optical system, square aperture, silicon Nipkow disk). These confocal microscopes, which only come with non-laser illuminators, are able to form images at a rate of several hundred frames per second under favorable circumstances.

TABLE 1: TEMPORAL COHERENCE OF MERCURY ARC AND LASER LIGHT

source	λ(mm)	bandwidth Å	coherence length(mm)
Hg (low P)	5461	100	< 0.03
Hg (high P)	5461	10	< 0.3
He Ne laser	6328	$10^{4 \text{ to } 5}$	~ 10^5

Reynolds et al, 1989.

TABLE 2: SPATIAL COHERENCE OF MERCURY ARC AND LASER LIGHT

source	(μm) size	(mm) distance	(μm) λ	angle	spatial coherence
Hg	10	500	1/2	2×10^3 (rad)	~30mm
Hg	1000	500	1/2		~0.3mm
laser	12cm	collimator 1/2			12 cm
laser	70cm	diameter 1/2			12 cm

Reynolds et al, 1989.

RELATION OF FLUROCHROMES WITH SPECTRUM OF MERCURY ARC

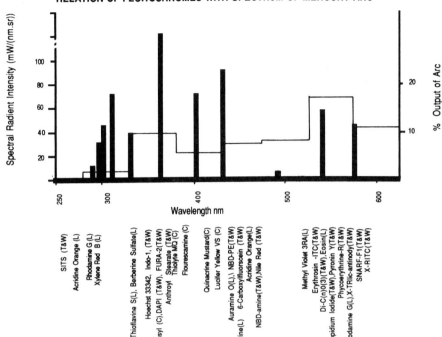

FIG. 1. Important fluorochromes and associated Mercury lines. Spectral data from OSRAM literature, Optical RadiationCorp. literature. Information on absorption maximum (I) Loveland (1970), (C) Chen, R.F. and Scott, C.H. (1985) Anayl. Let 18:393–421, (T&W) Tsien and Waggoner this volume.

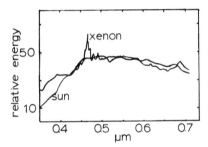

FIG. 2. Spectral distribution of xenon arc compared to sunlight (redrawn from Loveland, 1970)

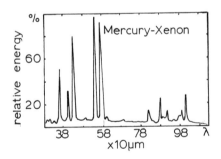

FIG. 4. Spectral distribution of mercury-xenon arc (data from Optical Radiation Corp.)

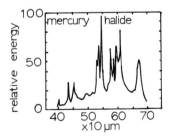

FIG. 3. Spectral distribution of mercury-halide arc (redrawn from Loveland, 1970)

While the laser serves the beam-scanning instruments well as an intense highly-collimated light source, unintended interference affects caused by the high coherence of laser light often present image interpretation problems in the non-fluorescent modes. Furthermore, only a few familiar wavelengths are available from the lasers provided and this may sometimes require the development of new fluorochromes and labeling methods (see Chapter 18) The next section will discuss the practical de-

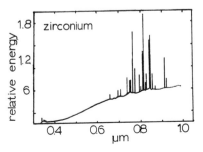

FIG. 5. Spectral distribution of zirconium arc (redrawn from Loveland, 1970)

tails of non-laser light sources and the chapter will end with a discussion of the proper adaptation of laser light for disk scanning confocal microscopy.

CHARACTERISTICS OF NON-LASER LIGHT SOURCES

The basis for choosing between non-laser sources are

- presence of the desired emission wavelength
- source (brightness) radiance
- source size
- source distribution
- source coherence
- stability

Wavelengths Available

Figures 1–5 show the spectra for sources using mercury, xenon, mercury-halide, mercury-xenon and zirconium arcs plotted with the same horizontal scale. The carbon arc (not shown) have a very intense line at 400 nm. The mercury and Hg-Xe arcs has many intense spectral line in the UV and visible. The xenon and zirconium arcs have spectral lines in the near IR.

Several reasons for choosing to operate at particular wavelengths were listed in the Introduction. The mercury arc lamp has intense lines in the blue and green portions of the spectrum making it the lamp of choice for disk-scanning confocal fluorescence microscopy. Image resolution can be improved in confocal fluorescence microscopy if one can choose the excitation wavelength from a continuous source (Cox, 1984).

Source Radiance

Radiance is the radiometric quantity related to the photometric brightness. Radiance is the radiant flux per unit area, solid angle. Arc lamps are many orders of magnitude, more radiant than tungsten filament lamps. The HBO-100, 100 W high-pressure mercury arc lamp is the most radiant of the commonly used lamps whatever the wattage because it has a very small source size (compared to the 200 W for instance). The larger arcs are only useful to illuminate larger areas of the specimen.

Source Stability

The quartz-halogen lamp has become commonly used in microscopy because its non-blackening nature maintains a constant envelop transparency and results in a constant level of output. Tungsten filament lamps, powered by regulated power supplies, are far more stable than arcs, making them useful for photometric measurements. Generally speaking arcs are less stable. (Fig. 6)

Loveland (1970) points out that light of the carbon arc can be made more reproducible than other arcs if the electrodes are first baked dry. The intensity of the xenon arc can be modulated rapidly in time as is the case in electronic flash for photography.

Source Coherence

Tungsten ribbon lamps give a broad spectrum of light with low spatial coherence. The coherence of arc lamps can be low if a large emission area is used as the source. The sun is usually considered an incoherent source but even it can behave as a coherent source if used for high-resolution imaging.

Source Distribution

Tungsten filament lamps can have the filament shaped to permit the best use the light-collection system. Filaments are often bent into disks or wide bands to match the input aperture of monochrometers. Arc lamps generally distribute the light source as a torus surrounding the axis between the two electrodes.

COLLECTING THE LIGHT AND RELAYING IT TO SPECIMEN

Illumination of the specimen: A basic part of microscopy

As for conventional microscopy, the type of illumination for confocal microscopy can be considered to be divided between transmitted (where light passes through the specimen) and incident (where light incident upon the specimen is detected on the same side as either reflected light or as an induced luminescence such as fluorescence or phosphorescence). Transmission confocal microscopes, though well-developed, are not widely used in biology because of the need to move the specimen. Most confocal microscopes in general use are based upon incident illumination where the objective also serves as the condenser and light passes through the single-objective in both directions.

The most common contrast modes of commercial confocal microscopes are epi-fluorescence and backscattered or reflected light. Illumination for the two contrast modes differs only in the use of excitation and emission filters, and a dichroic beam-splitter for fluorescence compared with a semi-transparent beam-splitter for reflection. All scanning mechanisms for confocal microscopes use an illumination method that fills the backfocal plane of the objective. Since our discussion centers upon the use of non-laser sources, we will consider the illumination for the two disk-scanning mechanisms.

Tandem scanning: Basic description

The tandem scanning mechanism consists of a spinning Nipkow aperture disk at the intermediate image plane of the objective. The thousands of apertures arranged in spirals both scan the object and sample the resulting real image. The double-sided optical system developed by Petran uniformly illuminates the area of the disk that is to be imaged onto the object. Through a series of mirrors and beam-splitters, another projection of the spots on the specimen is focused onto a conjugate set of holes on the diametrically opposed region of the symmetrical aperture disk (Fig. 7a). This series of mirrors and beam splitters permits the illuminating and sensing apertures to be distinct thereby reducing the amount of stray illumination reflected by the solid part of the illuminated area of the disk from entering the imaging side of system. Since the open area of the disk is only 1–2% of the illuminated area, the system is wasteful of light.

Single-sided disk scanning: Basic description

In the single-side disk-scanning optical system, the spinning Nipkow aperture disk is again located at the intermediate image plane of the objective, but the same apertures serve as both source and pinhole because the beam-splitter is above the disk

(Fig. 7b). The aperture disk is tilted and "black chromed" to prevent the reflections from the disk from being visible in the eyepiece. Furthermore, a polarizer, placed in the illumination path, a quarter waveplate above the objective, and an analyzer at the eyepiece form another system to reduce the effect of disk reflections. Because it lacks the series of mirrors needed in the double-sided system, the single-sided system is self-aligning and so has somewhat greater intensity transmission. However, the apertures again constitute such a small percentage of the illu-minated area that the system wastes much of the available il-lumination (see Chapter 10 for details).

How do you uniformly illuminate both the objective back focal plane and the intermediate image plane?

Kohler illumination has become the most common optical scheme of illumination in both transmitted and reflected conventional light microscopy (Fig. 8). It is used to uniformly il-

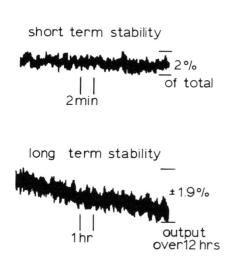

FIG. 6. Stability of 150 W xenon are (redrawn from Optical Radiation Corp.)

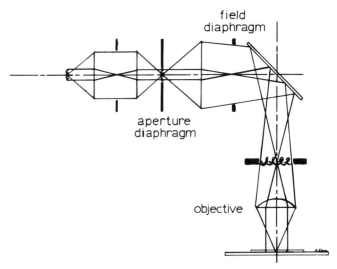

FIG. 8. Kohler illumination (after Piller, 1977)

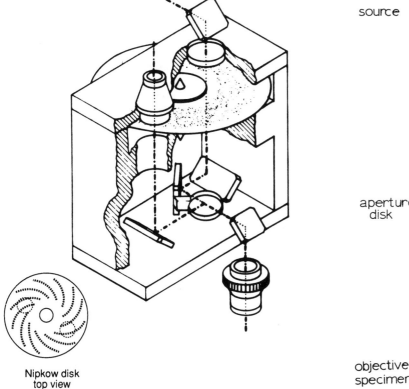

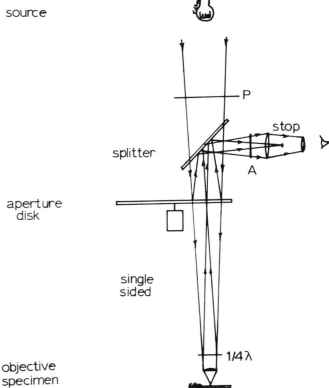

FIG. 7. Illumination scheme of single- (right) and double-sided (left) scanning disk confocal microscopes (after Kino and Xiao, 1989 and Chapter 10)

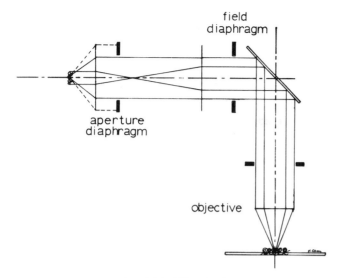

FIG. 9.   Critical illumination

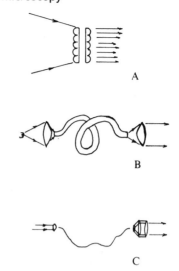

FIG. 11.   Scrambler for uniform illumination
A. Array of lenses (data from Oriel Corp. Catalog, Vol. II)
B. Light guide spiral (data from Leitz, Inc.)
C. Single fiber optic (after Ellis, 1979)

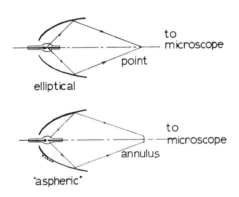

FIG. 10.   Use of elliptical and "aspheric" collectors (data from Optical Radiation Corp., and Oriel Corp. Catalog, Vol. II)

luminate the image field from a spatially complex source by imaging, a small portion of the source at the back-focal plane of the condenser (or objective in epi-illumination) so a diffuse image of the source is produced at the plane of the specimen. The field aperture (which effectively lies in an intermediate image plane) is imaged onto the specimen to limit the area illuminated without altering the angle of the illuminating light. In the case of highly non-uniform sources, a diffusing opal glass may used to further improve uniformity at the focal plane. The coherence of the illumination can be varied by varying the size of the source region imaged. Kohler illumination is not very efficient since it makes maximum use of neither the full source surface nor the full spatial distribution of the emitted light. The usual collecting schemes use lenses to collect from one side with possibly a spherical mirror on the opposite side. In the case of arc lamps the reflected image is moved adjacent to the direct image to increase the apparent source size (Piller, 1977).

Critical illumination requires a highly uniform emitting surface because it images this surface directly onto the image plane in the specimen on the stage (Fig. 9). Since it images the source,

it can utilize a larger solid angle than the Kohler illumination. It is, however, dependent upon a large uniform sources. The coherence of the illumination in this system is that of the source. If a large source is imaged, the coherence is quite low. Brightness variations caused by convection of the plasma in the arc lamp make it tiring to view the specimen if the plasma is imaged directly onto the specimen plane, but a time-average of the arc image is quite uniform.

A spherical mirror is often used on the back side of an arc, making use of light going in that direction to yield broader source. As is often noted, "You cannot get more light out of an optical system than you put into it," but one should try to collect as much of it as is available. An elliptical mirror can be used to capture light from the sides of an arc lamp source, thereby collecting a larger solid angle of the light emitted than is possible in the usual scheme (Fig. 10). The light projected by such a system can be as high as 85% of that emitted but unfortunately the projected ray bundle has a dark central spot. The coatings on such eliptical mirrors should be dichroic, letting the heat pass through. Such reflectors are sold by Oriel and Optical Radiation Company. If some scrambling is done and the image extended, this can be a desirable illumination scheme for disk-scanning instruments. This approach can be refined to provide a more uniform output by altering the elliptical surface to use the fact that we are not using the second focus of the ellipse. A module using these aspheric reflectors is made by Optical Radiation Company and ICL Technologies.

Scrambling and filtering the light

A major function of Kohler illumination systems is to make the illumination more homogenous, however, for many sources it does not "scramble" light sufficiently. Illumination light needs to be scrambled to decrease heterogeneity, spatial coherence and temporal coherence. Most scrambling methods use multiple reflection or scattering to accomplish this goal. Some methods useful for confocal microscopy are diagrammed in Fig. 11. They include:

- an array of simple lenses to image the source at infinity
- a large-diameter light-pipe bent into a single spiral (Leitz)
- a zoom lens coupling a small diameter fiber loop (loop is vibrated) (Ellis, 1979)

These will be discussed further in the final section.

If high quality microscopy is done on light-hungry microscopes, such as those using disk-scanning, more provisions have to be made to remove heat and other unwanted wavelengths before they enter the scrambler system. Ideally, only wavelengths critical to image formation should leave the source. Rather than using broad band mirrors, dichroic mirrors for specific wavelengths should be used to select the light going to the disk and also to reflect unwanted heat. In the single-sided version, this would decrease the load of light involved in flare and scattering from the disk as well as that involved in heating it.

Heat-absorbing glass is the most common heat filter used but a liquid heat filter, consisting of a liquid chamber filled with salt solution to screen out the unwanted wavelengths, has much higher heat capacity. Aside from heat removal, liquid filters can be easily made to function as bandpass or cutoff filters by changing the salt solution. An extensive description of solutions to be used has been described by Loveland (1970).

MEASURING WHAT COMES THROUGH THE ILLUMINATION SYSTEM

The procedures for measuring the light throughput with a photometer in any microscope have been thoroughly described in a step-by-step manner in the book *Photomicrography* by Loveland (1970). He even describes making a photometer for such a purpose. Using a modern photometer with a fiber-optic probe, one can even measure in the most difficult locations in the microscope. Such measurements are the only way to pinpoint those parts of the light path where preventable losses are taking place.

Young (1989) describes the use of a feedback-controlled light emitting diode to generate known amounts of light from small (5–50 microns) sources. Using this system he has been able to calibrate the input-output characteristic of a microscope system over four orders of magnitude.

Exposure time and source brightness

In conventional microscopy, every point of the image is formed in parallel. In scanning microscopy the image is formed by scanning a point or a group of points over the surface to be imaged and this scanning process takes a finite amount of time. If it is a raster scan, then the image is completed when the raster is completed and so the confocal microscope is a sampling system in both time and space. In the case of moving or changing specimens, the scan time must be short compared to the expected rate of change and this means that the source must be sufficiently bright to elicit from the specimen sufficient signal to make a usable image during the scan time. In other words, shorter scan times need brighter sources. In practice, it has been the inability of the arc sources to match the brightness of the laser that has prevented the disk scanning instruments from seriously challenging the laser instruments in viewing low intensity fluorescent specimens.

When comparing disk and laser scanning data rates, it is important to specify the area illuminated on the specimen because the former effectively collects the data in parallel while the latter collects only from one point at a time. Given comparable pinhole sizes and optical efficiencies, the crucial factor is the rate at which the narrow-band, excitatory radiation strikes a certain area of the specimen. The area chosen should be that from which signal can be usefully detected by the optimal detector for a disk-scanning microscope, a cooled CCD. If we assume a 512^2 CCD operating at the magnification needed to make 0.1 μm pixels (see Chapter 4), this suggests an area about 50 μm square on the specimen.

The illumination systems of the present, commercial, double-sided disk-scanning confocal microscopes can concentrate only 2–3 microwatts of narrow-band light into a 50 × 50 μm area while the single-sided instruments can produce 6 μw (personal communication V. Cejna, Technical Instruments, San Jose, CA). On the other hand, the laser sources on the LSCM can easily deliver 100× more power (without producing significant fluorescence saturation) and can consequently produce data from (and bleaching of!) the specimen at a proportionally higher rate.

On the other hand, because disk-scanning instruments use many simultaneous probes, the absolute limit on data acquisition presented by fluorescence saturation is far less of a limitation. As a result, the disk-scanning approach could eventually produce even higher frame rates than the laser instruments if sufficiently intense sources can be developed.

Significant improvements (~10×) are probably possible in the design of the illumination optics and, in addition, larger CCD sensors (~1000^2) would permit parallel detection of data from a larger area of the specimen maintaining the same pixel-size. This second strategy would increase the effective data acquisition rate by an amount proportional to the number of sensors in the detector, but it would do so only at the price of viewing ever larger fields of the specimen. In other words, unlike increased source brightness, it would not permit more rapid imaging of a particular cell.

Stationary specimens

When confocal microscopy is performed upon fixed specimens, there is no fundamental limitation on scan time and good optical sections can be obtained along the Z axis in all contrast modes. Each scanning mode has its own advantages and spatial resolution may be improved over conventional microscopy if the detecting aperture is sufficiently small. Most confocal microscopy so far has been done on such fixed specimens.

What if the specimen is moving or changing?

When some or all of the specimen is moving or changing, the design of most confocal microscopes are challenged (Boyde, 1985). As yet only prototype or home-built microscopes have auto-focus and specimen tracking. The general user only has access to the glide stage or a motorized Z axis. The scanning mechanism in the confocal microscope must to be speeded up to get an adequate sampling of a moving specimen. The faster the scanning, the more light is needed to provide statistical accuracy for each "image" frame. Because of the sampling nature of the scanning, we still have some ambiguity in time as

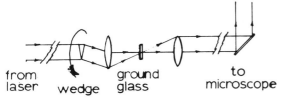

FIG. 12. Phase randomization scheme for laser use (after Hard, Zeh and Allen, 1977)

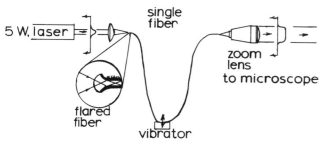

FIG. 13. Phase randomization scheme for laser (after Ellis, 1979)

to when a particular volume element is detected for inclusion into the image. The faster the movement or change studied, the more efficient the illumination system, or the more intensely radiant the source must be.

What is a reasonable duration for image formation? It really depends upon the nature of the specimen and the question being investigated. Traditionally we have considered only fixed and preserved specimens, but even Leeuwenhoek was struck by looking at living, moving specimens. The current interest in the mechano-chemical event of dynein, or of kinesin generating macromolecular movement are in this direction. The use of voltage sensitive dyes (milleseconds) by the neurobiologist and other cytologists await the capability for low-light-level imaging methods that view at faster than video rates to follow the two-dimensional spread of action and junctional potentials. The optical sectioning capability may even allow one to follow such potentials in a living ganglion.

INCOHERENT LASER LIGHT SOURCES FOR CONFOCAL MICROSCOPY

Even beam-scanning instruments, which already use laser light, would benefit if the coherence of the laser beam could be reduced. Although the coherence is not particularly troublesome in the fluorescence mode, it causes annoying interference effects in the backscattered light mode.

Besides being an intense light source, laser light is usually highly monochromatic and coherent (see Chapter 5). The monochromatic aspect could be useful in microscopy, allowing objectives to be designed as monochromats. There would be no need for the correction of chromatic abberations except in objectives for fluorescence microscopy. The extreme narrowness of the laser line would make the light easy to control, reflect or

exclude, using dichroic mirrors, etc. The extreme brightness means that much could be lost while leaving enough remaining. The high radiance of the laser also makes it an attractive light source for light-wasting disk-scanning microscope systems. It is only the coherence of laser light that is annoying. Interference fringes appear everywhere as a result of differing paths due to dust and other small optical path differences. The speckle that results from the interaction of these fringes causes the annoying bright and dark spots that can overlay the desired image, making small details uninterpretable.

Two methods have been proposed to minimize the effect of speckle. Hard, Zeh and Allen (1977) proposed a method to make laser light incoherent for microscope illumination in which phase-randomization was produced by introducing a rotating optical-wedge-and-ground-glass combination into the light path (Fig. 12). Since the wedge and the ground glass rotate, there is still some temporal coherence which becomes cyclic, and the need for the fixed placement and accurate alignment of the rotating device and the laser relative to the microscope make the method inconvenient.

Gordon Ellis (1979) proposed a second method to reduce the coherence of laser light for microscope illumination. The laser light is focussed into a flexible length of fine optical fiber (Fig. 13). The internal reflections in the bent fiber are constantly changing because the fiber is vibrated at high frequency and this makes the exit beam appear uniform in intensity (rather than a gaussian profile). The phase is scrambled due to the varying path lengths of the light passing through the fiber but the high radiance and monochromaticity are preserved.

Both methods minimize speckle by averaging in space and time. Speckle is not apparent if either the coherence length or the coherence interval is exceeded. Incoherent laser light can become an important light source for conventional or confocal microscopy. A large (5W) laser is needed and, at present, its great cost makes it out of reach for most microscopists, but the development of dye lasers with easy choice of wavelengths and low cost may overcome this hurdle.

REFERENCES

Boyde, A. (1985) Science 230: 1270–1272.
De Biasio, R., G.R. Bright, L.A. Ernst, A.S. Waggoner and D. L. Taylor (1987), J. Cell Biol. 105: 1613–1622.
Ellis, G.W. (1979) J. Cell Biol. 83: 303a.
Hard, R., Zeh, R. and R. D. Allen (1977) J. Cell Sci. 23: 335
Johnson, H. (1989) Advance Imaging (March): 22–23, 60.
Kino, G.S., T.R. and G.Q. Xiao (1988) Scanning Microscopy Technologies and Applications, E. Clayton, ed. Proc. SPIE 897: 31–42.
Loveland, L. (1970) Photomicrography, John Wiley and Sons.
Minsky, M. (1988) Scanning 10: 128–138.
Piller, H. (1977) Microscope Photometry, Springer-Verlag, New York. pp 253.
Reynolds, G.O., J.B. DeVelis, G.B. Parrent, Jr., B.J. Thompson, (1989) The New Physical Optics Notebook, SPIE Optical Eng. Press, Bellingham, Washington, pp 568.
Shapiro, H.M. (1988) Practical Flow Cytometry, 2nd edition, Alan R. Liss, Inc. pp 353.
Young, I.,T. (1989), in Methods of Cell Biology v. 30 ed. Taylor, D.L. and Y-L Wang ed., Academic Press, New York, p. 1–45.

Chapter 7

Objective Lenses For Confocal Microscopy

H. Ernst Keller

Carl Zeiss, Inc., One Zeiss Drive, Thornwood, NY 10594

ABSTRACT

No other component of the microscope is as instrumental in determining the information content of an image as the objective. The resolved detail, the contrast at which this detail is presented, the depth through the object from which useful information can be derived, and the diameter of the useful field are all limited by the performance of the objective. All other imaging components, such as relay optics, Telan systems, tube lenses, and eyepieces or projectives may have some corrective function but otherwise serve only to present the image generated by the objective to the detector in such a way that most of its information content can be recorded without degradation.

While this is true for any conventional microscope, it is particularly true for confocal scanning, where the objective becomes the condenser as well and needs to combine a high degree of optical correction with good throughput and a minimum of internal stray light or photon noise. In general, the demands on the performance of the objective for confocal scanning are identical to the needs for demanding video microscopy, photomicroscopy, densitometry, photometry, spectrophotometry and morphometry. However, this does not mean that confocal microscopy will not eventually call for special new lenses in which certain corrections may be sacrificed to enhance specific capabilities. In biological applications involving living cells, high photon efficiency is essential. To increase transmittance, field size and chromatic correction might be reduced to achieve highest numerical aperture at a reasonable working distance with a minimum number of lens elements. Another problem is the loss of correction for spherical aberration as the lens is focussed deep into an aqueous specimen. Reducing this effect may require automatic motor-driven correction collars.

Since the critical demands of light microscopy and confocal scanning microscopy have increasingly forced the performance of objectives to approach their theoretical limits, a brief refresher on aberrations, design concepts, materials etc. may be in order. An overview of optical aberrations in refractive systems—both inherent and induced by improper use of the microscope—and the basic performance characteristics of the different generic types of objectives will be presented.

The basic design concepts of microscope optics—finite versus infinite image distance, compensating versus fully corrected systems—need to be understood to properly match optical components. Optical materials and their properties for specific applications, cements and antireflection coatings all influence an objective's performance. Immersion liquids, coverglass, and mounting medium are part of the optical train and can strongly affect the quality of an image. All this we will try to put into qualitative perspective, particularly as it pertains to confocal scanning.

A detailed quantitative comparison of the performance of different microscope objectives must be based on accepted criteria and precisely defined testing methods. Many of the major microscope makers have developed their own proprietary methods, and no independent, fully "objective" test procedure exists at this time that will address and quantify all performance data of an objective.

How then should the user of a confocal microscope judge the performance of an objective? The pinholes in an evaporative coating are adequate to judge spherical aberration, astigmatism, coma, and flatness in transmitted light but do not work well in the epi-mode. Fluorescent beads in the $0.1~\mu m$ range are suitable replacements but the fluorescence soon fades. Diatomes have long been a standard because of their precise and regular spacings, and they can be viewed in the backscattered (reflected) light mode. How do we determine, at least qualitatively, how an image is degraded, for example, by focusing deep into a specimen or by pairing components which are not matched? These are all challenges that are not yet fully resolved. They point to a need for detailed testing procedures covering all aspects from source to detector.

Still, with our ability today to rapidly ray-trace lenses for their geometrical optical performance and to calculate wavefront aberrations, point-spread functions, and intensity ratios through the Airy disk, most objectives offered now are close to diffraction-limited, at least in the center of the image field. Field size and performance on the periphery of the field are both important in beam-scanning confocal microscopy. Long-term mechanical, thermal, and chemical stability of objectives used with lasers are a function of manufacturing tolerances and materials chosen.

Submicron tolerances for centration and spacing of lens elements in sophisticated, high-power objectives call for careful, gentle treatment by the user. A minor mechanical shock may generate enough stress on a lens element to seriously reduce the objective's performance in polarized light.

ABERRATIONS OF REFRACTIVE SYSTEMS

The ideal "diffraction-limited" objective will image an Airy disk from an infinitely small object point. Such an Airy disk is shown in Fig. 1, with its intensity distribution.

The diameter of the first dark ring D, generated by destructively interfering, diffracted wavefronts is

$$D = \frac{1.22\lambda}{n \times \sin\alpha}$$

($n\sin\alpha$ = numerical aperture) and determines the resolution (Fig. 2). Rayleigh set the limit for the smallest resolveable distance d between 2 points at

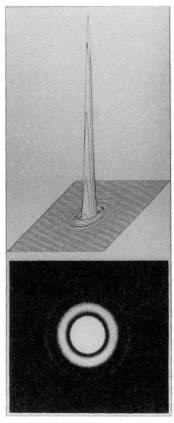

FIG. 1a. Airy disk and its intensity distribution.

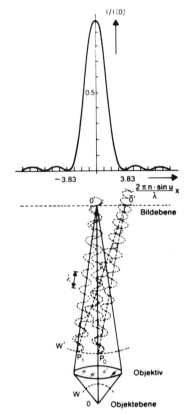

FIG. 1b. Generation and profile of the Airy disk or picture point.

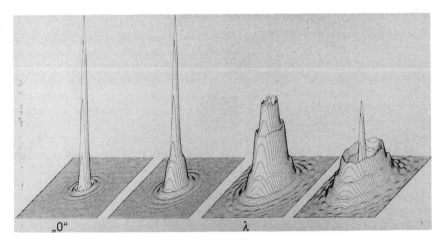

FIG. 2. Changes in intensity distribution with focus changes.

$$d = \frac{1.22\lambda}{2\,\mathrm{NA}}$$

or the radius of the Airy disk (λ = wavelength, n = refractive index of medium between object and objective, α = half-angle of collected rays from object point). This point-to-point resolution for a given objective in turn determines the magnification required to enable any given detector to record the resolved detail. For visual observation useful magnification is therefore 500–1000 times the NA of the objective.

Defocusing

Defocusing or inadequate focus will change the size and intensity distribution of the unit image point (Fig. 2). Since defocussing and depth of field are closely related, let us take a look at the 3-dimensional "image body", of the "diffraction limited" objective (see also Chapter 1).

Fig. 3 shows a cross-section perpendicular to the optical axis in the optimally focused image/object plane, again the Airy disk and its intensity distribution, while Fig. 4 represents a section in the optical axis and its intensity distribution. Defocusing

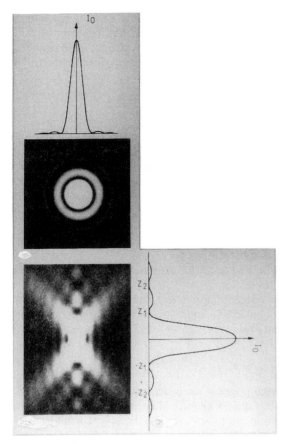

FIG. 3/4. Horizontal (focal plane) and vertical (optical axis) cross-section through image picture body.

results in alternating bright and dark spots in the middle of the Airy disc (Fig. 2). The extension of the central bright body along the axis is $4\lambda/(NA)^2$, but we can detect a change in the image with a defocus of only $\lambda/(NA)^2$ and call this the wave optical portion of the depth of field. Deviations from the "diffraction

limited" image point caused by lens aberrations can be grouped into wavelength independent (monochromatic) and chromatic aberrations.

Monochromatic aberrations

Spherical aberration

This axial aberration is generated by nonspherical wavefronts produced by the objective itself or improper use of the objective or tube length. Paraxial rays are focused differently from peripheral rays and a blurring of the image body results in asymmetrical intensity change when defocusing $\pm\Delta Z$ (Fig. 5).

Spherical aberration can be optimally corrected only for accurately specified object and image distances. It can, therefore, be easily induced by improper tube length caused by introduction of optical elements into the converging beam path of finitely designed systems or by the use of improper "windows," such as non-standard cover slips or poor-quality immersion oil between object and objective. Fig. 6 shows the changes in size and intensity distribution through the image point with increasing penetration into an object in watery medium with a Planapochromat 63/1.4 oil. The effect of this induced spherical aberration on the image point needs to be considered and either corrected for or at least understood before confocal microscopy can be optimally applied to 3D reconstruction.

With increasing NA, changes in the thickness or the refractive index of the "window" between the object and the objective become more critical, particularly with "dry" objectives. In the low-power, low-NA objective with relatively higher $NA_{imageside}$ where $NA_{imageside} = NA_{objectside}/Magnification$, small changes in tube length quickly lead to inferior images.

While for all types of objectives, the spherical aberration is corrected to less-than-perceptible limits, at least for visual observation, this holds true only if all optical specifications for a given lens are fulfilled. On high-NA dry objectives or on multi-

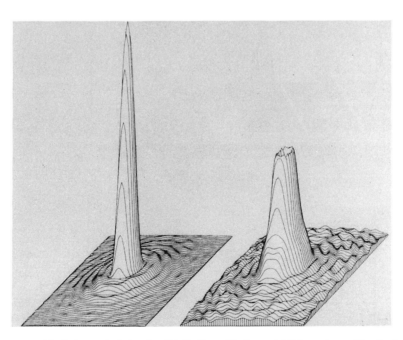

FIG. 5. Non-symmetrical change in intensity distribution with focus +/-Z in system with spherical abberation.

immersion objectives, the exact setting of the correction collar for the elimination of induced spherical aberration is essential.

Fig. 7 shows the change in depth resolution as a result of spherical aberration induced by coverslip thickness variations. Changes in the width of the intensity distribution for cover-glass thicknesses of 120 μm, 170 μm (nominal) and 220 μm severely reduce both the resolution and the depth discrimination of the pinhole detector.

Fig. 8 shows the changes in the half-width of the intensity distribution curve with changes in cover-glass thickness. With tolerances of $\pm$ 10 μm for top-quality cover glasses, the half-width changes by more than a factor of 2. With increasing numerical apertures ($>$ 0.5), particularly with dry and water immersion lenses, selection of cover glasses for correct thickness is important. Even oil immersion lenses like the Planapochromat 63/.14 perform optimally only with a cover-glass thickness of .17mm (see also Chapter 8).

Coma

For object points away from the optical axis so-called coma, a streaking radial distortion of the image point is generated (Fig. 9).

Fulfilling Abbe's sine condition

$$y' \times n' \times \sin \beta' = y \times n \times \sin\beta$$

(y = distance from axis; n = refractive index; β = viewing angle, all in image and object space, respectively) eliminates coma (aplanatic systems), but all potential factors that increase the effect of spherical aberration are especially critical to coma.

As coma is only evident off-axis, it is not important in specimen-scanning confocal microscopes. However, it can be important in laser-mirror systems which are often operated off the axis at high zoom to avoid axial specular reflections in the backscattered light mode.

Astigmatism

Two orthogonal wavefronts (tangential and sagittal) for off-axis points have different focal distances or radii. When a perfectly symmetrical image point in the center of the field is moved off-axis, it becomes either radially or tangentially elongated, depending on the focus. Intensity ratios diminish, and definition, detail, and contrast are lost with increasing distance from the center.

Fig. 10a shows the intensity distribution through one section of an astigmatic image point. With compromised focus between the radial and tangential extremes, a four-lobed Airy disk results (Fig. 10b).

Lens decentration in the objective or poor alignment of the system—objective, intermediate optics, and eyepiece—increases astigmatism.

Flatness of field

Image points of an extended flat object are focused onto a spherical dish. Central and peripheral zones are not simultaneously in sharp focus. Prior to the advent of flat-field objectives in the late 1930's (Zeiss), the "useable" field at the intermediate image plane was only 10–12 mm. With present-day flatfield or

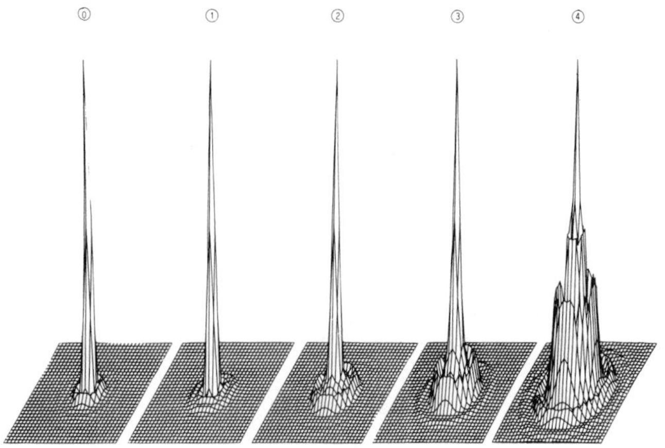

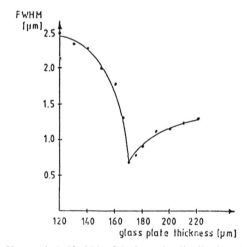

FIG. 6. Change in intensity distribution with increasing penetration into a watery medium with a Planapochromat. Penetration depth from 0 to 4 μm.

FIG. 8. Changes in half width of the intensity distribution with changing window thickness. Plan-Neofluar 63/1.2.

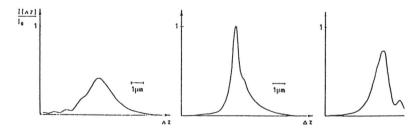

FIG. 7. Change in resolution and depth detection through windows of 120, 170, and 220 μm thickness with Plan-Neofluar 63/1.2 oil.

"Plan"-objectives, ocular fields of 18, 20 and 25 exhibit sharp detail from center to edge; however, this improvement has been obtained at the expense of increases in complexity, cost, and reduced transmission.

In Fig. 11 the field curvature for an Achromat and a Plan-apochromat are compared. Also shown is the astigmatism of the two orthogonal image spheres. Δ represents the depth of field unit $\lambda/(n.\sin\alpha)^2$.

It needs to be mentioned here that the term Plan or "F" for flatfield is no guarantee for a perfectly flat image with no astigmatism. No standards have been established. Also, the flatness in the final image may be affected by the correction of the eyepiece or other intermediate optics.

In confocal scanning through thick materials, the dish-shaped section obtained with the non-flat objective may be of little consequence to the biologist, as long as there is no astigmatism, and one is mindful of the distortion this produces in 3-D data sets. However, in material science and for many critical applications, such as high-resolution imaging in semiconductor inspection, flatness of field is important.

Distortion

The actual off-axis image point is usually either closer (barrel) or farther away (pin-cushion) from the axis than the ideal image point. Barrel or pin-cushion distortion results and the true geometry of an object is no longer maintained in the image. Although less critical in biomedicine than in material science, distortion is reduced to < 2% of the radial distance from the axis in most objectives.

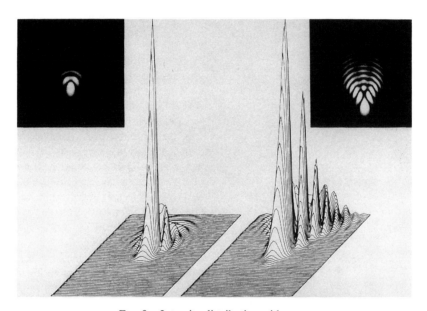

FIG. 9.   Intensity distribution with coma.

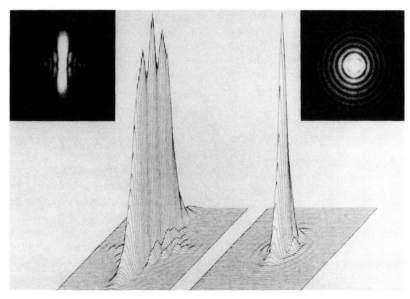

FIG. 10a, b.   Intensity distribution with astigmatism.

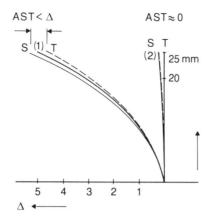

FIG. 11.   Flatness of field and astigmatism for (1) Achromat and (2) Planapochromat.

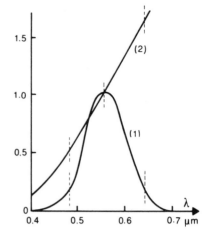

FIG. 13.   Spectral emission of tungsten source (2) and spectral sensitivity of eye (1).

Fig. 13 shows the spectral emission of a typical light source combined with the spectral sensitivity of the eye. If we set the intensity for 550 at 100%, the intensity in the center of the disk for 480 nm is approximately 10%, for 640 nm approximately 30%. In confocal scanning, the emission of the source and the spectral sensitivity of the detector need to be considered along with the emission peak and bandwidth of the specific fluorophor. Chromatic aberrations are both produced and corrected by the different dispersions of the glasses used. Glasses of "normal" dispersion have a close-to-linear decrease in refractive index with increasing wavelength and are used for Achromats. Only two wavelengths can have the same focus. The remaining "secondary spectrum" produces the greenish or purple fringes on images of sharp edges.

For objectives with better chromatic correction, glasses of "abnormal" partial dispersion are needed. Here the refractive index changes with wavelength more rapidly in either the blue or red region.

Abbe used fluorite (CaF_2) to reduce the secondary spectrum, and more recently glasses have become available with similar properties. This has resulted in the high degree of chromatic correction for an Apochromat (Fig. 12), where up to 4 wavelengths can have the same image location.

With Apochromat and Semiapochromat or Fluorite, the diffraction-caused spreading of the intensity distribution through the disc referred to above can also be virtually eliminated, as Fig. 14 illustrates. An Achromat still has substantial intensity in the first fringe, while the Apochromat approaches the theoretical resolution limit. The longitudinal chromatic aberration is less than or approaches $\lambda/(NA)^2$, the wave-optical depth of field.

Since the Apochromat requires elements of abnormal dispersion, their characteristics may not be ideal for some specific applications, such as fluorescence excitation in the near UV or polarizing microscopy. For this reason a fluorite objective is often more suitable, and Fig. 14 illustrates how close it comes to the performance of the Apochromat.

For confocal scanning of fluorescence images, the objective with best or identical correction at excitation and emission wavelengths will perform best, in terms of both transmission energy and resolution (see Chapter 3).

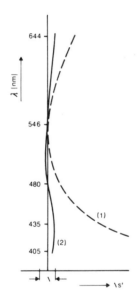

FIG. 12.   Chromatic correction of (1) Achromat and (2) Apochromat.

Chromatic aberrations

Wavelength dependent aberrations are caused by a) the dispersion in glass, and b) the different diameters of the unit image point and the unit image body for different wavelengths. This latter, diffraction-based aberration is barely noticeable in the center of the disk, but it may be seen on the edges of the first fringe, where it influences the resolution. We will look at this later.

Longitudinal chromatic aberration

The result of changes in lens focal-length with changing wavelengths. The image plane for only one wavelength or narrow wave band is in sharp focus; for other wavelengths, the image plane is defocussed. Fig. 12 compares the longitudinal chromatic correction of an Achromat with that of an Apochromat. In order to judge the influence of $\Delta s'$ for a given lens on the image quality, the spectral emission of the source as well as the spectral sensitivity of the detector need to be considered since both determine the brightness in the center of the disk.

The peak sensitivity for the eye is at 550 nm, with a spectral range of ~480 to ~650 nm.

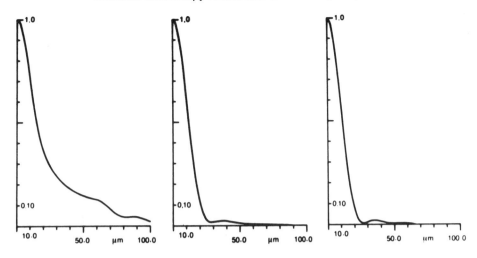

Fig. 14.   Intensity distribution for Achromat, Plan-Neofluar, Planapochromat.

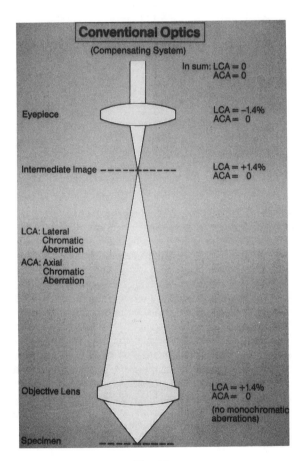

Fig. 15.

Fig. 16.   Zeiss's ICS optics concept.

Lateral chromatic aberration (LCA) or chromatic magnification difference

The magnification for different wavelengths changes, sharp edges in the image show blue or red fringes. The blue component at 436 nm may be imaged 1.4% larger than the red component at 630 nm. The LCA normally is greater for objectives of short focal length and can range from 1.1% to 1.9% of the radial distances. In confocal scanning of fluorescence images, this can cause poor registration between the excited and detected off-axis image points. Proper matching of all components is essential to assure full compensation of the LCA.

In most conventional microscope systems, all objectives are calculated for a constant amount of LCA, which then is compensated for by the eyepiece. This compensating system is illustrated in Fig. 15. Nikon in 1976 introduced CF optics, adding additional lenses to all their objectives to correct for LCA in the objective alone. In Zeiss' ICS (Infinity Color-corrected System) optics, no correction for LCA takes place in the objective.

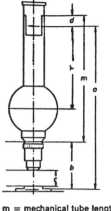

m = mechanical tube length = 160mm
a = object-to-image distance = 195mm
b = object distance of objective= 45mm
d = intermediate image distance
     of eyepiece = 10mm
c = working distance of the objective
r = distance mounting shoulder monocular
     tube to intermediate image

FIG. 17. Standard dimensions of conventional microscope.

The tube lens uniquely compensates for the full range of LCA of different objectives, generating a fully corrected intermediate image with 25 mm diameter in all techniques (Fig. 16). This in turn means less elements in the objective and a choice of more suitable glass types, particularly for the Plan-Neofluars, where only one selected heavy flintglass and no fluorite is used. This virtually eliminates auto-fluorescence in the objective, improves extinction ratios for polarizing microscopy and assures high light throughput and good contrast.

All off-axis aberrations can adversely affect the performance of beam-scanning systems. Potentially most critical is the lateral chromatic aberration in the confocal fluorescence mode, where the excited off-axis object point can be sufficiently shifted from the pinhole, reading only emitted, longer wave-length radiation, that a substantial energy loss may be registered.

Example: A 100× oil objective may scan a 100 × 100 μm field on the object with 500 pixels per scan line. The approx. 0.2 μm diameter blue pixel without lateral chromatic correction is shifted 1.9% of the distance from the center of the field against its red corresponding pixel. For the 50 μm distance from the center, a displacement of almost 1 μm or 5 pixel diameters would occur. Depending on the size of the pinhole, the consequences are obvious.

FINITE VERSUS INFINITY OPTICS

Most conventional microscopes are built around the German DIN (now ISO) standard, which calls for 160 mm tubelength, 45 mm parfocal distance, and 195 mm object-to-image distance (Fig. 17). This concept applies to many transmitted light techniques and has served us well for over 100 years.

Objectives with finite image-distance directly form a real intermediate image, either corrected (Nikon) or with residual LCA, to be compensated for by the eyepiece. Infinity-designed objectives require a tube lens to form this real intermediate image. While the tube lens can be employed to also correct for residual aberrations, the intrinsic design advantage of infinite image-distance (Fig. 18) is its relative insensitivity to optical components, such as filters, analyzers, compensators, DIC prisms, and reflectors in the telescopic space between objective

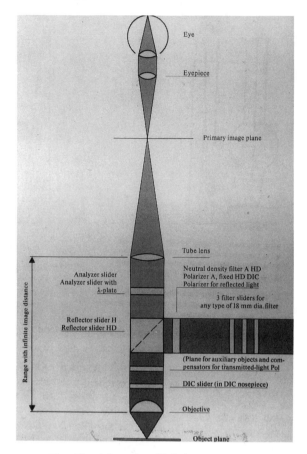

FIG. 18. Advantage of infinity correction.

and tube lens. Infinity or parallel beams are not affected by such components, as long as they themselves are plane parallel. The location of the image point remains constant, both axially and laterally, as does alignment between objective and tube lens.

In the converging beam path of the finitely designed system similar elements would cause axial, and possibly lateral, shift. This not only causes aberations but will make it difficult to get good image registration in multi-parameter techniques (double or triple fluorescence).

By adding so-called Telan systems, an "infinity space" is generated and these problems are eliminated (Fig. 19). But now we have two additional optical elements—one negative and one positive—and with them the potential for more flare and stray-light, which can be particularly troublesome with the coherent laser. Phase randomizing the laser may reduce signal distortions caused by internal specular reflections.

One added advantage of the infinity correction is that objective rather than stage focus can be easily accomplished, as is the case in some inverted and some upright microscopes.

The following major microscope manufacturers offer these design concepts:

- Cambridge (Reichert): Infinity for transmitted and reflected light
- Leitz/Wild: 160 mm for transmitted optics, infinity for reflected light
- Nikon: 160 mm for transmitted optics, 210 mm for reflected light
- Olympus: 160 mm for transmitted optics, infinity for reflected light
- Zeiss ICS: Infinity for transmitted and reflected light

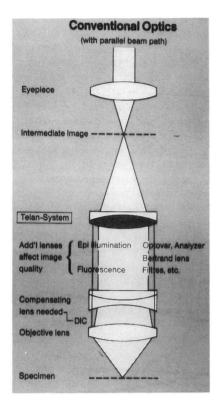

FIG. 19.

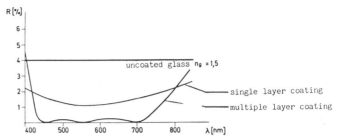

FIG. 20. Single vs. multilayer coatings.

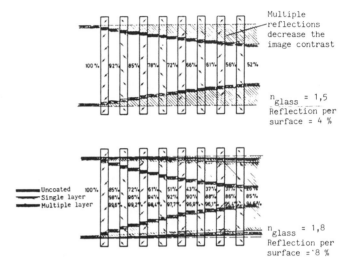

FIG. 21. Reflections on surfaces of n = 1.5 (above) versus n = 1.8 (below). At n = 1.5, the 8 elements with their 16 surfaces reflect 4% each resulting in a throughput of only 52%. At n = 1.8 the uncoated 16 surfaces would pass only 26%. The single layer antireflection coating increases the transmission to 85%, the multilayer coating to 94.6%. This increase in throughput and corresponding reduction in internal scatter and "noise" substantially enhances the contrast in an image because it makes both bright features brighter and dark features darker.

OPTICAL MATERIALS

Without going into the details of the more than 200 optical glasses available to the optical designer and their properties, such as refractive index, dispersion, transmission, contaminants—potential auto fluorescence, chemical and thermal resistance, and overall homogeneity, I will highlight certain properties that—while highly desirable for superb optical performance—may also compromise other requirements, such as high transmission in the near-UV range or high extinction factors in polarizing microscopy. Some new materials, such as lanthanum fluoride glass, approach the properties of natural fluorite and do away with its drawbacks, such as organic contaminants and a crystalline structure, which seriously affect an objective's performance in fluorescence and polarizing microscopy. The full apochromatic correction, however, still requires both natural fluorite and glasses that have reduced transmission in near UV.

The semi-apochromat, is therefore often the ideal compromise. It can be a true multi-purpose objective, combining excellent correction with good contrast and higher numerical aperture with high spectral throughput. The transmission for most Zeiss Plan-Neofluars (which contain no natural fluorite), for instance at 365 nm, is better than 50%, normalized for 550 nm. The transmission in this case is measured through the full aperture using an integrating sphere.

Cements between doublet or multiple lens elements can have spectral absorption properties that may render an objective not useable for specific applications. Their thickness is usually less than 10 μm.

Chemical and optical properties are usually proprietary. Decementation between lenses caused by heat and different coefficients of expansion is rare. Lasers of < 100 m W energy in

near-UV and visible range will cause no damage if their power is evenly distributed over the entire entrance pupil.

ANTI-REFLECTION COATINGS

As the sophistication of objectives increases, more elements are required, accentuating the need to eliminate internal reflections for higher transmission, better contrast, and less flare, particularly in incident or reflected light applications. Single-layer AR coatings dating back to the 1940s have since been refined and supplemented by multilayer coatings, increasing the transmission in the visible spectral range through an air-glass interface from ∼ 96% (not coated) to ∼ 99% (single layer coating) to ∼ 99.9% (multilayer coating) (Fig. 20 and 21).

Coating materials can be magnesium fluoride and a multitude of proprietary materials, all of which have their own optical properties potentially affecting the transmission of the system in given spectral regions. In general, the interference characteristics of AR coatings are spectrally limited, and constructive interference for highest transmission in the visible range means destructive interference in harmonically related frequencies outside the transmission band.

For specimens of very low reflectivity, the weak back-scattered signal may be overwhelmed by noise resulting from internal reflections in the objective lens. In this case, a so-called Antiflex system can be a great advantage. Here we illuminate with polarized light and observe through an analyzer at 90% to the polarizer. Internal stray light reflected specularly by optical surfaces retains its direction of polarization and is blocked by the analyzer. A ¼ wave plate is actually incorporated into the front element of the objective and with its vibration direction diagonal to the polarizer and analyzer. For a given wavelength (usually 550 nm) this generates circularly polarized light, in effect rotating the plane of vibration of both the illumination and the back-scattered light by 45° for a total of 90°. Light reflected from the object is now oriented parallel to the analyzer and can pass freely for detection. This system is used for the so-called reflection contrast or reflection interference technique but is most effective in all reflected light studies of weakly reflecting objects.

CONCLUSION

We can conclude that many modern microscope objectives are well suited for confocal scanning as long as they are used within their design specifications. In particular, as laser-based confocal scanning microscopy comes of age, requests for special new lenses for specific applications will certainly be made. In addition to the call for objectives with highest numerical aperture, longest working distance, and maximum throughput in the visible and/or near or far UV (as previously mentioned), this may be the time to "dream" about other exotic lens fea-

tures. We might imagine an an oil-immersion objective of high NA with automatic correction for the spherical aberration introduced by the penetration depth in a watery medium. (We should mention here that in more extreme cases of this application, the full NA of the objective will not be utilized because of total internal reflection, at least for illumination or excitation. For instance, the illumination NA of a Planapochromat 63/1.4 e.g. would be reduced to 1.33.) We can also conceive of a tuneable objective, a lens whose chromatic correction can be "tuned" to the specific excitation and emission wavelengths in use to produce the best image quality and throughput. If such tuneability is impossible, perhaps special lenses will be designed for use with specific fluorophores.

An even more exotic dream for a substantial increase in signal intensity might be realized in using two matched lenses on top and bottom of the specimen and equipping the lower one with a reflector to return the spot into itself, thus combining reflected and transmitted confocal scanning.

These are just a few thoughts on possible future developments in this area. No doubt, specialists in optical design will quickly return us to reality and make us do with somewhat less than our dreams.

Many thanks to a number of scientists at Carl Zeiss, West Germany, for their help in preparing this paper and for many of the illustrations. Special thanks to Mr. Franz Muchel, head of the mathematics group at Carl Zeiss, whose recent paper (Zeiss information sheet #100, 1/89, 20–27) on the new ICS optics has been particularly helpful.

Chapter 8

Size and Shape of The Confocal Spot: Control and Relation to 3D Imaging and Image Processing

G.J. Brakenhoff, K. Visscher and H.T.M. van der Voort

Department of Molecular Cell Biology, Section Molecular Cytology, University of Amsterdam, Plantage Muidergracht 14, 1018 TV Amsterdam the Netherlands

ABSTRACT

A confocal microscope can be considered as a 3D sampling instrument for collecting data from spatial structures, especially biological ones. Optimal data collection in confocal microscopes requires the adaptation of the dimensions of the sampling volume to the lateral and axial raster parameters employed during data collection. It is shown how, in principle, the collection volume can be partly manipulated by the use of variable pinholes both in the illumination and detection paths. The effective confocal spot will depend on the optics used, the degree of aberration, and the alignment of the instrument. Measurements of the axial response both in fluorescence and reflection for some high N.A. lens systems as a function of the above factors are presented. The use of variable pinholes in computer-controlled instruments is discussed, especially in relation to operation in fluorescence. It is indicated that proper interpretation and processing of 3D confocal data requires at least approximate knowledge of the applicable 3D response function.

INTRODUCTION

Confocal microscopy is a well-established technique for the investigation of three-dimensional structure in biological and industrial materials. (Brakenhoff et al., 1985, 1988; Carlsson et al. 1985; Wijnaendts van Resandt, 1985; Steltzer et al., 1987). The basis for this success is the optical sectioning capability of this type of microscopy, which enables one to study the 3D structure of intact specimens in their natural environment. The principle of confocal microscopy has been described before (Sheppard et al., 1977; Wilson et al., 1984). For first demonstrations of the improved imaging see Brakenhoff et al. (1979) and of optical sectioning Brakenhoff et al. (1980), Wijnaendts van Resandt (1985) and Carlsson (1985).

The lateral resolution together with its sectioning capability, makes a confocal microscope in fact a three-dimensional imaging instrument. The measured value of a certain imaging parameter at a specific data point in space is an average over the specimen weighted with the applicable spatial confocal response function. It is represented by the product in specimen space of an overlapping illumination intensity and detection sensitivity distribution. These are generated in the confocal point by the projection of the laser illuminated pinhole and the back projection of the detector pinhole, respectively. This 3-dimensional response function constitutes in fact an optical probe with spatial dimensions, which, as a first approximation and for the purposes of this paper, can be described by its lateral and axial full width at half maximum (FWHM).

In reflection, the generation of the detected signal by the object is, unfortunately, considerably more complicated. Unlike in fluorescence where the incoherence of the emitted radiation permits the use of the approach described above, in reflection we have to consider the object as a collection of scattering elements. The total scattered signal after illumination will be sensitively influenced by the structural detail in the object on a scale below the resolution of the microscope. As an example one may think of two scatterpoints in the object at the same lateral position but axially separated either a $1/4$ or $1/2$ wavelength apart. Due to interference of the scattered light we will detect no signal in the $1/4 \lambda$ case and, in the $1/2 \lambda$ case, four times the intensity of a single such scatter point. Therefore the detected signal in reflection will only be predictable for certain well-defined objects, such as a mirror plane or a single scatter point. In this chapter we will use the response to the former to evaluate the axial response of a few lens systems as a function of operating conditions.

In the confocal microscope coupled to a computer system, data are usually digitized on a raster grid of 256×256 or 512×512 pixels per plane with 8 to 32 2D-planes per 3D image. Together with the lateral magnification and the axial spacing of the section planes, this grid determines the spatial sampling of the object. If the collected data are to represent the spatial structure of the object at a certain parameter, the lateral and axial dimensions of the confocal spot ideally should be of the same size as the lateral and axial dimensions of the collection raster (or double this size if we want to satisfy the Nyquist criterium). If it is smaller, then the object may be misrepresented, because parts of the object are not addressed by the microscope. If the optical probe is too large we will have oversampling in view of the optical resolution and expose the object to more radiation than necessary (see Chapter 4).

Below we indicate how to use variable pinholes both on the illumination and detection side of the confocal microscope for controlling within certain limits the lateral and spatial extension of the effective sample volume. The approach is to indicate approximately the effects that can be expected. A proper treatment should be based on modelling the actual imaging at high N.A. in the full vector approach, as done for certain cases by van der Voort (1989).

PINHOLES AND OPTICAL PROBE FORMATION

We will examine separately how the illumination distribution and detection sensitivity distribution can be controlled by pinholes in the respective illumination and detection paths. As indicated above, the optical probe for confocal image formation is the convolution of both.

The 3D shape of the illumination distribution may be controlled by varying the effective Numerical Aperture with which the confocal lens is used. As indicated in Fig. 1 we can do this by using a variable pinhole in the illuminating laser beam as a diffracting element. Setting the pinhole at a diameter d_i will produce a beam with a FWHM divergence of $\lambda/2d_i$. If the confocal illumination lens is positioned at a distance L from the pinhole, an area with a radius of approximately $L\lambda/2d_i$ on the lens will be illuminated. If this radius is smaller than the radius A of the lens, then the effective NA for the illumination is $n\sin\alpha = nL\lambda/2d_if = n\lambda M/2d_i$ with M = L/f the (de)magnification of the confocal lens. The dependence on numerical aperture of the FWHM of the lateral Δr_i and axial Δz_i extension of the illumination energy distribution in focus is given by the well-known relations (Born and Wolfe, 1975)

$$\Delta r_i = 0.61\,\lambda/n\sin\alpha \text{ and } \Delta z_i = 2\lambda/n\sin^2\alpha.$$

We find then, that as long as the illumination beam does not fill the confocal lens, the confocal illumination spot dimensions depend on pinhole diameter as

$$\Delta r_i = 1.2\,d_i/nM \text{ and } \Delta z_i = 8d_i^2/n\lambda M^2. \qquad (1)$$

To control the spatial extension of the detection sensitivity function we also use a variable pinhole, but its effects on detection differ from those of the illumination pinhole. For detection we always use the confocal lens at its full angular aperture α_o. First, at very small detection pinholes diameters d_d, the dimensions of the detection sensitivity function are determined by the diffraction-limited imaging of the confocal lens with full angular aperture α_o. Then the respective FWHM lateral and axial widths Δr_d and Δz_d of the detection sensitivity function will have the diffraction determined minimum values of

$$\Delta r_d = \Delta r_{dm} = 0.6\lambda/n\sin\alpha_o \text{ and } \Delta z_d = \Delta z_{dm} = 2\lambda/n\sin^2\alpha_o.$$

At intermediate values of d_d, that is, with $d_d/M \approx \Delta r_{dm}$ (M the magnification factor for the detector), we see a gradual increase of the confocal detection spot dimensions, until finally at still higher values, the imaging can in fact be described from the geometrical point of view. In the latter limit, we find for the FWHM values of the respective lateral and axial detection response widths

$$\Delta r_d = d_d/M \text{ and } \Delta z_d = \sqrt{2}\,d_d/M\tan\alpha_o. \qquad (2)$$

In addition, other properties are associated with the use of variable pinholes. On the illumination side, the intensity in the confocal illumination distribution is independent of pinhole size as long as the lens pupil is not filled, that is, when $\lambda L/2d_i <$ A and A is the confocal lens radius. This is because closing the pinhole d_i in the illuminating laser beam will cause the power passing the pinhole to decrease proportionally to d_i^2. However, as the irradiated area in the focused confocal spot decreases due to the increased filling of the pupil, which is also proportional to d_i^2; the intensity in the confocal spot will be constant and independent of d_i. After the pupil is filled, the power in the confocal light distribution will fall off as d_i^4: d_i^2 due to reduction of the effective pinhole size and another d_i^2 as the confocal lens

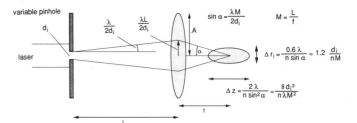

FIG. 1. Confocal illumination arrangement with a variable pinhole. The effective dimensions of the confocal illumination spot can be controlled by varying the filling factor of the lens by means of a variable pinhole inserted in the laser beam. The optical situation is considered to be an immersion system in which the confocal spot is formed in a medium with a refractive index n.

intercepts a smaller amount of power from the widening beam. On the detection side, we would like to stress the fact that while the detection pinhole is used to vary the dimensions of the detection sensitivity distribution, the outcoming radiation is always collected with full N.A. This assures that signal collection efficiency is always optimal for a given choice of spatial detection conditions, a property especially important in fluorescence, where the available light flux is often limited.

PRACTICAL USE OF VARIABLE PINHOLES

The relations for the lateral and axial dimensions of both the illumination and detection distributions (equations 1 and 2) can be used in various ways. If, for instance, the signal-to-noise level is too low, one can sacrifice some resolution by opening the detection pinhole to increase the signal. Then, without much additional loss of resolution, one can also increase the illumination distribution width to the same width as the detection distribution. This will increase the signal even further as a larger volume in the specimen participates in the fluorescent generation. As indicated above, the probe intensity stays constant hence the local irradiation load on the specimen does not change. However, in the combined use of the illumination and detection pinhole, the detected signal will increase at a rate roughly proportional to the 4th power of the loss of resolving power. Owing to the different dependence of $\Delta z_{i;b}$ and $\Delta r_{i;b}$ on d_i and d_d, we can optimize either the axial or the lateral resolution, as required by the situation. On the other hand, one can also use this approach to set either the lateral or the axial imaging properties to a desired value and estimate the consequences this will have for the other factor.

The full potential of the use of variable pinholes becomes clear when this approach is considered for imaging at various magnifications, in conjunction with factors like saturation and bleaching in fluorescence. This is especially true when a computer-controlled instrument is considered. For example, at low zoom magnifications, image collection on a certain 3D grid may be such that the sampling volume is smaller than the sampling grid dimensions. Then, apart from the undesirable undersampling of the object (see Chapter 4), the specimen may be bleached or damaged on a pattern corresponding to the sampling grid. This effect can be prevented if the size of the illuminating spot is increased automatically when low magnification is used. The increase in collection volume with the larger detection pinhole will increase the detected signal amplitude, permitting a further reduction of total specimen exposure at low magnification for a given signal to noise ratio in the image.

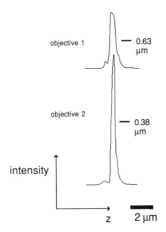

FIG. 2. Confocal reflection response of two different 100×, N.A. = 1.3 immersion objectives under otherwise identical conditions. The detected intensity of the two objectives is stated in arbitrary units but the curves are mutually comparable. Wavelength: 488 nm.

An attractive aspect of the use of a variable pinhole in a computer controlled instrument is that the functions mentioned above can be performed automatically as a function of magnification and z-sample distance. Also, the type of object may be taken into account through a user-set option which determines the priorities in the program that controls the instrument. For instance, in sensitive or weakly fluorescent specimens, as mentioned above, it is advisable to open up both the lateral detection and the illumination distribution width. In thick objects, this will lead to an impermissible loss in contrast due to a great increase in the axial extension of the illumination distribution caused by reduced illumination on the pupil. However, in thin objects, which actually "do" their own sectioning, the larger pinholes would be the optimal course of action for sensitive specimens. For bleach-sensitive specimens at low magnifications, one would give priority to the larger illumination spot dimensions to avoid specimen damage. For sturdy, thick specimens, the necessary sectioning dictates a small illumination spot. For intermediate cases, experience may lead to optimal algorithms to balance the various factors.

EXPERIMENTAL AXIAL CONFOCAL RESPONSE

In practice, the optical performance of a confocal microscope may differ from the results in the idealized case of diffraction-limited imaging assumed above. These may be associated with the optical properties of the optics employed or with instrument-determined conditions such as alignment or size of pinholes, etc. For this reason, the effective optical probe may not have the shape one would expect theoretically. We will present here some measurements that will illustrate the necessity for selecting and testing the optics employed in confocal microscopy and will stress the importance of an accurate alignment. They will also demonstrate the dependence on detection pinhole size of the axial resolution in both reflection and fluorescence.

Fig. 2 shows the confocal reflection response to a mirror object scanned in the axial or Z-direction. The responses of two 100× N.A. = 1.3 immersion objectives corrected for a nominal tube length of 160 mm. are compared. The optical situation is very simple: the confocal lens, one beamsplitter and the illu-

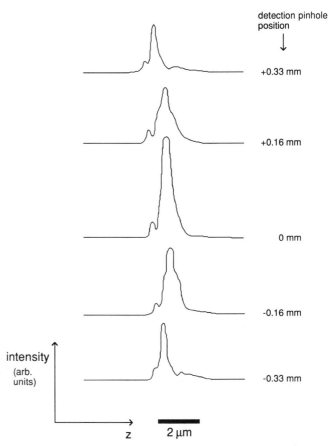

FIG. 3. Axial confocal response in reflection to a mirror object as a function of detection pinhole position, measured with objective 1. Other conditions are the same as in Fig. 2.

mination and detection pinholes at the conjugate image planes of the confocal spot. The pinholes were perfectly x-y-z aligned (see below) and had a diameter during this measurement equal to 1/4 of the diffraction-limited Airy disk (projected in object space). For the purposes of this measurement, they can be considered as a point source and point detector. The width of the response of objective 2 is close to the expectations for the ideal system, while the broadening of the objective 1 response clearly shows the effect of aberrations, probably mainly spherical aberration. Note also that the detected peak signal in the well corrected system is 2.5 times higher than that in the non-optimal one.

Sensitivity to proper alignment is demonstrated in Fig. 3. It is well known that correct lateral alignment of the illumination and detection pinholes is very important and most instruments provide facilities for this. We have found that precise axial adjustment is also essential. This fact runs contrary to expectations as movements along the axial direction at the intermediate image plane, where the pinholes are located, are demagnified into confocal object space by the magnification factor of the objectives squared. Fig. 3 shows the dependence of the axial mirror response of objective 2 on the axial position of the detection pinhole. Position 0 mm designates the optimal axial pinhole position and the other curves are taken with the pinhole moved axially by the indicated distance. The positive direction corresponds to a movement of the pinhole towards the confocal lens. These axial movements translated into confocal object

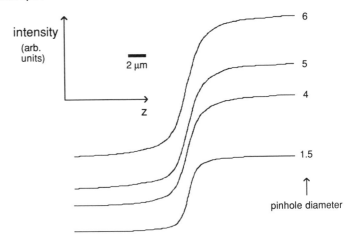

FIG. 5. Axial confocal response to a fluorescent step object as a function of pinhole size (see text). Excitation: 488 nm., detection: above 520 nm. Other conditions are the same as in Fig. 3.

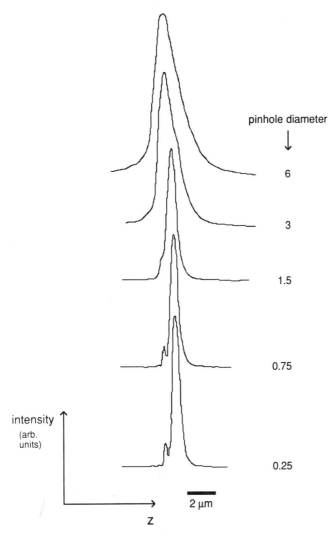

FIG. 4. Axial confocal response in reflection as a function of pinhole size (see text). Other conditions are the same as in Fig. 3.

COMMENTS AND CONCLUSIONS

We have indicated some potential applications of variable pinholes and how they can be employed for the optimal 3D sampling of fluorescent specimens in a confocal microscope. It seems especially fruitful to equip computer-controlled instruments with facilities of this type.

After image collection in confocal microscopy, an awareness of the shape of the optical probe with which the data were acquired is essential for interpreting the data correctly. As shown by Van der Voort (1989) the apparent intensity with which object elements will appear in the image depends on the object structure and and orientation. The reason for this is that the shape of the optical confocal probe in space is not spherical but ellipsoidal along the Z-axis. Both the direct interpretation of 3D confocal data by observers and the quantitative interpretation during image processing and analysis should take into account the actual shape of the confocal optical probe in order to deduce correct conclusions from the data.

space correspond to shifts of ± 33 nm. It is surprising that relative position shifts of the detection and illumination distributions over distances of about one tenth of the applicable wavelength under immersion conditions produce changes in axial response as large as those measured. At present we do not have a good explanation for this behaviour.

The axial response in reflection, as a function of detection pinhole size, is shown in Fig. 4. The detection pinhole size, after projection in confocal object space, is expressed in units of FWHM of the diffraction-limited Airy distribution. We see that the axial width of the response function, over the indicated range of pinholes, increases by a factor of more than 3. Similarly, we see in Fig. 5 that the steepness of the response into a fluorescent step function at the surface of a 1-mm-thick slab of fluorescent material, is also strongly reduced at larger detection pinholes. Only the shape of the curves in Fig. 4 and 5 should be regarded. The signals for each curve have been adjusted such that the responses have approximately equal amplitudes in these figures. Curves such as those above have been published before, for instance, for fluorescence by Wijnaends van Resandt (1985); however, presented as a function of pinhole size, they emphasize the importance of control over the effective optical probe, which determines the imaging in confocal microscopy

REFERENCES

M. Born and E. Wolf. Principles of Optics. 5th ed. Pergamon Press, Oxford, 435–448 (1975).

G.J. Brakenhoff, P.J. Blom and P. Barends. Confocal scanning light microscopy with high aperture immersion lenses. J. of Micros. 117: 219–232 (1979).

G.J. Brakenhoff, J.S. Binnerts and C.L. Woldringh. Developments in high resolution confocal scanning light microscopy (CSLM). In: Scanned Image Microscopy ed. E.A. Ash, Academic Press, London (1980).

G.J. Brakenhoff, H.T.M. van der Voort, E.A. van Spronsen, W.A.M. Linnemans and N. Nanninga. Three-dimensional chromatin distribution in neuroblastoma nuclei shown by confocal scanning laser microscopy. Nature, 317: 748–749 (1985).

G.J. Brakenhoff, H.T.M. van der Voort, E.A. van Spronsen and N. Nanninga, Scanning Microscopy, 2:33–40 (1988).

K. Carlsson, P.E. Danielson, R. Lenz, A. Liljeborg, L. Maylüf and N. Ashlund. Three- dimansional microscopy using a confocal scanning laser microscope. Opt. Lett. 10:53–55 (1985)

M. Minsky, U.S. Patent 3013467, Microscopy Apparatus, Dec. 19, 1961 (filed Nov. 7, 1957).

M. Petran, N. Hadrawsky and A. Boyde. The Tandem Scanning Reflected Light Microscope. Scanning 7:97–108 (1985).

C.J.R. Sheppard and A. Choudhury. Image formation in the scanning microscope. Optica, 24:1051 (1977).

E.A.K. Steltzer and R.W. Wijnaendts van Resandt. Nondestructive sectioning of fixed and living specimens using a confocal scanning laser fluorescence microscope: Microtomoscopy. Proc. SPIE 809:130–137 (1987).

R.W. Wijnaendts van Resandt. Optical fluorescence microscopy in three dimensions: microtomoscopy. J. Micros. 138:29–34 (1985).

H.T.M van der Voort and G.J. Brakenhoff. 3-D image formation in high aperture fluorescence confocal microscopy: a numerical analysis. J. Micr. to be published, 1989.

T. Wilson and C.J.R. Sheppard, Theory and Practice of Scanning Optical Microscopy, Academic Press, London (1984).

Chapter 9

The Intermediate Optical System of Laser-scanning Confocal Microscopes

Ernst H.K. Stelzer

Confocal Light Microscopy Group, European Molecular Biology Laboratory (EMBL), Meyerhofstrasse 1, Postfach 10.2209, D-69oo Heidelberg, Federal Republic of Germany (FRG), Tel +49 6221 387 354, FAX +49 6221 387 306

This text tries to explain some of the basics of intermediate optical systems in confocal microscopes. Most of the considerations are very simple and based on geometrical optics. The author therefore saw no need to present lengthy mathematical equations. The simple calculations that are part of the text should be sufficient to understand which calculations are relevant for the design of confocal microscopes.

It is the purpose of this chapter to describe and compare the various intermediate optical systems used and to help understand the function of the mirrors, lenses and other components that are required. This chapter concentrates on laser-based single spot scanning instruments, disk-scanning systems are covered more fully in Chapter 10.

DESIGN PRINCIPLES OF CONFOCAL SYSTEMS

Overview

The basic optical layout of a confocal fluorescence microscope is found in Figures 1 and 2. A laser beam is focused into a pinhole. The spatially filtered light is deflected by a dichroic mirror and focused into the fluorescently labeled specimen. The fluorescent light is emitted in all directions, a part of it is collected by the lens and focused into a pinhole in front of the detector. Light that is emitted from locations in front or behind the focal point in the object is focused into points either in front or behind the detector pinhole. Since these beams are expanded in the plane of the pinhole, only a fraction of the light enters the detector. The detector pinhole hence discriminates against the out-of-focus contributions from within the object.

Another description is that the lens forms an image of both the source and the detector pinhole in the object. If the diffraction limited images overlap, the instrumental setup is confocal. This description emphasizes symmetry considerations.

Since this arrangement observes only one spot in the object and the main interest is to form an image, the sampling light spot must be either scanned through the object (beam scanner) or the object must be moved through the light spot (object scanner).

Additional important elements in the confocal arrangement are the extra filter set, the scan unit, the intermediate lens and the detector.

Microscope Objectives

The basic geometrical optics of the confocal microscope are diagrammed in the three parts of Fig. 1. Fig. 1a outlines the major elements of the confocal microscope in terms of the objective lens and its image and object planes (a more complete description is found in Chapter 7). The relations between the various parameters are described in DIN 58 886/58 887 (Naumann/Schröder 1987, pp. 356). The user of the microscope (in practice) needs to know only the magnification and the numerical aperture of the lens. Most of the other properties (e.g. the diameter of the entrance aperture) can be easily calculated. The sketch in Figure 1 shows an ideal setup as it is well known from many papers on confocal microscopy (Bacallao & Stelzer 1989). The microscope objective is, however, a thick lens and the locations of its principal planes are not known. Also important is that the image and object distances are fixed. If the full correction of the lens is to be exploited, these distances must be used. This fixes the positions of the image and the object planes relative to the position of the microscope objective.

All microscope objectives are corrected telecentrically (Fig. 1b). The entrance and exit pupil are both at infinity in the object and image space respectively. Telecentric systems are space invariant and linear. Space invariant means that the lateral and the longitudinal magnification of the optical system are constant throughout the whole space. The shape of the point spread function is independent of the absolute location of the point source. **All beams pass the telecentric plane with an angle that is characteristic of the position of the light spot in the object plane.** This property is very important and the conjugate telecentric planes, like the conjugate image planes, are shown in overviews of the optical paths of conventional microscopes. The knowledge of these positions is important when it comes to extending optical paths, as we will see later.

Position of the Pivot Point

If a scanning mirror is used to move the sampling light spot in the object plane, where should it be located? A single mirror is capable of affecting only the angle of propagation of a laser beam. What is needed is to find the position along the optical path where a change in angle will result in a linear motion of the focused spot on the specimen. From the description above, it should be obvious that the pivot point (the center of the rotation) of the mirror must be in a conjugate telecentric plane of the microscope objective. If we had a one-dimensional scanner we would place the center of the scan mirror in the center of a conjugate telecentric plane. The stationary beam falling on this mirror would be deflected and, according to the deflection angle, the spot would move to different positions in the object

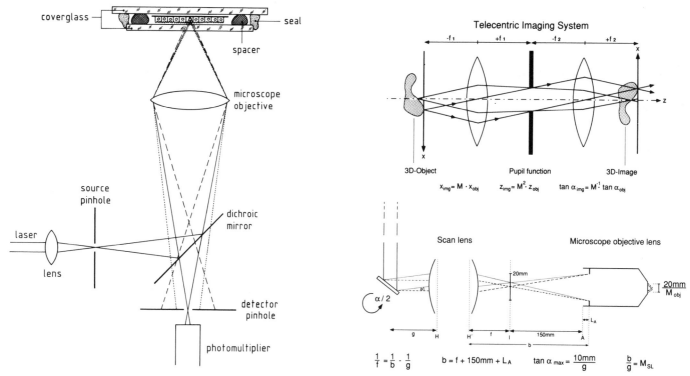

FIG. 1. *Basic Confocal Optics* a) (left) The optical system of a confocal fluorescence microscope. The microscope objective forms an image of the source pinhole and an image of the detector pinhole in the object. Both pinholes are positioned on the optial axis in an image plane of the objective lens. The images of the two pinholes therefore overlap in the object. b) (top right) Telecentricity in light microscopy. A telecentric system is arranged like a Keplerian telescope with a stop in the common focal area of the two lenses. The most important result of such a setup is that the magnification factor determines all the properties of the system and that the magnification is spatially invariant (following Streibl 1984, p. 16). Observing e.g. two points in focus and then out of focus shows that the center distances will not vary. Telecentric arrangements are therefore found in all optical measurement devices since they are insensitive to defocusing. c) (bottom right) Calculations in a confocal microscope. This sketch illustrates which calculations must be made when designing a confocal beam scanning laser microscope. The distance b between the entrance aperture of the microscope objective A and the principal plane H' of the scan lens is fixed to $b = f + 150mm + L_A$. Since $1/f = 1/g + 1/b$ we calculate g the distance between the pivot point of the mirror and the principal plane H of the scan lens. This allows us to calculate the magnification $M = b/g$ and the scan angle of the mirror $tan \, \alpha_{max} = 10mm/g$. The assumptions are a) that the image has a size of $20mm$ and b) that the microscope objective is corrected for $150mm$. These assumptions are valid if we use standard microscope objective lenses. The main problems are to determine the distance L_A and the positions of the principal planes H and H' which must be requested from the manufacturers. Since the focal length of the scan lens is the only free parameter, the design must now be tuned to have a magnification in the order of 0.5 to 2 (specified magnification of a photographic objective lens) and a scan angle that is quite high so that the galvanometers are used to their best. Hints: A focal length of $f = 100mm$ is usually a good starting point, $H' - H$ is usually negative and L_A is on the order of $20mm$.

plane. Any conjugate telecentric plane is an image of the telecentric plane of the microscope objective. An intermediate optical system would form an image of the scan mirror in the entrance aperture of the microscope objective. Not every arrangement is, however, valid. As pointed out above the microscope objective must be used with fixed object and image distances or else it will not function correctly. If the (incident) laser beam is collimated, the intermediate optical system must have its focal plane coincide with the image plane of the microscope objective (Fig. 1c).

The imaging outlined so far can be described in another way. Every spot in the object plane has a conjugate spot in the image plane. As the light spot is moved in the image plane the conjugate light spot is moved in the object plane. To scan the object plane light spots must be produced in the image plane. If the beam falling into the intermediate optical system is collimated, a spherically corrected beam will be achieved only if the focal plane of the lens and the image plane of the microscope objective coincide. The position of the light spot in the image plane then depends on the scan angle.

This concept can be easily expanded to include more than one mirror and hence to scan in two perpendicular axes. As

pointed out the mirrors must be placed in conjugate telecentric planes. Any number of these planes may, however, be easily generated by adding additional optical systems. The image of a second mirror must then be formed on the first mirror. If the two mirrors move the beam in orthogonal planes, the object is scanned along its x- and y-axes.

Position of the Detector Pinhole

The images of the source and the detector pinhole overlap in a confocal microscope. The position of the illuminating light spot in the image plane is therefore also the position of the image of the light spot formed in the sample. Hence, the pinhole in front of the detector must be placed in a plane that is conjugate to the image plane of the microscope. In a scanning system this means that we need an optical arrangement that will form an image of the image plane. The scan system will move this image across the pinhole and the light of only one point in the object will enter the detector. If everything is set up correctly this point will be the point on the object that is being illuminated by the laser. In most cases the pinhole will be placed in the focal point on the optical axis of a lens. This

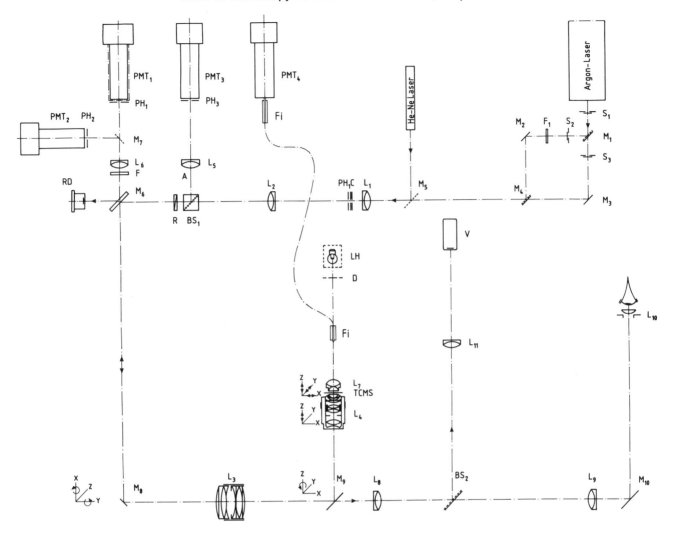

FIG. 2.   Schematic drawing of a typical confocal beam scanning laser microscope. The light source is an Argon ion laser. A set of two dichroic mirrors (M1 and M4) and a filter (F1) separate two lines (488nm and 514.5nm). One shutter (S1) switches the light off. Two other shutters (S2 and S3) are used to select either of the two excitation beams. The expanded and spatially filtered beam (lens L1, pinhole PH1 and lens L2) passes a polarizing beam splitter (BS1) and is deflected by a dichroic mirror (M6) into the scan unit (M8). The scanned beam falls through an intermediate lens (L3) into a microscope objective (L4) and forms a light spot moving across the object (TCMS). The fluorescent light emitted in the object is collected with the same lenses. The lens (L6) behind the dichroic mirror (M6) focuses the light into a pinhole in front of a photomultiplier. The lambda/4 plate (R) polarizes the light circularly. The light reflected in the sample is therefore vertically polarized when it enters the beam splitter (BS) and deflected in the direction of the photomultiplier. Other confocal beam scanning microscopes have in principle the same optical arrangement. Differences are discussed in the text. Use this figure to understand the placement of the optical elements and the position of the scan unit. The small x/y/z axes and the arrows next to some of the elements indicate which freedom the moving parts have.

lens and the intermediate optical system discussed above form a conjugate image plane. The image is spherically corrected only on the optical axis.

PRACTICAL REQUIREMENTS

Illumination

Starting in the object plane, the basic requirement is to have a light spot as small as possible. The spot size should be determined only by the wavelength of the incident (exciting) beam and the numerical aperture of the objective lens, i.e., the system should be diffraction limited. According to Goodman (p. 103, 1968), *"An imaging system is said to be diffraction limited if a diverging spherical wave, emanating from any point-source object, is converted by the system into a new wave, again spherical, that converges toward an ideal point in the image plane."* Since

we have real elements this requirement is definitely not fulfilled. Every optical element will cause a deviation and will thus increase the spot size. The actual spot size can be measured in the image plane of the microscope objective. In general, it should not be larger than the spot size in the object plane times the magnification of the lens (e.g. a 1.3/100× lens at a wavelength of 500 nm would have a spot diameter in the image plane of approx. 42 micron). Another important requirement to achieve the diffraction limit is that the entrance aperture of the microscope objective is uniformly filled with a spherical light wave (if the microscope objective is corrected for infinity a planar wave must fill the aperture of the microscope objective). Since every optical element modifies the wavefront one goal of the optical system is to generate a light spot in the image plane that is smaller than actually required. This is equivalent to over-illuminating the microscope aperture (the deviation from the diffraction limit with a wavefront error is nicely demonstrated on page 2–6 of the Melles Griot Optics Guide 4; real performances of lenses are found in Chapter 5 of MG4). Efficiency in the illumination path is not of great importance as lost light can be easily made up by using a more powerful laser.

Detection

To achieve the diffraction limit in the detection path is of course as important as in the illumination path. It seems, according to Wilson & Carlini (1987) and Chapter 11, that the pinhole may be larger than in the ideal case with only a modest decrease in the out-of-focus discrimination of the confocal set up. Increasing the pinhole diameter is complementary to over-illuminating the entrance aperture of the microscope objective and can be used to correct the same errors that were mentioned in the discussion of the illumination path. If, however, the optical arrangement of the detection path is close to the ideal case, nothing should be gained by increasing the pinhole size. Especially, and this is a good test, the intensity of the signal from a point object should not increase by more than a factor of two with a larger pinhole diameter. The idea is that we observe the image of a single point that is in focus. A well corrected confocal arrangement will collect all the available light and focus it into the pinhole. By increasing the size of the pinhole in front of the detector we would in addition collect the light that is emitted from around the point object but should not get any more light from the sample.

The detection efficiency is always crucial in fluorescence microscopy. The basic rule is to have as few optical elements in the detection path as possible. Sticking as closely as possible to this rule helps in avoiding losses due to reflection or absorption and prevents unwanted variations of the wavefront.

Distortion

Another important aspect is to keep the geometric distortion introduced by the inaccuracies of the scanning process as small as possible. The distortions can arise from deficiencies in either the mirror positioning system or the intermediate optics. The movement of the scanning mirror is known only approximately and it is very common to run the horizontal galvanometers in a sine function that is linear to 4% only in a range of +/-30 degrees. The scanning system and the way it is used obviously define the geometrical distortion to a very large degree. These factors also influence the efficiency of the illumination and the average energy penetrating a unit area. Finally, great care must be taken when the intermediate lens is selected. The optimal solution is an f-theta lens (for a description of scan lenses see MG4 Chapter 8).

Several laser scanning systems have been developed based on the principles outlined so far . The general rule is that the costs of optical perfection and low geometric distortion require greater complexity which in turn results in a reduced photon efficiency. The following discussion is offered to assist in evaluating the tradeoffs.

EVALUATION OF ILLUMINATION/DETECTION SYSTEMS

Influence of optical elements on the properties of light

All the optical elements of the confocal arrangement influence the beam. The light beam is characterized by

- the energy spectrum E(lambda),
- the plane of polarization P(lambda),
- the modal distribution,
- the beam waist diameter,
- the beam divergence,
- the direction of the beam, and
- the position of the beam relative to the optical axis.

In a fully corrected optical system, the designer considers all these parameters but in confocal microscopy this is usually not necessary. After all, a laser confocal microscope does not form a complete image and the wavelength used at any one time is only a small fraction of the total optical bandwidth. Several rules govern the properties of the incoming beam, i.e. the properties of the beam entering the entrance aperture of the microscope objective and another set of rules determines the properties of the beam entering the detector. The optical elements in either illumination or detection path are used to "shape" the beam, i.e. to take care that the beam will have the desired properties. The actual problem is that neither set of optical elements is perfect and to a varying degree they influence more than one of the properties of the beam.

Errors Caused By Optical Elements

A shift of the beam is caused by every flat optical component that is tilted relative to the optical axis and every lens that is not correctly centered. If the optical layout is designed for parallel beams, shifts are usually compensated in the detection path. In the illumination path a shift can result in vignetting. On the other hand, in laser arrangements with collimated beams flat surfaces are purposely tilted by a degree or half a degree to avoid interference effects caused by specular reflections. If the tilts are too large, refraction and dispersion can cause a visible, wavelength-dependent shift of the beam. If the tilt is in the range of one degree the shift is in the order of 6 micron/mm of glass

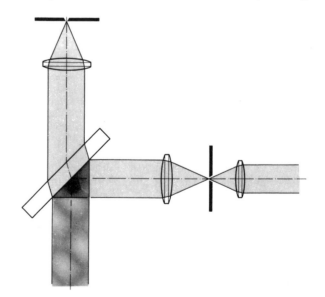

FIG. 3. An optical arrangement of class 1. The laser beam comes in from the right hand side, is spatially filtered, expanded and deflected by a dichroic mirror. The laser beam falling into the dichroic mirror is collimated. The fluorescence emission passes the dichroic mirror and is focused into a pinhole. The property of this beam is equivalent to that of a collimated laser beam. Due to refraction effects, the thickness of the dichroic mirror causes a shift of the beam. The diaphragm on the right hand side is the source pinhole, the upper diaphragm is the detector pinhole. Both pinholes are in conjugate image planes.

while, in the tilt range of 45 degrees, the shift is in the order of 330 micron/mm.

In the confocal microscope, a deflection of the beam is very critical and practically uncorrectable. Deflections are caused by flats with surfaces that are not perfectly parallel or by lenses that are tilted relative to the optical axis. As pointed out above, in telecentric systems the deflection determines the position of the light spot in the object plane. Every deflection of the beam in addition to that in the scan arrangement therefore causes a shift of the observed area. Typical planarities achieved today are below 1 second of arc. If the thickness varies 1 micron over a length of 25 mm and the collimated beam is focused with a 90 mm lens, the shift in the focal plane is 2 micron. Since the critical shift depends on the diameter of the pinhole an estimate of what is tolerable depends to a large extent on the magnification of the microscope objective used. The dichroic mirror is in this respect the most critical part in a confocal fluorescence microscope. Even slight changes cause the image of the source and detector pinhole not to overlap any more. This is all the more important as a fluorescence microscope must operate with several excitation lines and this means that the dichroic mirror is frequently changed. It must be changed without affecting the angle and the different dichroic mirrors must have similar surface characteristics.

The change of the state of polarization does not seem to be very critical. However, a number of optical elements, especially many dichroic mirrors, have a reflection coefficient that is polarization dependent. Also a lot of the microscope objectives have polarization dependent imaging characteristics. Changing a dichroic mirror can therefore have suprising effects on the image and on the amount of light that penetrates the sample. In practice, it seems best to work with light that is either circularly polarized or phase randomized (see Chapter 8).

Every element in the detection path causes an intensity loss. If the elements are coated (broad band anti-reflection coating in transmission, broad band high reflection coating for mirrors) the energy losses can be as low as 0.5–0.01% per surface.

The largest intensity losses are caused by the different filters. Narrow-band interference filters used to select a laser line transmit between 50 and 80% depending on the batch, the manufacturer and the bandwidth. Dichroic filters reflect between 80 and 90% of a single laser line and transmitt more than 80% of the light 20 nm above the maximum reflection. Long pass colour filters transmit more than 90% of the light 20 nm above the 50% cut off wavelength. The filter specifications are set by the laser line used and the emission and excitation spectra of the fluorophore and therefore a compromise cannot be avoided. Carefully adapting the filters to a dye or an experiment with more than one dye is worth a lot of trouble and time. The goal is to use a long-pass glass filter or a broad band interference filter that comes close to the emission maxima in the detection channels. If possible a change of the laser wavelength (an Argon ion laser offers lines from 458nm to 528nm) or even a different dye should be considered. Dyes change their properties after they are coupled to antibodies **and** after they are incorporated into the target.

Evaluation of Optical Arrangements

Figures 3 through 5 show different optical arrangements for confocal fluorescence microscopes. They all show the heart of

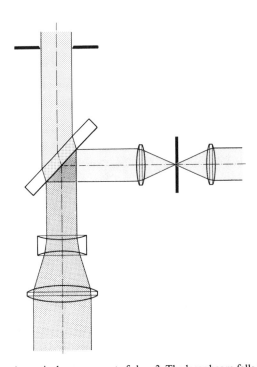

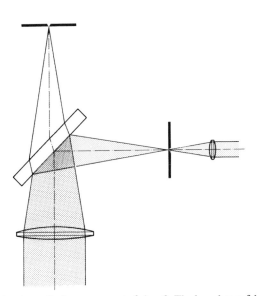

FIG. 4. An optical arrangement of class 2. The laser beam falls in from the right hand side. The beam is focused into a pinhole and spatially filtered. The divergent beam is deflected on the surface of a dichroic mirror into a lens. After passing this lens the beam is collimated. The same lens is used to focus the fluorescence emission into a pinhole. The two lenses form a beam expander as in class 1, the dichroic mirror is however placed inside the beam expanding unit. The fluorescence light upon passing the dichroic mirror is shifted off the axis and the overall geometric length is reduced.

FIG. 5. An optical arrangement of class 3. The laser beam falls in from the right hand side. The beam is deflected by a dichroic mirror. The fluorescence emission passes the dichroic mirror and enters a detector that is some distance away. Due to refraction the thickness of the dichroic mirror causes a shift of the beam. The lens required in a class 1 design is unnecessary due to the large distance between the image plane and the detector. The beam expander (shown as a Galilean telescope) is in the part that is common to the detection and the illumination paths. The role of the spatial filter is discussed in the text.

such an instrument, the assembly that is used for the separation of the excitation, and the emission bands. This section will discuss these arrangements and evaluate them in the terms discussed above.

Figure 3 The excitation light enters from the right hand side. The pinhole is in the focal point of the first two lenses. The collimated laser beam is spatially filtered and expanded. The expansion is determined by the ratio of the focal lengths of the two lenses and should be chosen to fill the entrance pupil of the microscope objective. The spatially filtered beam is again collimated and deflected by the dichroic mirror in the direction of the scan unit. The fluorescent light emitted in the sample passes the dichroic mirror and a third lens focuses the beam into a pinhole in front of the detector. The dichroic mirror causes a shift of the emission beam. This shift is intrinsic and "corrected" by displacing the third lens. Since the light beams are collimated, any shifts of the beam can be corrected. The arrangement is, however, not able to correct a tilt of the dichroic mirror which must therefore be carefully controlled. A polarizing beam splitter and a lambda/4 plate could be placed between the beam expander and the dichroic mirror without decreasing the efficiency of the detection path (see figure 2). This setup is optimal since it uses a small number of elements which guarantees a high detection efficiency and it uses each optical element as it should be used, e.g. a collimated beam passes the dichroic mirror, and a planar wavefront enters the intermediate lens.

Figure 4 The excitation beam enters from the right hand side. The pinhole is in the focal point of both lenses. The arrangement of the two lenses is that of a beam expander. A divergent beam is deflected on the surface of the dichroic mirror in the direction of the scan unit. The second lens is also used to focus the fluorescence emission into the pinhole in front of the photomultiplier. A convergent beam therefore passes the dichroic mirror. The fluorescent beam is therefore modified in two ways, it is shifted and the geometric length is reduced. This arrangement is therefore not able to correct either a shift of the beam or a tilt of the beam due to the dichroic mirror. It is also not possible to insert a beam splitter arrangement to make use of the reflected light. The arrangement is sparse and therefore efficient but the dichroic mirror is used with a convergent beam. This is not correct, since the transmission/reflection properties of the dichroic mirror depend on the angle of illumination, and so the spectral response will now be different for axial and non-axial rays.

Figure 5 The excitation beam enters the arrangement from the right hand side. The beam is deflected in the direction of the scan unit. The fluorescent light passes the dichroic mirror and enters a detector that is some distance away. The beam is shifted in the dichroic mirror. Any further shift of the beam is corrected in this arrangement. A tilt of the dichroic mirror is not correctable. The setup is obviously efficient as it uses the minimal number of optical elements and a collimated beam passes the dichroic mirror. The advantage of not having to use a lens is only partially true as one needs to achieve large distances (more than one meter) before the beam may enter the photomultiplier. This is done by placing three, four or more mirrors into the detection path. The large number of mirrors makes the device at least in principle more sensitive to mechanical vibrations. However, the distance between two con-

jugate image planes over the diameter of the detector is a constant to a first approximation and hence the performance of this arrangement should be equivalent to that described as class 1 (see Fig. 3). The lens in front of the pinhole will decrease the path length but it also decreases the effective area of the detector and hence makes the introduction of a pinhole necessary.

The use of a beam expander (as shown in Figs. 3 and 4 but not 5) is in principle debatable. The beam can, of course, be expanded elsewhere in the system. (e.g. in a scan lens such as the eye piece.) It is, however, complicated to spatially filter the beam in the detector path. The main problem is that the laser may not run in TEM_{00} mode (see Chapter 5). If that is the case the beam must be spatially filtered and then it may also be expanded in the same process. If the laser does run in TEM_{00} mode, the light need not be spatially filtered. In this case a spatial filter should not matter as all light would pass it. Filtering the light and making sure that a planar wavefront is produced is definitely wise. An argument in favor of a spatial filter is that it removes the effects of all the optical elements before the filter, such as bandpass filters, mirrors, etc.

Not shown in the figures are filters and special equipment for double fluorescence experiments. Although all these could be placed in front of the lens it is better to put them behind the detector pinhole and to use area detectors. It is therefore not necessary to include these parts in this discussion. (A practical problem may be a low efficiency in one of the channels. If two pinholes are used one can be larger to improve the signal while the other is still optimal.)

Evaluation of Scanner Arrangements

Figures 6 through 9 show four different arrangements of x/y scanners for confocal microscopes. This section will describe

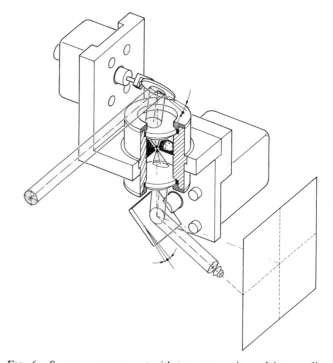

FIG. 6. Scanner arrangement with two scan units and intermediate imaging optics. Two mirrors are used to scan the beam along the x- and along the y-axis. The intermediate optics is arranged such that it forms an image of one mirror on the other mirror. If the last mirror is in a telecentric plane then both mirrors are in conjugate telecentric planes of the microscope.

and evaluate them. It should be noted that not all of the optical arrangements described in the paragraph above can be combined with all of the scanner arrangements.

Figure 6 This arrangement uses two mirrors and relay optics. The two mirrors move perpendicularly, so the combined movement produces a movement of the light spot in a plane. Since the relay optics form an image of the first mirror in the second mirror, both mirrors will be in conjugate telecentric planes of the microscope as long as the second mirror is in such a telecentric plane. This arrangement is optically perfect. The reason to avoid it is that the requirements for the relay optics are very strict. They must produce perfect images and this is done at the expense of efficiency. To have a well-corrected image across a large spectrum requires more optical elements than to have a well-corrected image across a small spectrum. A simple solution that is intrinsically achromatic, using two concave mirrors, has been realized by W.B. Amos (personal communication).

Figure 7 Two mirrors can also be used without any relay optics. The two mirrors move in perpendicular axes. The mirrors are placed as closely as possible and the telecentric plane is located in the midpoint between the two mirrors. This arrangement approximates perfect telecentricity the closer the two mirrors come together. The actual error depends on the magnification of the intermediate optical system but in a real case is in the order of 4 mm over 100 mm. The advantages are obviously the sparsity of the arrangement and its small size.

Figure 8 The arrangement described above can be improved by moving the axis of one mirror off the beam axis. This mirror then effectively shifts as it rotates. The combined movement improves the position of the mirror in the telecentric plane by a factor of 25 (personal communication, Kjell Carlsson, Carlsson & Liljeborg 1989). The combined movement also changes the path length as the y-scanner moves to the next line. This scanner arrangement may therefore not be used with the optical arrangement described as class 2 (see Fig. 6).

Figure 9 The simplest solution is to use a single mirror. A galvanometer is mounted on a scan unit. A galvanometer performs the fast movement and, by moving the galvonometer assembly, the orthogonal slow movement is achieved. One mirror is easily placed in a telecentric plane of the microscope and the efficiency is only limited by the reflection coefficient of the mirror (Stelzer et al. 1988).

Scanner arrangements can be evaluated in a number of terms. The main issue for a confocal fluorescence microscope is efficiency. Other requirements could be the speed with which an object is scanned, the precision with which an object may be scanned, the size of the scan unit, the long term stability/repeatability of the scan movement or the possibility to randomly access volume elements (voxels).

Disk Scanners

As pointed out above, the pinholes in a beam scanning device are located at the conjugate image planes of a conventional microscope. The pinholes can be placed at the first image plane directly. In the so-called tandem scanners (Petran et al. 1968) part of a rotating disk with holes in it is placed in the first image

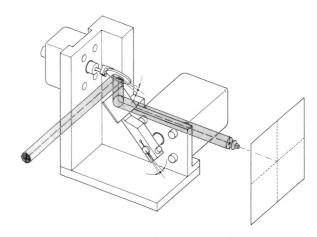

FIG. 8. Scanner arrangement with two scan units. Two mirrors are used to scan the beam along the x- and along the y-axes. While one mirror is turned around the center of its axis, the other has a pivot point that is off-axis. This latter movement compensates the missing intermediate imaging optics. The two mirrors are therefore in an approximate conjugate telecentric plane of the microscope.

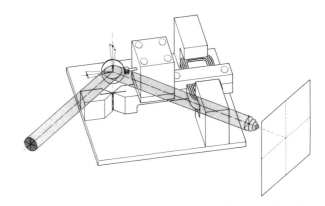

FIG. 9. Scanner arrangement with one scan unit. One mirror is used to scan the beam along the x- and along the y-axis. This mirror is easily placed in a conjugate telecentric plane of the microscope. This solution is easily accomplished by mounting a galvanometer on a scan unit whose center of rotation is in the center of the mirror.

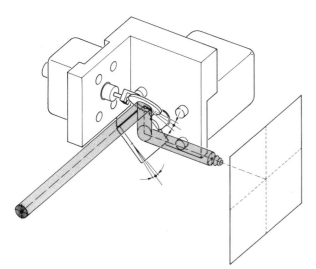

FIG. 7. Scanner arrangement with two scan units. Two mirrors are used to scan the beam along the x- and along the y-axes. The mirrors are placed as closely as possible. The geometric midpoint of the two mirrors is placed in a conjugate telecentric plane of the microscope. Both mirrors are therefore only approximately in a telecentric plane.

plane. The holes serve both as sources and as detector pinholes. They are arranged in such a way that the object is uniformly covered by the holes as soon as the disk rotates. The distances between the holes should guarantee no overlap in the detection and the illumination path. Since a hundred or more "beams" scan the object, images are generated much faster than with a single beam scanning device. As tandem scanners form a real image, a solid-state camera may be placed in the final image plane of the microscope to detect the data with a quantum efficiency probably 4–8 times better than that of a photomultiplier. The main problem is the low brilliance of a conventional light source. The pinhole array covers only 1.5–2.5% of the intemediate image plane and so only 1/60 to 1/40 of the excitation light passes the disk. The brilliance of the source can be easily increased by using higher powered lamps or by using a laser as the light source but heating problems eventually limit the effectiveness of this approach.

Another problem is the diameter of the pinholes. As these should match the specifications of the objective lens (e.g. 30 micron in diameter for a $63\times/1.4$), one disk can be used for only a few lenses. In a disk scanner that operates in the first image plane, the source and detector pinholes cannot be optimized independently. Finally, the diameter of the pinhole must be matched by a reasonable thickness of the pinhole which, at least in principle, is in conflict with the stability of the disk at high speeds. A more detailed description of disk scanners is found in Chapter 10.

Object Scanners

The first operating confocal microscopes where stage scanners (Minsky 1958; Brakenhoff et al. 1979; Marsman et al. 1983; Stelzer & Wijnaendts 1985). One source and one detector pinhole are placed in conjugate image planes. The optical arrangement is stationary and the object is scanned through a single beam that is located at the center of a lens. The only geometric distortion in the image is derived from the imperfectly controlled movement of the object. Object scanners therefore offer the best image for data processing purposes. The devices are very efficient because the optical requirements are simple. Disadvantages are the low scanning speed ($10 - 150$ lines/second) and the special preparation techniques that are necessary to achieve low moving masses. A real problem may be mechanical resonances. The force on the objects is usually very low (in comparison to gravity) but may still distort living specimens suspended in aqueous media.

Attachment to Microscopes

A conventional microscope offers several ports through which a confocal set up could be attached to it and through which the excitation beam can enter and the emission beam can leave the instrument. Commonly used are the video port, the ocular and the port for the photographic film camera. Having mentioned efficiency as one of the main issues in confocal fluorescence microscopy it should be obvious that one should use those ports in which the beams penetrate the smallest number of optical elements. Inverted microscopes traditionally (but not necessarily) have a long distance between the object and the ocular or video port and there are often many relaying lenses in the optical path. If for other reasons the inverted microscope

is the system of choice, these parts should not be used. Instead, the instrument should be modified to permit confocal operation using a separate path. For example, in the Nikon CF series or the new Zeiss series in which the objective lenses (plus a tube lens) are chromatically corrected, the attachment could be performed through the first image plane. The video port of the ZEISS AXIOPHOT gives direct access to this plane. A confocal setup may be interfaced to this plane and no optical elements decrease the efficiency. The advantage of scanning through video ports and eye pieces (an example of an f-theta lens) is that this solution requires no modification of the microscope.

Merit Functions

Functions that determine the performance of an instrument can be object-dependent and object-independent. One merit function is the product of all transmission and all reflection coefficients (see Tables 1 and 2) weighted with the emission and absorption spectra of the fluorophore. This function is object dependent. The sum over all surface errors and the sums over all tilts, thickness variations and deviations from planarity are object independent. Object dependent functions can be used to measure the performance of an instrument and to compare the data with that generated at later times or by other instruments.

TABLE 1. TYPICAL INTENSITY LOSSES IN AN ILLUMINATION PATH SIMILAR TO THAT SHOWN IN FIGURE 2.
Light losses in the microscope are not covered in the table since they cannot be influenced by the designer

Element	Per Unit	Cumulative
Laser head exit	0%	100%
Bandpass interference filter	10–30%	70%
SMPP optical glass fiber	50%	35%
Expander lens	0.5%	35%
Deflector	0.2%	35%
Polarizing beam splitter	2%	34%
Quarter wave plate	0.5%	34%
Dichroic mirror	2–10%	31%
Scan mirror #1	2%	30%
Scan mirror #2	2%	29%
Final entering microscope		29%

"Per unit" refers to the loss in intensity due to that element, and **"Cumulative"** is a pessimistic estimate of the intensity that will reach that element.

TABLE 2. TYPICAL INTENSITY LOSSES IN A DETECTION PATH SIMILAR TO THAT SHOWN IN FIGURE 2.
The table does not cover the quantum efficiency of the detector (90–95% loss with a photomultiplier tube) and the efficiency of the electronics

Element	Per unit	Cumulative
Exit microscope	0%	100%
Scan mirror #1	2%	98%
Scan mirror #2	2%	96%
Dichroic mirror	5–30%	67%
Dichroic mirror	0.5–25%	50%
Filter	0.5–80%	25%
Achromatic lens	0.5%	25%
MM optical glass fiber	70%	22%
Final entering PMT		22–75%

"Per unit" refers to the loss in intensity due to that element, and **"Cumulative"** is a pessimistic estimate of the intensity that will reach that element.

This is not so easy with the other four merit functions; however these can be used in the design phase of an instrument to decide which development path should be followed.

The sum over all surface errors can include all elements beyond the source pinhole. This function determines how much the beam will deviate from a perfect planar wavefront and hence how well the beam may be focused and how much the objective lens must be over-illuminated. A wavefront error of a quarter lambda reduces the midpoint of the spatial frequency range by almost 50% (MG4 2–6).

REQUIREMENTS FOR MULTI-FLUORESCENCE EXPERIMENTS

Multi-fluorescence experiments are those in which specimens are observed that have more than one labeled target. Such experiments can be performed by observing each target separately or by observing two or more targets at the same time. In the first case, special filter combinations would be selected for each excitation line and each emission band. In the second case, one excitation line would cause the emission in two or more bands that must be separated in the detection path.

The main problem in the first case is obviously to move several filter sets without changing the illumination **or** the detection path. Any change would result in non-overlapping pixels. What can be tolerated depends on the resolution of the objective lens used. As pointed out above, the images of the source and the detector pinhole must overlap in the object plane. This requires that the dichroic mirrors each occupy the same orientation and position. Observing each fluorophore separately on the other hand provides the necessary degrees of freedom needed to make optimal choices of the filter sets which excite only one dye and do not affect the other.

Separating two emission bands for simultaneous measurement after excitation with a single line is possible only with a relatively low efficiency since the bandpass of the two filter sets being used will cut off a lot of each others' spectrum. Also, if a single excitation wavelength is used, one of the dyes will always be excited more efficiently than the other. The advantage, however, is that the two pixels are definitely in register because a single spot of incident light spot is the source of both detected signals. If the color separation filters are placed behind the pinhole, this setup is also unaffected by changes of filter sets.

A problem that cannot be delt with so easily is the crosstalk between channels. Possible sources are spectral (because of the limited performance of the filters) and electronic (due to the low bandwidth of the amplifiers which may be used to sample the two wavelengths on alternating pixels).

SPECIAL OPTICAL ELEMENTS

Multi-mode optical glass fibers

Instead of placing the detector photomultiplier directly behind the pinhole, the light may also be fed into a multi-mode optical glass fiber. These fibers have diameters of 200–1000 micron and, in the visible range, transmission factors in the order of 99.9% per meter. If the output is index-matched to the entrance window of the detector, the only important loss occurs in the fiber entry (0.3–4%). A good reason for using MM glass fibers is a reduction in weight or size and the simplified packaging of the microscope. Another important reason is the cool-

ing of the detector, which is not so easy in an environment with an uncontrollable humidity, but relatively simple if the detector is in a separate box some distance away. Cooling of detectors reduces PMT dark current but is even more important when using solid state detectors.

Single-Mode Polarization-preserving Glass Fibers

A development that has become available as a product only recently is the single-mode glass fiber which can be used in the illumination path (e.g. Schott, York, PI). These fibers must, however, preserve both the mode of the laser output (TEM$_{00}$) and the polarization of the light. With a core diameter of 4–5 micron, an SMPP fiber easily replaces the detector pinhole as the spatial filter. The main problem is its relatively high loss of 50–60% and of course its sensitivity to vibrations (mechanical noise). The main advantage stems from the fact that, in contrast to a pinhole, the entrance and the exit are physically displaced. The exit is unaffected if the entrance follows the beam and vice versa. In practice this feature adds (depending on the setup) three or four degrees of freedom. Fiber launchers that are tiltable under piezocontrol are interfaceable to a computer. Changing the location of the entrance pinhole allows one to follow the beam if the line selecting bandpass filter is changed or it can be used to regulate the power of the excitation beam. The variation of the position of the exit pinhole can be used in multi fluorescence experiments to correct errors due to filter changes in the detector part (see also Figure 10).

Polarizing Elements

The combination of a polarizing beam splitter and a lambda/4 plate is very useful. How to use it is described in Fig. 2. The

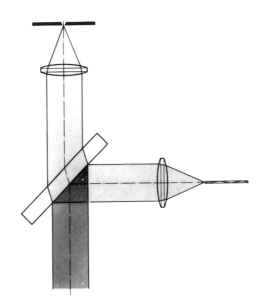

FIG. 10. An optical arrangement of class 1 using an SMPP optical glass fiber. The fiber tip is in the focal point of a lens. Upon exiting the glass fiber the laser beam is collimated. Complete plugs for laser light delivery systems consist of the tip and a short-focus achromatic lens. The fiber plug is tilted around the center of this lens. In this arrangement the lens is replaced by one with a larger focal length. This lens is fixed in space. Tilting the fiber plug will now shift **and** turn the fiber tip. Therefore the angle under which the beam leaves the lens is changed.

horizontally polarized beam passing the beam splitter is completely unaffected but then circularly polarized by the quarter wave plate. The light reflected or backscattered in the sample is deflected on the dichroic mirror, turned another 45 degrees in the quarter wave plate and, now vertically polarized, is deflected by the polarizing beam splitter. This beam can be used to generate reflection contrast. It should not be forgotten that the signal derived from the specimen is probably backscattered and not reflected. From a physical point of view backscattered and reflected light have different properties. This signal will only be available if in the process of contrast generation the light preserves its polarization. The arrangement does not affect the efficiency of the detection path and there are good reasons to believe that a circularly polarized beam is better focused by standard objective lenses than a linearly polarized beam (Van der Voort et al., 1988, and Chapter 8).

Mechanical Scanners

Scanners **wobble** above and below a line and they **jitter** along it. The wobble tells how well a scanner remains on the line and the jitter how well the scanner remains on the pixel of that line. In a scanning microscope these galvanometer specifications can determine the actual resolution limit of the microscope. Let us assume an optical scan angle of $\pm 3°$ i.e. a complete mechanical scan of $6°$ (100 mrad). The number of pixels per line is 2500. This means the jitter (and the wobble) must be lower than *(105 mrad/2500=) 40 micro rad*. This is about 1–2 times smaller than e.g. the specification of the General Scanning GF120DCT which is *50–100 micro rad*. Our experience is that specifications of scanners are conservative, that their actual performance is better and therefore the scanners are sufficient for microscopical purposes. The actual test is to use them at very low scan angles, which are e.g. encountered with high N.A., low magnification lenses. The minimal angle with our system is $\sim 20\mu$ rad/line.

Another problem is the mirrors of the scan units. Due to the low reflection coefficients of the standard components, they are custom made for fluorescence microscopical applications. These mirrors require conflicting specifications as they should be small, light-weight, mechanically stable, flat to fractions of a wavelength and the reflecting surface should be centered on the axis of rotation of the scan unit. The compromise depends to a large degree on the application of the confocal fluorescence microscope and the arrangement of the scan unit.

Our emphasis has always been efficiency and the instruments are tuned to perform best with high N.A., high magnification lenses. This does not require a large beam diameter. This case is similar to low N.A., low magnification but different from high N.A. and low magnification which requires a large beam diameter to fill the entrance aperture and large scan mirrors.

Acousto-optical Scanners

Acousto-optical deflectors (AOD) have the advantage of being much faster than mechanical scanners (16 kHz and more in contrast to about 400 Hz for galvanometer scanners). They do not have any moving parts to wear out but simply replacing the faster of the two scanners in one of the arrangements described above is not possible. The dispersion of the refracting material requires a chromatic correction that is available only at the expense of additional elements in the detection path. A completely modified arrangement is imaginable in confocal fluorescence microscopy. The incident beam is first deflected in the AOD and then by the slower galvanometer scanner. The dichroic mirror is placed **between** the two scanners. In the appropriate optical arrangement both scanners are in conjugate telecentric planes. The fluorescence emission is deflected by the slower scanner and again deflected in the direction of the detector by the dichroic mirror, so it never reaches the AOD. A lens focuses the beam into a slit in front of the detector. A slit must be used because the movement along one axis is not compensated. This solution is not "completely confocal" (it is confocal along one axis), but it seems to work sufficiently well (personal communication Draaijer; Draaijer et al. 1987; see also Chapters 11, 19).

In comparison to mechanical scanners AODs have a small deflection angle of 2.7–3.5 degrees (about 12 degrees are needed), a limited resolution (750–1000 lines), a non-circular aperture (up to 3 mm by 40 mm) and a low diffraction efficiency (50–70%). These parameters depend on each other. A higher resolution can be achieved, but at the expense of a spatial variation of the diffraction efficiency (10% at 2000 lines). Finally, an AOD must be adjusted for every excitation wavelength (a general reference is Gottlieb et al.). An interesting alternative is an instrument devised by Goldstein (1989).

CONCLUSIONS

The most important issue in confocal fluorescence microscopy is photon efficiency which determines the rate at which photo damage occurs and the speed at which an image may be recorded. As long as the arrangement maintains the necessary diffraction limit, the general rule is the more sparse an optical path is the more efficient will it be. The scan system must be chosen in accordance with the photon efficiency. Since a number of different scanning microscopes have been realized, each of them employing different optical and scan arrangements, time should show which are the most efficient and the most versatile to use. My personal preferences are the optical arrangement shown in Figure 3 and the scanner arrangments shown in Figures 7 and 8.

Sparsity, relative simplicity and a good illumination efficiency are advantages of single beam scanners over disk scanners. It is also not true to say that the technology is yet technique is stable: the large number of companies and the short product lifetimes indicate that much can still be done. The disadvantage of single beam scanners is that they must use relatively inefficient detectors to achieve high recording speeds and saturation

TABLE 3.   SCAN RESOLUTION REQUIRED FOR DIFFERENT MICROSCOPE OBJECTIVE LENSES

Microscope Objective				Image Plane		Scanner
N.A.	Magn.	Res.	Res.	Lp/MM	Lp/image	microrad/line
1.32	100	0.208	20.8	48	960	115
1.4	63	0.196	12.4	81	1616	68
1.4	40	0.196	7.9	127	2545	43

(Microscope Objective: **N.A.** is the numerical aperture, **Magn.** is the magnification, **Res.** is the resolution in the object plane in micrometer. Image Plane: **Res.** is the resolution in the image plane in micrometer, **Lp/mm** is the number of line pairs per mm, **Lp/image** is the number of line pairs per image. Scanner: **microrad/line** is the change of the optical deflection required per line in the image.)

effects (see Chapter 16) in the fluorophore are also important but these cannot be dealt with by the designer of confocal microscopes. They depend on the dye, the biological application and the achievements that can be made in future biochemical developments.

Ceterum censeo that conventional fluorescence microscopes are excellent devices. Biologists who feel that they do not get the improvement they expect from confocal fluorescence microscopy should take a very good look at a conventional device and consider the acquisition of a CCD camera (Hiraoka et al. 1987 and Chapter 17). Conventional fluorescence microscopes also have excellent out-of-focus discrimination that is sufficient for many problems. Using a CCD camera, a powerful (and nowadays cheap) computer and appropiate software to discriminate against unwanted flare light will in many cases be a simpler and perhaps equally efficient solution to many biologically relevant problems (Agard & Sedat 1983; Fay et al. 1989 and Chapter 17).

ACKNOWLEDGEMENTS

I thank Brad Amos, Kjell Carlsson, P.C. Chen, Arie Draaijer, Reinhard Jörgens and Sture Wahlsten for interesting information and comments on the manuscript. Pekka Hänninen, René Müller, Clemens Storz and Jim Pawley where so kind to critically review the manuscript.

REFERENCES

Agard, D., and J. Sedat (1983), Nature **302**, 676–681.
Bacallao, R., and E.H.K. Stelzer (1989), "Methods in Cell Biology" **31**, Academic Press, San Diego, 437–452.
Brakenhoff, G.J., P. Blom, and P. Barends (1979), J. Microsc. 117, **219-232.**
Carlsson, K., and A. Liljeborg (1989), J. Microsc. **153**, 171–180.
Draaijer, A., and P.M. Houpt (1988), Scanning 10, **139-145.**
Fay, F.S., W. Carrington, and K.E. Fogarty, J. Microsc. **153**, 133–149.
Goodman, J.W. (1968), "Introduction to Fourier Optics", McGraw-Hill, San Francisco.
Goldstein, S. (1989), J. Microsc. **153**, Rp1-Rp2.
Hiraoka, Y., J.W. Sedat, and D.A. Agard (1987), Science **238**, 36–41.
Marsman, H.J.B., R. Stricker, R.W. Wijnaendts-van-Resandt, G.J. Brakenhoff, and P. Blom (1983), Rev. Sci. Instrum. **54**, 1047–1052.
Minsky M. (1957), U.S. Patent #3013467, Microscopy Apparatus.
Minsky M. (1988), Memoir on inventing the confocal scanning microscope. Scanning 10, **128-138.**
MG4 is the Melles Griot Optics Guide 4 (1988). The catalogue from Melles Griot is very informative and contains numerous excellent comments on optical elements and performance characteristics.
Schröder, G. "Naumann/Schröder: Bauelemente der Optik — Taschenbuch der technischen Optik", Carl Hanser, München Wien, 1987.
Petran, M., M. Hadravsky, M.D. Egger, R. Galambos (1968), J. Opt. Soc. Am. **58**, 661–664.
Stelzer, E.H.K., and R.W. Wijnaendts-van-Resandt (1985), SPIE **602**, 63–70.
Stelzer, E.H.K., R. Stricker, R. Pick, C. Storz, and P. Hänninen (1989), SPIE **1028**, 146–151.
Wilke, V. (1985), Scanning **7**, 88–96.
Van der Voort, H.T.M., and G.J. Brakenhoff (1989), SPIE **1028**, 39–44.
Wilson, T., and A.R. Carlini (1987), Optik **72**, 109–114.

Chapter 10

Intermediate Optics in Nipkow Disk Microscopes

G. S. Kino

Edward L. Ginzton Laboratory, Stanford University , Stanford CA 94305–4085

THE TANDEM SCANNING REFLECTED LIGHT MICROSCOPE (TSRLM)

The confocal laser scanning scanning optical microscope (LSCM) has the major advantages that it yields a very short depth-of-focus, its transverse definition and the contrast of the image are better than with a standard microscope, the device is very well-suited for optical cross-sectioning, and with the use of a laser beam, the intensity of illumination can be very high. At the same time, it is possible to choose the wavelength of the illumination very easily [Wilson et al, 1984].

The major disadvantages of the LSCM are associated with the mechanical scan required. This limits the frame time of the image to a few seconds. In all cases, the image is formed too slowly to be directly observable by eye. Thus, image processing in a computer is needed and the simplicity of the standard microscope is lost. Over twenty years ago, Petran and Hadravsky demonstrated the Tandem Scanning Reflected Light Microscope (TSRLM), an alternative method to obtain a real-time image with some of the advantages of the confocal scanning microscope [Petran et al, 1968, Petran et al, 1985]. The basic idea was to use, instead of a single pinhole, a large number of pinholes. The pinholes are separated by a distance large enough so that there is no interaction between the images on the object formed by the individual pinholes. The complete image is formed by moving the pinholes so as to fill in the space in between them.

In the original system, the pinholes were drilled in a thin sheet of copper and laid down along a path consisting of a multiple set of interleaved Archimedean spirals. Several hundred pinholes are illuminated at one time [Petran et al, 1968, Petran et al, 1985]. Since only about one percent of the area of the disk is transparent, a relatively intense light source is required; typically a mercury arc lamp is used for the source. In their second (improved) system, shown in Fig. 1, the light passes through the disk to the objective lens of the microscope located a tube length away from the disk. Thus, a diffraction-limited image of each pinhole is formed on the object. A major problem is to prevent the reflected light from the disk from reaching the eyepiece where it would cause enough glare to obscure the image of the object. Therefore, in the TSRLM, the light reflected from the object is passed back through the objective lens, a beam-splitter, and a set of mirrors to a conjugate set of pinholes on the opposite side of the disk which is then viewed using a Ramsden eyepiece.

In the TSRLM each pinhole is of the order of 30–80 μm diameter, spaced approximately ten pinhole radii apart. In the original system, the disk was spun at a few hundred rpm to obtain a real-time scanned image. As with any confocal microscope, only the light from the region near the focal plane passes back through the pinholes; in addition, a very small proportion of the defocused reflected light passes back through nearby pinholes.

The advantages of real-time imaging and the good cross-sectioning ability of the microscope are apparent to anyone seeing it for the first time. The disadvantages are a poor light budget and the considerable difficulty in alignment due to its mechanical complexity. Several mirrors must be carefully positioned in the x and y directions and two tilt angles adjusted so that the reflected light is imaged onto the correct pinholes. Recently, a commercial version of this microscope has been developed in which the optical system has been somewhat simplified, and the disk is made of silicon with square holes etched in it with an anisotropic etch. Relatively large pinholes of 40–70 μm diam are used so that the alignment is not too critical. For the same reason, the depth-of-focus is somewhat worse than it would be with an equivalent LSCM with optimal pinhole size unless very high magnification (200×–300×) objectives are used.

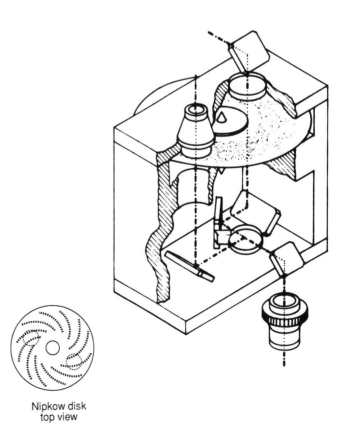

Nipkow disk
top view

FIG. 1.   The tandem scanning reflected light microscope.

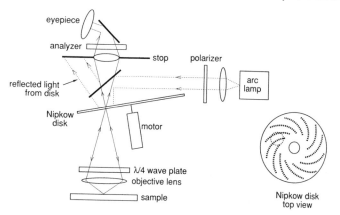

FIG. 2. The real time scanning optical microscope.

THE REAL-TIME SCANNING OPTICAL MICROSCOPE (RSOM)

It was apparent that the improvement needed in the TSRLM is to be able to detect the light through the same pinhole from which a given area of the specimen was illuminated. In this case, alignment would not be a problem and a large number of optical components could be eliminated. The problem is to eliminate the light reflected from the disk. This has been done in the Real Time Scanning Optical Microscope (RSOM), illustrated in Fig. 2, by adopting the following principles [Xiao & Kino, 1987, Xiao et al, 1988]:

- The disk is made by photolithographic techniques and consists of specularly reflecting black chrome, with a reflectivity of a few percent, laid down on a glass disk. The highly polished chrome yields a well directed reflected beam, which is easier to eliminate with a light trap than a diffusely scattered beam.
- The disk is tilted and a trap is placed at the position where the light reflected from the disk is focused, thus further differentiating against the reflected light.
- To eliminate the remaining reflected light, the input light is polarized by a polarizer and the light that is received at the eyepiece is observed through an analyzer, with its plane of polarization rotated at right angles to that of the input light. A quarter-wave plate is placed in front of the objective lens so that light which has passed through the objective to the sample and back will have its plane of polarization rotated by 90 degrees and thus can be observed with the eyepiece.

A typical system uses a disk with 200,000 pinholes, 20–25 micrometers in diameter, rotated at approximately 2000 rpm. Provided the light intensity is sufficiently high, this produces a 700 frames/sec 5000-line image of high quality. The depth of focus of this image is comparable to the best mechanically-scanned LSCM as is its transverse resolution. There are, however, some more subtle differences in the performance of the two types of microscopes because the real-time system uses relatively broadband light.

A Köhler illumination system is used, so that if the disk were not present, a point source would be focused to a point at the back focal plane of the objective lens; in practice, a mercury vapor short arc source is imaged on the back focal plane of the objective [Born & Wolf, 1975]. With the disk present,

this implies that the central axes of the diffracted beams passing through individual pinholes all pass through the center of the back focal plane of the objective lens. Thus, the illumination, and hence the definition of the system are made as uniform as possible over the field of view.

IMAGES OF THE EYE

As an example of the high quality images obtainable, images of the lens and cornea of a rabbit eye obtained with the RSOM are shown in Fig. 3. These images were video recorded with an MTI SIT video camera connected to an IBM AT computer with a Data Translation frame grabber board, averaged 5 times and processed to remove some glare from internal reflections in the microscope (a simple subtraction of a constant value of signal), then photographed from the video monitor. All of these pictures were taken with a 50 × 1.00 N.A. Leitz water immersion objective with a tube length of 160 mm. A later version of this microscope, (which is now in operation), should be capable of obtaining direct, real-time images, easily observable by eye, of at least the quality of the ones shown here.

The images in Fig. 3a show the detail of the outer epithelial surface. The bright spots are dead cells sloughing off from the surface. Figure 3b shows the intact surface epithelial cells. Moving the focus a few microns further into the cornea shows the convoluted basement membrane (Fig. 3c). As the focus was moved into the cornea, we saw a cluster of cells inside the stroma, and a nerve can be clearly seen (Fig. 3d). Upon focusing further inside the sample, the surface of the endothelium can be seen (Fig. 3e) about 400 μm below the tear film. Figure 3f shows the fibrous structure of the lens of the rabbit eye.

It can be seen from these results that images of excellent quality can be obtained with the RSOM. The microscope can be used to create a series of thin optical sections from these 5 μm thick endothelial cells from the level of the microvilli on their posterior surface down to their anterior surface adjacent to Decemet's membrane.

PINHOLE SIZE

Two important criteria in the design of the real-time scanning optical microscope are the choice of the optimum size and spacing of the pinholes in the disk. If the pinholes are too small, there is a serious loss in light intensity; if they are too large the range and transverse definitions suffer. With too large a pinhole size, the light entering the pinholes is diffracted into a relatively narrow beam which may not fill the pupil of the objective lens, and hence causes it to behave like a lens with a smaller aperture. Similarly, the beam returning from a point reflector through the objective does not fill the pinhole. Thus, the transverse and range definitions are not as good as for a pinhole of infinitesimal size.

It follows from the Rayleigh-Sommerfeld scalar diffraction theory, using the Fraunhofer approximation, that at a distance h_1 (the tube length of the objective) from a circular pinhole, the field y_1 at the pupil plane of the objective at radius r_1 from the axis varies as [Goodman, 1968, Kino, 1987, Kino & Xiao, to be published]:

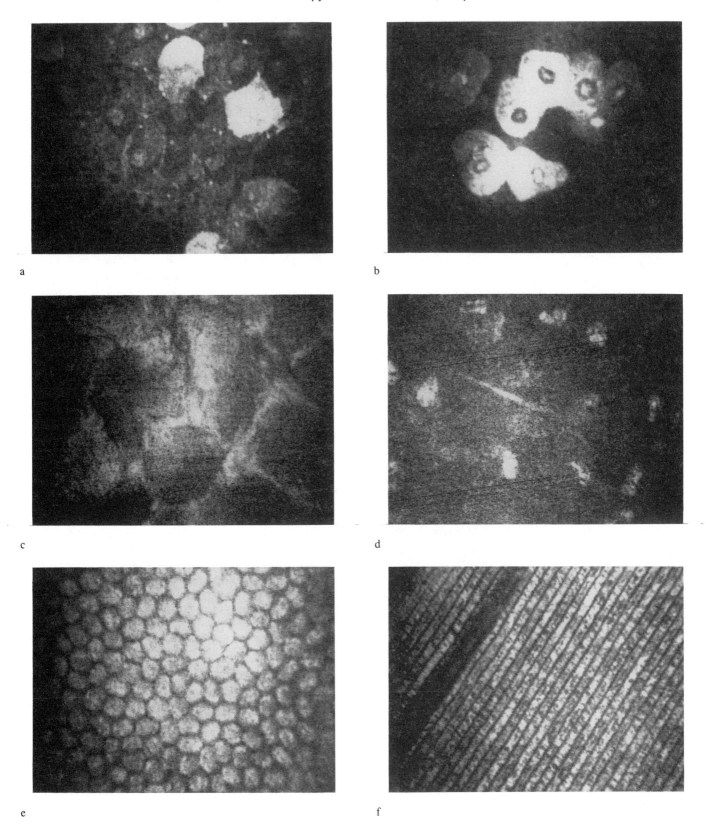

FIG. 3. (a, b, c and d) Images of the cornea. a. Exfoliating (bright cells) and the intact surface of the epithelial cells (darker cells). The cells are about 20–30 μm in diameter, about 4 μm thick at the nucleus and about 2 μm thick at the periphery. b. An image of the intact surface epithelial cells with the focal plane at the center of the nucleus. c. An image of the convoluted basement membrane (basal lamina) between the basal epithelial cells and the stroma. The bright areas of the image are centered in the focal plane and the darker areas are slightly below the focal plane. d. An image of the anterior region of the stroma showing a submicron diameter nerve fiber and sections through the cell processes of several stromal keratocytes. e. An image of the corneal endothelial cells about 400 μm below the tear film. f. This image of the rabbit ocular lens made on a freshly excised ocular lens. The separation between adjacent fibers is about 2 microns and the submicron transverse bands are readily observed. The dark object on the lower right side (see arrow) is the nucleus. /The image is from the bow zone of the lens, about 200 microns below its surface.

$$\psi_1 = A\psi_0 \frac{J_1(kr_1/h_1)}{kr_1/h_1} \tag{1}$$

where ψ_0 is the field at the pinhole, $k = 2\pi/\lambda$, A is a constant, and λ is the optical wavelength in free space.

Using this formula, we may make a rough estimate of the optimum pinhole radius a(opt) by choosing the radius at the half power points of the beam diffracted by the pinhole to be equal to the pupil radius b of the objective. This leads to the result:

$$a(opt) = \frac{0.25\lambda h_1}{b} \tag{2}$$

where h_1 is the spacing between the pinhole and the objective (the tube length). For a tube length $h_1 = 160mm$, $\lambda = 540nm$, and $b = 2$ mm; this leads to a pinhole radius a(opt) = $10.8\mu m$. More exact results will be given in graphical form below. It is apparent from Eq. (1) that if the pinholes are made too large, the fields at the pupil plane will be highly nonuniform and may even reverse in sign across the pinhole. This condition gives rise to a highly undesirable, nonuniform focused spot at the object.

When the size of the pinhole is infinitesimal, the normalized intensity of the signal reflected from a perfect mirror a distance z from the focal plane is given by the approximate formula:

$$I(z) = \left[\frac{\sin k_2 z(1-\cos\Theta_0)}{k_2 z(1-\cos\Theta_0)}\right]^2 \tag{3}$$

where $k_2 = nk$, n is the refractive index of the medium, and the numerical aperture of the objective is N.A. $= n\sin\Theta_0$.

We may derive from Eq.(3) a very useful formula for the spacing d_z of the half power points of the response:

$$d_z = \frac{.45\lambda}{n(1-\cos\Theta_0)} \tag{4}$$

The definition of resolution depends to a large extent on what type of object is imaged and what criteria are important to the observer. For integrated circuits, we are often interested in measuring profiles of stepped surfaces. For biological applications of confocal microscopy, we are often more interested in distinguishing two neighboring point reflectors. When a confocal microscope images a point reflector, the intensity I(z) of the optical signal at the detector varies with distance z from the focus as follows:

$$I(z) = \left\{\frac{\sin\left[\frac{k_2 z(1-\cos\Theta_0)}{2}\right]}{\frac{k_2(1-\cos\Theta_0)}{2}}\right\}^4 \tag{5}$$

It should be noted that this formula is different from that for the reflection from a plane mirror and gives a range resolution approximately 1.4 times greater than that given by Eq. (4) for the reflection from a plane mirror. Fortunately, the intensity of the signal due to small scatterers far from the focus falls off far more rapidly with distance than does the reflection from a plane mirror. Consequently, a large number of small scatterers some distance from the focus give very little glare.

The magnitude of the normalized intensity I(z), given by Eq. (3) for a 0.95 aperture, has been compared with a nonparaxial scalar theory. It is found that even with a 0.95 aperture, the difference between the two results for the resolution d_z is small.

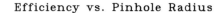

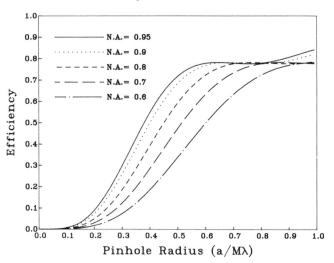

FIG. 4. Plots of the efficiency η as a function of $a\lambda/M$ for different numerical apertures.

For an infinitesimal pinhole size, $\lambda = 546$ nm and a numerical aperture of 0.95, the depth resolution given by Eq. (4) is $d_z = 353nm$, while a more exact calculation yields $d_z = 375nm$; thus, there is a 6% error in the use of Eq. (4) which reduces to a 2% error for NA = 0.9. It follows that the analytic form of Eq. (4) is a very convenient one. A similar calculation from Eq. (5) for the range resolution of a point scatterer predicts a resolution of $d_z = 498nm$. With a liquid immersion lens and a larger aperture, the resolution would be correspondingly smaller.

Exact calculations from a nonparaxial scalar theory have been made for the range resolution, d_z, the transverse resolution, and the power efficiency for a disk with finite pinholes of radius, a, and an objective lens of magnification M. Ideally, if several different lenses are to be used in a turret mount, the pinhole size has to be changed for each lens, unless the magnification and N.A. are kept constant. However, if the optimum pinhole size is chosen for the highest magnification lens, which is usually the lens with the highest numerical aperture, then the pinhole diameter will be larger than optimum for the lower N.A. lenses, where the loss in resolution may not be so critical.

The pinhole efficiency η is defined by the relation:

$$\eta = \frac{P}{P_0} \tag{6}$$

where P is the power reflected back through a pinhole from a perfect mirror at z = 0 and P_0 is the power transmitted through an individual pinhole from the source. The total efficiency of the system, as discussed below, also depends on the total area of the pinholes relative to the area of the beam incident on the disk.

Plots of the efficiency η with respect to the parameter $a/\lambda M$ are given for different numerical apertures in Fig. 4 (the result for a refractive index n can be found by multiplying the abscissa by n). For a typical RSOM with n = 1, M = 65×, $\lambda = 546nm$, $\sin\Theta_0 = 0.9$, and a = $10\mu m$, $na/\lambda M = 0.28$. The reflected power passing back through the pinhole is 22% of the incident power on the pinhole. Plots of the calculated depth resolution d_z as a function of $a/\lambda M$ for different numerical apertures are given in Fig. 5. It will be observed that, as might be expected, the res-

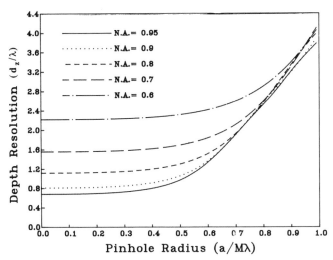

FIG. 5. Plots of the normalized depth resolution d_z/λ as a function of $a\lambda/M$ for different numerical apertures.

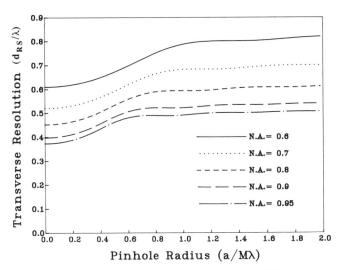

FIG. 6. Plots of the normalized transverse resolution dRS/λ as a function of $a\lambda/M$ for different numerical apertures.

olution becomes worse as the pinhole size is increased. It will be noted that the case treated by Wilson et al for the confocal microscope is that for a collimated beam illuminating the objective, which is equivalent to a transmitting pinhole of infinitesimal size, but a receiving pinhole of finite size [Wilson & Carlini, 1987]. Thus, their results are different from ours; pinhole size is far more critical in the RSOM since the diameters of both the transmitting and receiving pinholes vary together.

The transverse response of an RSOM or TSRLM is more difficult to calculate than that of an LSCM, since we need to determine the image seen by a stationary observer through a rotating set of pinholes. We therefore need to define a time-averaged point spread function. We have assumed that an observer looks at one point in space and determines the signal arriving at that point as the point reflecting object is moved a distance r from the axis. The point object is illuminated by a set of moving pinholes, and the image is observed through this same set of rotating pinholes. First, the variation of the illumination of the point object as the position of the illuminating hole is changed is found as the position of the illuminating hole is changed, and then the average signal received at a point of observation on the axis of the objective lens at the plane of the pinholes is determined. This is the time-averaged pointspread function.

A plot of the resolution between half power points d_{RS} as a function of the parameter $a/\lambda M$ for different numerical apertures is given in Fig. 6. It will be observed that the resolution is degraded by a factor of approximately 1.4 as the pinhole size is increased from infinitesimal to very large values. When the pinhole size is large, the system becomes a standard microscope. When it is infinitesimal, the point spread response becomes that of a perfect confocal microscope.

PINHOLE SPACING

As the spacing between the pinholes is decreased, the area of the pinholes approaches the total area illuminated. In this case, the intensity of the image no longer falls off rapidly with

the defocus distance z, and part of the defocused light reflected from the object can return through alternative pinholes to the eyepiece. If the proportion of incident light transmitted through the pinholes is α, then the beam is highly defocused, the reflected beam power still passes through the pinholes and cannot be eliminated in either the TSRLM or LSCM. It should be noted that if there are reflections from the lenses themselves, even good AR coated lenses, or from the surface of a biological sample or the coverslip, it is important to keep the parameter α low so that weakly reflecting internal features in a transparent material will not be obscured by glare. For this reason alone it is advisable to keep the area of the pinholes within the illuminating beam to be less than a few percent of the total area illuminated by the source, although compromises are sometimes made to obtain stronger illumination.

A second problem is that if the pinholes are too closely spaced, there is interference between their images on the object, and speckle effects will be apparent when a narrowband light source is employed. Consider, as an example, the speckle effects when the beam passing through the disk is reflected from a mirror at the focal plane. The main contribution to the signal passing back through a pinhole is from the beam transmitted through it and reflected back to it, but there are other contributions from the sidelobes of the beams transmitted through the neighboring pinholes and reflected back to the central pinhole. Normally, if the pinholes are more than three to five radii apart, the interference effects only show up with narrowband laser illumination. The use of a diffuser or phase-randomizer placed in front of the laser source could help in this regard (See Chapters 2 and 6). With a mercury arc source, the bandwidth of the illumination is usually adequate to eliminate this effect. However, another closely related form of interference has been observed from an object with two reflecting points at the same spacing as the image of the pinholes on the object. In this case the two points can give rise to signals from the corresponding pinholes in the form of fringe patterns; the phenomenon is a kind of Moiré effect.

ILLUMINATION EFFICIENCY AND REFLECTION FROM THE DISK

We have shown that one source of loss in the TSRLM or LSCM is due to loss of light at the pinhole itself. This contributes a factor η. There is also a major source of loss due to the filling factor α defined as the fraction of pinhole area to total illuminated area. Thus, the illumination efficiency of the TSRLM or RSOM, due to these effects alone, is decreased by a factor $\alpha\eta$. The beamsplitter provides an additional source of light loss (a factor of 0.25); this factor is the same as would be expected in a standard reflecting microscope, but can be eliminated by the use of polarizing beamsplitters, or in the case of a fluorescence microscope, a dichroic beamsplitter. In the RSOM, the polarizer provides one more source of loss (a factor of 0.5). Thus, both microscopes have an illumination efficiency typically less than 1%, which is the reason for using an arc source rather than the filament lamp used in a standard microscope. Since the pinhole size employed in the TSRLM is typically 40–80 μm, the factor η is approximately 0.8, and the picture is approximately three times brighter than for an RSOM with 20μm pinholes and the same value of the parameter α. In this case, the transverse resolution is close to that of a standard microscope, while the range resolution will be somewhat worse than for the RSOM.

A comparison of these microscopes with the LSCM shows once again that the basic problem with the TSRLM and with the RSOM is a lack of light. With a 75 watt arc source we could expect, at best, about 40 mw to illuminate the disk, of which a proportion $\alpha\beta\eta$ is utilized, where β is the loss due to the beamsplitter and polarizer. Thus, if P_{ill} is the light power that could reach the disk directly, the power reaching the detector from a perfect reflector would be $P_{det} = \alpha\beta\eta\,P_{ill}$. If we imagine that the detector is a TV camera with 250,000 elements, and the integration time is 1/30sec, the energy reaching one pixel of detector in this time is:

$$W_{det} = 1.3 \times 10^{-7}\alpha\beta\eta\,P_{ill}$$

For an LSCM, the maximum power P_{las} that can be used on one small spot on the order of 0.3μm in diameter is on the order of $P_{las} = 0.5$mw. If it takes 10sec to scan one frame, and there are 250,000 pixels on the screen, the scan time for one spot is 10/250,000sec or 40μsec. The energy reaching one element of the detector through a beamsplitter (0.5 reduction) is therefore:

$$W_{LSCM} = 20 \times 10^{-6}\,P_{las}$$

As examples, we take $P_{ill} = 40$ mw, $\eta = 0.03$, $\beta = 0.5$, $\alpha = 1$, and hence $W_{det} = 7.7 \times 10^{-11}$ Joules or about 2.7×10^{8} photons, and $P_{las} = 0.5$mw with $W_{LSCM} = 1 \times 10^{-8}$ Joules. Thus, there is far more energy available in the LSCM than in the TSRLM, let alone the RSOM, which will be somewhoat more inefficient if it is used with its optimum definition. The use of a 1 watt laser as an illuminating source with a rotating diffuser could possibly eliminate this disparity. Nevertheless, with well-designed beamsplitters and condensers, and sensitive cameras, there should be enough light available for direct observation with a TSRLM or RSOM of weakly reflecting biological materials, as has proven to be the case.

Fluorescence imaging is more difficult than direct imaging, both for the laser-illuminated CSOM and the Nipkow disk mi-croscopes, because of the low light level. One problem with the Nipkow disk microscopes is chromatic aberration of the objective lens; the better the range resolution, the greater the effect of chromatic aberration. Thus, it is difficult to work with the ultimate resolution of the lens. An advantage of fluorescence imaging in the RSOM and TSRLM is that reflections from internal elements on the microscope become less important because color filters eliminate the reflected light. In addition, a dichroic beamsplitter can eliminate the beamsplitter loss. The main problem here has been to obtain enough light. It has therefore often been necessary to use long exposure times for photography or to use extremely sensitive TV cameras. However, recent designs seem to provide enough light for direct viewing by eye of fluorescent images.

INTERNAL REFLECTIONS

When weakly reflecting biological materials are being observed, small reflections from the system itself can be of vital importance. In an RSOM, the reflections from the disk are often the most important source of glare. If the disk transmits 1% of the light, and the reflection from cells in a sample, such as the lens of the eye, is only 0.01%, it is necessary to have the power reflection coefficient of the disk considerably less than 10^{-6}. By using the measures already described, it is possible, with care, to satisfy this criterion. However, there are other internal reflections common to both the RSOM and TSRLM which are

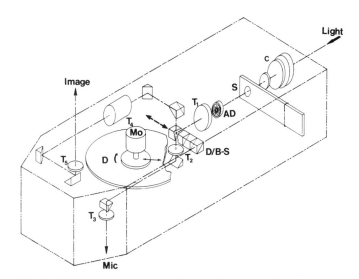

FIG. 7. Major components and light path in K2-BIO single-pass disk confocal attachment. Light from a mercury arc source is collected (C) and then passes through a shutter (S) before being focussed onto an aperture diaphragm (AD). From there the light proceeds through a four-position beam splitter (D/B-S; out, 50%, dichroic 1, dichroic 2), through transfer lens, T_1, and onto the aperture disk (D). The disk is rotated by the motor (Mo) and can be moved (small arrow) to three positions, (out, 35 μm holes: 2% transmittance, 20 μm holes: 1% transmittance). The disk, resides in an intermediate image plane formed by T_2 and T_3 and, therefore, the pinholes in the disk are focussed into spots at the in-focus plane of the microscope (Mic). Returning light from the spots illuminated on the sample passes through T_3 and T_2 to be focussed on the bottom side of the disk. Light from the plane-of-focus passes through the pinholes (from which it came) and then proceeds through T_4 and T_5 to the eye or other image recorder. Not shown are the polarizer, 1/4 wave plate and analyzer used to suppress reflections of the illuminating light from the disk, as shown in Fig. 2.

associated with the lenses, beamsplitters, and so on. These reflections need to be dealt with carefully; with good design and great care in assembly, they can usually be made sufficiently low not to cause a major problem.

Internal reflections are not such a serious issue in fluorescence microscopes. If color filters or dichroic beam splitters are employed, the incident light reflected from internal parts does not reach the eyepiece. However, the problem in this case is to obtain sufficient light. Stratagems such as careful design of the condenser, using a high intensity 200 watt mercury vapor light source, decreasing the hole spacing and hence increasing the fill factor of the disk to several percent, make it possible to increase the incident light intensity on the object by more than a factor of 10. Coupled with the decreased saturation effects due to the lower peak intensity of light employed in this microscope (compared to the LSCM) the TSRLM and the RSOM should be very important devices for use in fluorescence imaging.

A recent embodiment of these design principles is the K-2 BIO (Technical Instruments, San Jose, CA), a single-pass disk scanning attachment for use on biological samples using fluorescence or back-scattered light. This device (Fig. 7) fits between the microscope body and the binocular eyepiece unit of any standard microscope. The disk can be removed for non-confocal operation or placed so that regions of the disk having 20 or 35 μm holes are present in the intermediate image plane for confocal studies.

ACKNOWLEDGEMENT

This work was supported by the National Science Foundation under Contract No. ECS-88–13558 and the Office of Naval Research under Contract No. N00014–87-K-0337.

REFERENCES

Born, M. and E. Wolf, *Principles of Optics,* Pergamon Press (1975).

Goodman, J.W., *Introduction to Fourier Optics,* McGraw-Hill (1968).

Kino, G.S., *Acoustic Waves: Devices, Imaging, and Analog Signal Processing,* Prentice-Hall, New Jersey (1987).

Kino, G.S. and G.Q. Xiao, "Real-Time Scanning Optical Microscopes," to be published in *Scanning Optical Microscopes,* Ed: T. Wilson, Pergamon Press, London, England.

Petran, M., M. Hadravsky, M.D. Egger, and R. Galambos, "Tandem Scanning Reflected Light Microscope," J. Opt. Soc. America **58,** 661–664 (1968).

Petran, M., M. Hadravsky, and A. Boyde, "The Tandem Scanning Reflected Light Microscope," Scanning **7,** 97–108, (1985).

Wilson, T. and C.J.R. Sheppard, *Scanning Optical Microscopy,* Academic Press (1984).

Wilson, T. and A.R. Carlini, "Size of the Detector in Confocal Imaging Systems," Opt. Lett. **12**(4), 227–229 (1987).

Xiao, G.Q. and G.S. Kino, "A Real-Time Confocal Scanning Optical Microscope," Proc. SPIE, Vol. 809, Scanning Imaging Technology, T. Wilson & L. Balk, Eds. 107–113 (1987).

Xiao, G.Q., T.R. Corle, and G.S. Kino, "Real-Time Confocal Scanning Optical Microscope," Appl. Phys. Lett. **53** (8), 716–718 (1988).

Xiao, G.Q., Kino, G.S. and Mastera, B.R., "Observation of the Rabbit Cornea and Lens with a New Real-Time Confocal Scanning Optical Microscope." Scanning, accepted for publication (1989).

Chapter 11

The Role of the Pinhole in Confocal Imaging Systems

T. Wilson

Department of Engineering Science, University of Oxford, Parks Road, Oxford, OX1 4UU

INTRODUCTION

Confocal scanning microscopes are particularly attractive by virtue of their enhanced lateral resolution, purely coherent image formation and optical sectioning (Wilson and Sheppard, 1984). It is probably the latter property which is most useful as it gives rise to the ability to image a thick specimen in three-dimensions. This is possible because the optical system images information only from a thin region in the neighbourhood of the focal plane. This permits us to store many image slices in a computer to give a three dimensional data set which describes the object. There are now many sophisticated computer software systems available to display this data in various ways. Obvious examples include the extended focus technique (Wilson and Hamilton, 1982) in which we merely add up (integrate) the images from various depths to provide an image of greatly extended depth of field. We may also produce images where object height is coded as brightness or combine the whole data set to provide an isometric view of the object, Figure 1. It is also possible to use false color to label features of interest or, by simple processing, to obtain stereoscopic pairs (van der Voort, 1985). Other forms of image display are discussed in Chapter 10.

Figure 2 shows a schematic of a confocal scanning optical microscope. The only difference between a confocal and a conventional scanning microscope is that the confocal arrangement uses a point detector rather than a large area one. All the considerable advantages of confocal microscopy derive from the small size of this detector. The success or failure of a particular microscope implementation in achieving true confocal operation depends on the correct choice of pinhole size and shape to approximate as closely as possible the ideal point detector.

In many applications, however it is not possible to use as small a detector as we would like because of signal to noise problems. This is particularly true in fluorescent imaging. In the following, therefore, we will discuss the origins of the optical sectioning property and show how it deteriorates as detector geometries of finite size are employed. We will begin by considering brightfield microscopes and conclude with a discussion of fluorescent systems.

THE OPTICAL SECTIONING PROPERTY

The physical origin of the property is shown in Figure 3. When the object is in the focal plane (dashed lines) the reflected light is focussed on to the pinhole and a large signal is detected. On the other hand, when the object is positioned out of the focal plane, a defocussed spot is formed at the pinhole, and the measured intensity is greatly reduced. The strength of the optical sectioning, that is the rate at which the detected intensity falls off with axial distance, is clearly a function of both the detector size and the object feature. If we begin our discussion by considering an ideally small point detector we can readily calculate the images of idealised objects. We will consider the images of a single point, a line and a plane. We show, in Figure 4, these images as a function of a normalised axial distance u, which is related to real axial distance, z, via

$$u = \frac{8\pi}{\lambda} \sin^2(\alpha/2) z \qquad (1)$$

where λ is the wavelength and $\sin\alpha$ the objective lens numerical aperture. The results for the case of the point and line are shown for focussing directly on top of the feature. In particular we see that the sectioning is twice as weak in the case of a point object as a plane for $I(u) = O$ whereas; at the half intensity resolution, $u_{1/2}$, the values are at about $u = 4$ and $u = 3$ respectively. (These benchmark values will be useful in interpreting later graphs where $u_{1/2}$ is a parameter).

In the paraxial approximation we can write the axial image of a plane as

$$I(u) = \left(\frac{\sin u/2}{u/2}\right)^2 \qquad (2)$$

We see, therefore, that the strength of the sectioning depends on the size and shape of the specific object feature imaged. In order to have a convenient experimental measure of sectioning we will concentrate on the planar object. In practice we will scan a perfect reflector through focus in a reflection microscope and note the form of the response. We define a metric of the sectioning as being the full-width-half-maximum of this response. Equation (2) is a paraxial expression: fortunately it is possible to derive a high angle equivalent which is more accurate at high numerical aperture, (Sheppard and Wilson, 1981b), and based on this theory it is possible to predict optical sectioning strengths as shown in Figure 5.

THE OPTICAL SECTIONING PROPERTY WITH A FINITE-SIZED CIRCULAR DETECTOR AND COHERENT LIGHT

It is clear from Figure 3 that the strength of the sectioning will become less as the detector size is increased. In the limit of a very large detector the sectioning disappears altogether. Figure 6 illustrates the effect. Here the pinhole size is denoted by a normalised radius, v_p, which is related to real radius, r_p, via

$$v_p = \frac{2\pi}{\lambda} \sin\alpha r_p \qquad (3)$$

We see that the curves corresponding to vp=0 and vp=1 are indistinguishable on the scale of Figure 6, which implies that the strength of the sectioning is relatively insensitive to pinhole size up to some limit (Wilson and Carlini, 1987a). This is borne out in practice in Figure 7 where we see that the response of the microscope is essentially indistinguishable for pinholes of 5 μm and 10 μm diameter. These results were obtained (Wilson and Carlini, 1988a) using red light (6328 Å wavelength) from a helium neon laser and a 32× 0.5 numerical aperture objective lens. The effect of introducing larger detector pinholes is shown in Figures 8(a) and 8(b). It is seen that the curves become distinctly broader by the time a 150 μm diameter aperture is used.

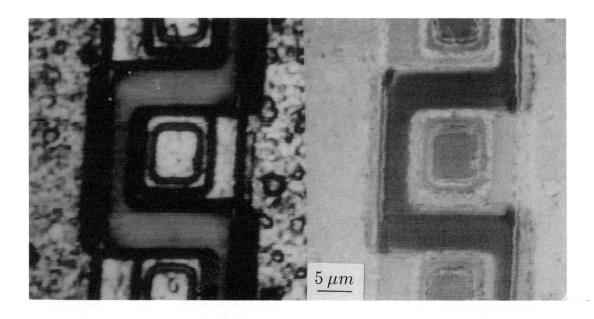

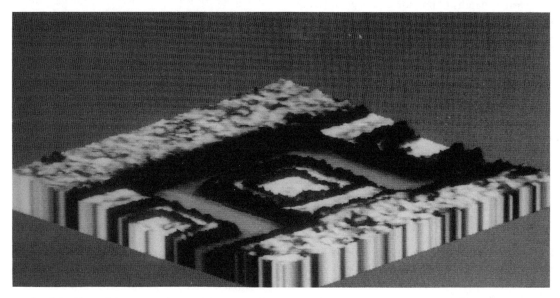

FIG. 1.   An example of the kind of data processing available in confocal microscopy. The top left hand image shows an extended focus image of a portion of a particularly deep transistor. The top right hand image is the corresponding height image where object height is coded as image brightness. The bottom image is a computer generated isometric image of the same microcircuit.

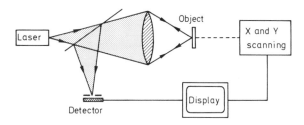

FIG. 2.   The optical arrangement of a confocal scanning optical microscope.

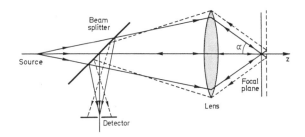

FIG. 3.   The physical origin of the depth discrimination property.

However, we can still expect that a degree of depth discrimination will be present in instruments using such large pinholes.

We can also see that although the curves of Figs. 7 and 8 show the same trends as the theoretical curves, they do not agree perfectly. In particular the experimental results are somewhat asymmetric and the side lobes do not go down to zero. This could have a variety of causes (Wilson and Carlini, 1988). The most likely one is that the pupil function is not perfectly uniform across the aperture. The simple theory assumes that this is given by a circ function. However, interference techniques (Mathews, 1987) and curve fitting (Corle et al., 1986) show that this is not the case and that the transmission of the pupil falls off towards the edge, Figure 9. This is due partly to the variation in Fresnel reflection coefficient at the edge of the pupil and is particularly apparent with large NA objectives.

It is interesting and important to note that any small apodisation or shading in the lens pupil has a dramatic effect on the axial behaviour, but only a minor one on the lateral response.

In conventional microscopy this is not so important as there is no depth sectioning property, and it explains why they give relatively good images with less than ideal lenses. As a dramatic example we may consider the situation in which the central portion of the lens pupil is blocked off, leaving a very thin annular region to transmit the light. It is straightforward to show that the intensity in the focal plane of this lens is given by $J_o^2(v)$, which when plotted is somewhat similar in shape to the $(2J_1(v)/v)^2$ form of the Airy disc in a full aperture lens. When we come to consider the axial response, however, the situation is vastly different. The full aperture case gives the response to a perfect reflector of $\mathrm{sinc}^2(u/2)$, equation (2), whereas in the case of a narrow annular pupil $I_{plane}(u) = $ constant! This suggests that

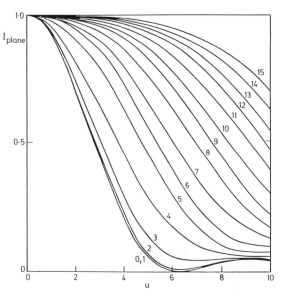

FIG. 6.   The variation of I_{plane} (u) versus u for a variety of detector pinhole sizes, v_p.

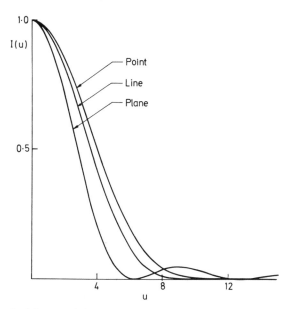

FIG. 4.   The on-axis images of point, line and plane objects as a function of normalised axial distance u.

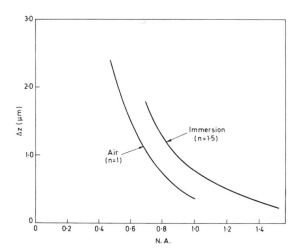

FIG. 5.   The optical sectioning strength as a function of numerical aperture. The curves are for red light (0.6328Å wavelength). Δz is the full-width-half-intensity of the I_{plane} (u) versus u curves.

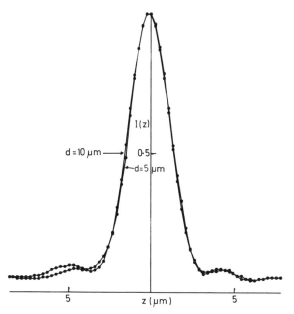

FIG. 7.   Detected intensity as a function of axial position as a plane mirror is scanned axially through focus in a scanning microscope employing 6328 Å radiation and a 32 x, 0.5 NA objective lens. The curves are for detector apertures of 5 μm and 10 μm.

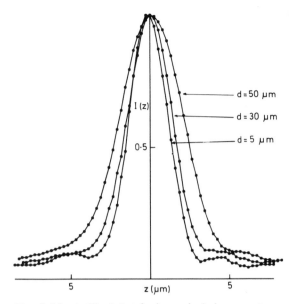

FIG. 8. (a)   As Fig. 7, but for increasingly large apertures.

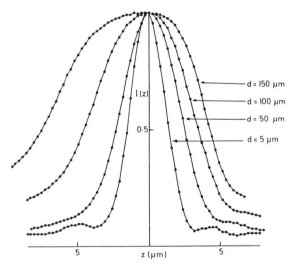

FIG. 8. (b)   As Fig. 7, but for a much larger range of aperture.

we may well be able to use apodisation, by inserting pupil-plane filters, to tune the axial response of a confocal microscope without dramatically sacrificing or altering the lateral resolution. If we now compare the half-widths that theory predicts, as in Figure 6, with our measured results we obtain the curves of Figure 10. We confirm here that for pinhole radii less than about 2.0 optical units the strength of the sectioning remains constant. The experimental data are shown as dots and the theoretical prediction as the full line. We note that we have excellent agreement at low values of normalised pinhole diameter but less good agreement when larger pinholes are used. This is to be expected, as the experimental results are far from symmetrical here, which makes the measurement of $u_{1/2}$ somewhat difficult. In displaying the results we merely divided the half-width of curves, such as Figure 8 by two.

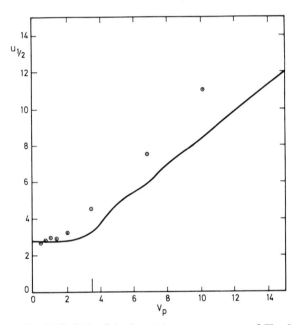

FIG. 10.   Half-width of the I_{plane} (u) versus u curves of Fig. 5 as a function of normalized detector radius, v_p. The theoretical curve is shown as the full line and the experimental results as the dots for a numerical aperture of 0.44.

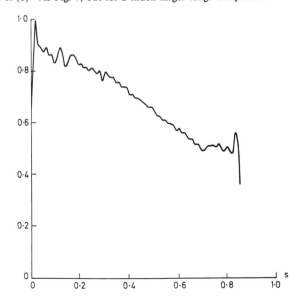

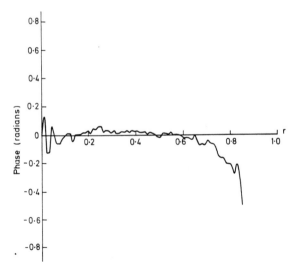

FIG. 9.   The modulus (a) and phase (b) of the pupil function of a 0.5 numerical aperture lens. The radial coordinate is a measured in terms of the angular position from the focus, q, via s = $(\sin(\theta/2)/\sin(\alpha/2)2$.

LATERAL RESOLUTION AS A FUNCTION OF EFFECTIVE DETECTOR SIZE

We have concentrated on the axial response because this is the key advantage of confocal microscopy. However, the lateral imaging also deteriorates if finite-sized detectors are used. In particular, the imaging immediately becomes partially coherent which makes image interpretation and calculation more difficult. As a specific example we will take a single point object and ask what happens to the half width of the image as the pinhole is made larger. We already know that on this basis the confocal system is approximately 1.4 times superior. Figure 11 shows the behaviour for intermediate sizes of pinhole. We see that by inadvertently choosing a detector corresponding to $v_p \approx 4.0$ optical units we would obtain imaging inferior to the conventional microscope. The most important implication, however, is that to obtain the true confocal resolution improvement a value of v_p less than about 0.5 optical units should be chosen. If we compare this value with that predicted by Figures 6 and 10 we see that the lateral resolution is much more sensitive to pinhole size than the axial resolution. Indeed, the curves corresponding to $v_p = 0$ and to $v_p = 1$ are indistinguishable on the scale of Figure 6, whereas the lateral resolution has already started to deteriorate by $v_p = 1$. To put these optical units in context we note that the first dark ring of the Airy disk occurs at $V_p = 3.7$ optical units and marked with a carat on Figs 10 and 11.

THE ROLE OF ABERRATIONS

Another reason for the asymmetry in the responses of Figure 8 is the presence of aberrations in the objective lens. In order to see which aberrations are important we can introduce a very simple model by writing the pupil function in the presence of defocus, u, primary spherical aberration, A, primary coma, B, and primary astigmatism, C, as

$$P(u,p\theta) = \exp\frac{1}{2}jup^2 \exp2\pi j[Ap^4 + Bp^3\cos\theta + Cp^2\cos^2\theta] \quad (4)$$

We can now write (Wilson and Çarlini, 1989)

$$I_{plane}(u) = \int_o^{2\pi} \int_0^1 P(u,p,\theta)P(u,p,\pi-\theta)pdpd\theta \quad (5)$$

from which it is clear that primary coma has no effect on the axial imaging of a perfect reflector. (It does, of course, have an effect on the imaging in general.) Figure 12 indicates the effect of a combination of spherical aberration and primary astigmatism on the axial imaging. This theoretical curve, although derived from a paraxial theory, does, nevertheless, show the main features of a typical objective response.

It is important to get a feel for the effect of aberrations, because the three dimensional imaging capabilities of confocal microscopes almost inevitably mean that we must focus deep into a specimen, and hence run the risk of unavoidably introducing spherical aberration. The effects of aberrations may be investigated by using an objective lens fitted with an adjustable collar to compensate for imaging through various thicknesses of cover glass. Aberrations can then be introduced merely by suitably adjusting the collar or moving the pinhole axially, and curves similar to Figure 8 could be obtained for various detector

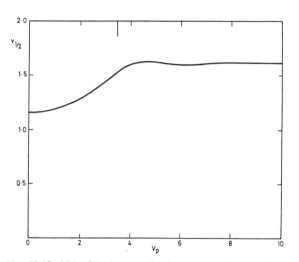

FIG. 11.   Half-width of the images of a single point object as a function of detector pinhole size.

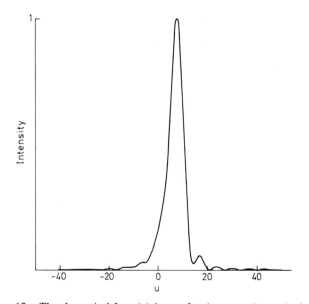

FIG. 12.   The theoretical I_{plane} (u) image for the case when spherical aberration (A = 0.5) and primary astigmatism (C = 0.3) are present.

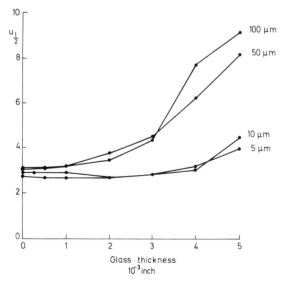

FIG. 13.   The half-width of I_{plane} (u) curves versus the degree of aberration introduced. The abscissa is essentially proportional to A. Curves are shown for diferent pinhole sizes.

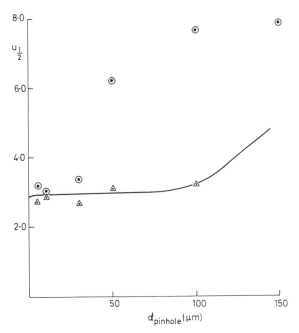

FIG. 14. The half-width of I_{plane} (u) curves as a function of detector aperture diameter. The full line is theoretical and the dots experimental. The triangles correspond to zero aberration setting whereas the circles result from setting the correction collar to t = 4 thousandths of an inch.

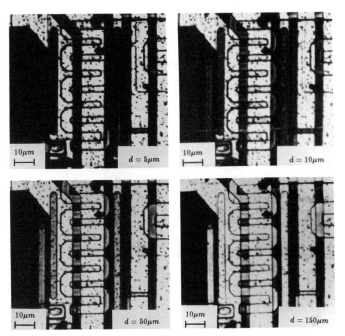

FIG. 15. A series of images of an EPROM taken with 5 μm, 10 μm, 50 μm, 150 μm sized detector pinholes.

sizes at a specific value of deliberately introduced aberration. The general trend which is observed is that the curves become wider and the side lobe levels increase as the amount of aberration worsens.

An alternative representation of the data is shown in Figure 13, where the half width of the I_{plane} (u) response is plotted as a function of the total aberration present. The aberration is measured as the glass thickness for which the objective lens collar is set to correct. In this case it is related to t, the cover glass thickness. A family of such curves is presented, each plot relating to a different size of detector pinhole. In all cases worsening aberrations caused a rise in the measured half-width. However, at the larger pinhole sizes, the effects are considerably more marked. These aberrations (but not lateral chromatic aberration) are therefore seem to be more significant for the larger detector pinhole sizes, which may be relevant in some scanning disk systems.

A final representation of the data is shown in Fig.14. Again the solid line represents the theory. We should, however, mention that these experimental results were obtained with a reflecting objective. Thus the theoretical line is not strictly applicable, although it is clearly representative of the behaviour.

Another kind of aberration which can be introduced unintentionally comes about by using an objective lens with a tube length different from that for which the microscope system was designed. This can have a very dramatic effect on the axial response and although it is possible to correct this somewhat by inserting appropriate correcting lenses, it is important to be aware of the problem (see Chapter 7).

IMAGES WITH A FINITE-SIZED DETECTOR

We now move on to the important question of how the actual images change visually if a finite sized pinhole is used. We use

a portion of an EPROM control circuitry as a test specimen because it has features with well defined height. Our earlier results suggest that for our particular objective lens, that the depth discrimination should not significantly degrade until we use pinhole sizes greater than, say, 30 μm. This is borne out in practice, Figure 15, and we see that by the time a 150 mm diameter pinhole is used the image becomes very similar to a conventional image, Figure 16.

The effect of noise on the crispness of the images may also be seen. In general the smaller the pinhole, the superior the image. This is particularly true of situations where the pinhole is too large to give an improvement in the single point resolution. We shall return to this point later.

EXTENDED-FOCUS AND AUTO-FOCUS IMAGING WITH A FINITE-SIZED DETECTOR

The existence of the depth discrimination property has suggested the extremely simple extended-focus technique (Wilson & Hamilton, 1982) as a method of obtaining an in-focus image of a thick three-dimensional specimen. It consists of adding up (integrating) a series of images obtained at different focal settings. An alternative method, the auto-focus technique, consists in principle of scanning the object axially at each picture point, noting the maximum value of the detected signal and displaying this value at the appropriate picture point to produce the image. The methods clearly have much in common and may be produced simultaneously. Figure 17 shows the images created from data obtained using different sized pinholes and illustrates, as might now be expected, that acceptable, although inferior, images can be obtained even when very large detector pinholes are used.

HEIGHT IMAGING WITH A FINITE-SIZED PINHOLE

An inevitable consequence of the auto-focus technique is the ability to produce a surface profile of a specimen merely by

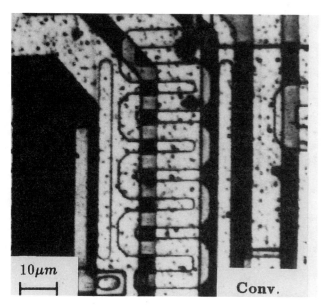

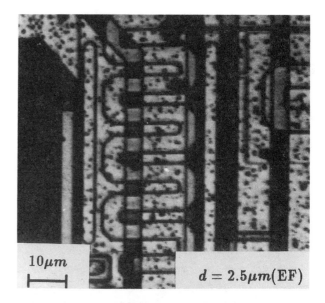

FIG. 16.   Conventional scanning microscope images of the EPROM.

noting the axial position at which the maximum signal is detected at each picture point (Hamilton & Wilson, 1982a, b). This information may be displayed as an isometric projection, or alternatively, in the form of an image where the brightness of each picture point corresponds to the height of that portion of the specimen above, or below, some datum level. Figure 18 shows such images created from the previous data, and we see that although acceptable images may be obtained with reasonably small detector sizes, the quality does drop off quite dramatically when larger sized apertures are used.

In general, then, we can conclude that the sectioning quality is observably inferior with finite sized pinholes. However, if the pinhole is not extremely large, this reduced sectioning does not prevent us from obtaining acceptable three-dimensional reconstructions with techniques such as extended focus or auto focus.

ALTERNATIVE DETECTOR GEOMETRIES

We have concentrated so far on circular detectors, but there are other detector geometries which can be used. These include squares (Awamura et al, 1987) and slits (Koester, 1980). In some sense these are all compromises to the ideal point but, in the case of the slit in particular, they permit a larger signal to be detected. This increase in signal is particularly important in the fluorescence case, which we shall discuss later.

We begin by considering a square detector of side $2\,a_p$. If we now require that the area of this detector be equal to a circular one of radius v_p, i.e. $a_p = \sqrt{\pi}\,v_p/2$, then we find that the I_{plane} (u) versus a_p curve is virtually indistinguishable from the circular case of Figure 6. If we again measure the sectioning strength via the half widths of these curves we see that in the circular case the sectioning is constant for v_p less than about 2.5, or in the square case for a_p less than about 2.2. Thus, as far as axial response is concerned, finite sized square apertures exhibit substantially similar behaviour to finite sized circular detectors.

If we now move on to consider the sectioning strength of a slit detector, we find for a point source and an infinitely narrow

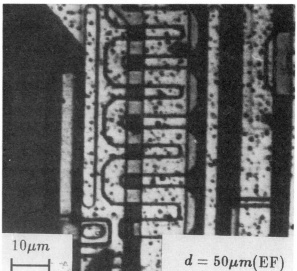

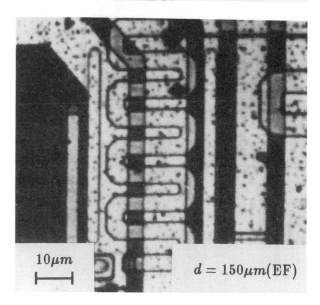

FIG. 17.   A series of extended-focus images created from data obtained with 2.5, 50 and 150 μm sized detector pinholes.

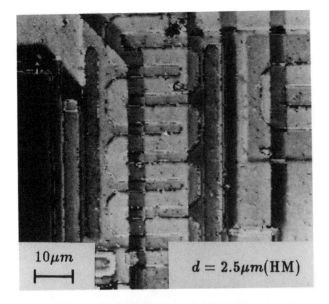

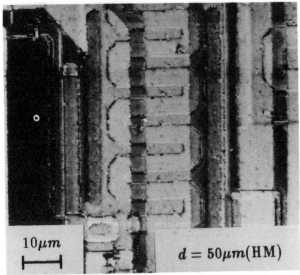

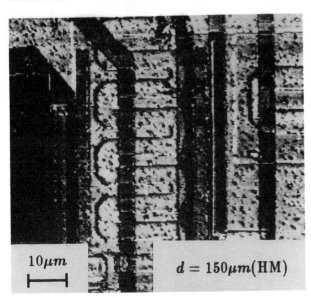

FIG. 18. A series of height images created from data obtained with 2.5, 50 and 150 μm detector pinholes. The maximum signal criterion was used to form these images.

long slit that the response is given by Figure 19 (Wilson, 1989). There is no simple mathematical expression for this curve; the main observations are that the sectioning is less strong, and that response has no zeroes and takes much longer to die away, Figure 20. The question of the correct choice slit width can also be addressed, and a whole family of curves similar in trend to Figure 6 may be derived. Again, if the half width is taken as the metric of sectioning, the curve of Figure 21 results from which we see that we really need to try to use a slit of width less than about one optical unit to achieve maximum sectioning. This means that we must use a slit considerably smaller than the circular pinhole in order to obtain optimum sectioning and in addition there will be directional effects.

A problem with using a slit detector is that the image of a circularly symmetric object will not necessarily be circularly symmetric. If we take as an example a simple point object, we find that the image may be written (Wilson and Hewlett, 1989)

$$I(t,w) = \left(\frac{2J_1(\sqrt{t^2 + w^2})}{\sqrt{t^2 + w^2}} \right)^2 \left(\frac{3\pi}{8} \frac{H_1(2t)}{t^2} \right) \tag{6}$$

where J_1 and H_1 are first order Bessel and Struve functions

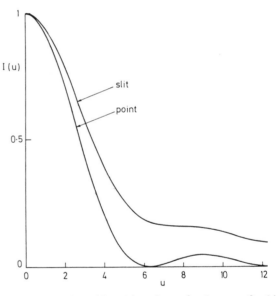

FIG. 19. The variation of I_{plane} (u) against u for the case of a thin slit and a point detector.

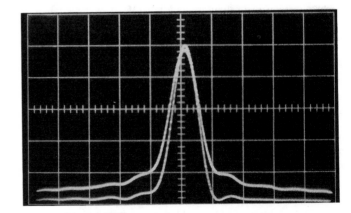

FIG. 20. Experimental I_{plane} (u) curves taken with point and slit detectors. One large division here represents 2.0 mm axial movement.

respectively. The variables t and w are optical co-ordinates in the x and y directions respectively. The slit in this case was oriented parallel to the y-axis. Figure 22 shows the difference in the focal plane behaviour. If we introduce defocus into the system, the difference becomes even more pronounced, as the images of Figure 23 indicate. Here the image of the square shaped pad has been dramatically washed out in a direction parallel to the orientation of the slit. Notwithstanding this example, it is possible to obtain very good three dimensional reconstructions from data sets derived with slit detectors. Indeed, images very similar to those presented in Figure 1 are possible (see Chapter 19).

Another form of detector which is becoming more important as semiconductor technology advances is the detector array. This is exciting because it permits us, in principle, to choose whatever detector distribution we want. In particular the detector sensitivity can be neagtive at some points. This freedom permits us to realise confocal microscopy in a completely different way. As an example if we were able to build a detector with intensity sensitivity $2J_1(av)/(av)$ then we would find that for a > 2 the axial image of a planar object would be exactly as given by equation (2). Although this may not be the best way of achieving confocal operation it does point to the new possibilities which open up.

The fact that, by using a detector array, we can sample the field at all points in the detector plane gives us more information and should enable us to produce better images which correspond more closely to specific object features. An example of this is the "type III" microscope [Schutt et. al.,1988]. The idea here is that instead of displaying, at each picture point, the intensity we detect on the optic axis we display instead, the maximum signal we measure in the detctor plane. This scheme is thought to be particularly sensitive to phase edges in biological tissue.

Other applications would be to obtain two images simultaneously, but taken with different sized detectors. This can be used to tune the optical sectioning strength and produce images which are very sensitive to surface height [Wilson and Hamilton, 1984].

Of course a scanning microscope scheme which uses a completely different form of detector is the tandem sacnning microscope [Egger and Petran, 1967]. Here the image is built up in real time by illuminating the object with a very large number of confocal spots simultaneously. This is achieved by using a rotating Nipkow disc. The design question here is how to choose the geometry of the apertures and their position in the disc. Circular, square and slit-shaped apertures have all been used. The additional constraint in this kind of microscope is that the apertures must be placed sufficiently far apart that no cross talk occurs between adjacent ones. The image formation in these systems is actually slightly different from that in confocal systems [Sheppard and Wilson, 1981a].

A constraint on these systems is that the image is viewed directly by eye and hence the apertures must not be so small that diffraction effects dominate (in this regard the diffraction effects from square holes may be particularly complex). This suggests that, in practice, these systems will not be truly confocal. However the very presence of the apertures does give optical sectioning and hence three-dimensional imaging is still available, but often with lower axial resolution. Figure 24 shows a comparison between the sectioning obtained in a confocal laser scanning microscope with a detection pinhole of normalised V_p and an incoherently-illuminated, tandem scanning (labelled direct view) microscope with equal sized circular pinhole. The ordinate represents the ten percent width of the I_{plane} (u) curves. The differences between the two systems is discussed in more detail elsewhere (Wilson, 1990) and Wilson and Hewlett (1989) and also Chapter 10.

NOISE

We have not yet said anything about the role of a finite sized detector in reducing the amount of flare and scattered light present in the image. We can consider the scattered light to be made up both of light which is scattered by elements of the optical system irrespective of the object and of that which re-

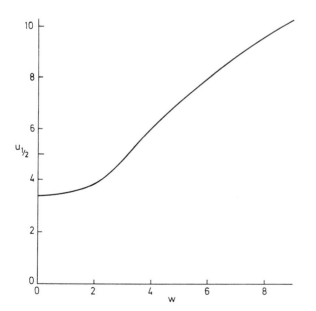

FIG. 21.   The half-width of the I_{plane}(u) curves for a slit shaped detector of half-width w optical units.

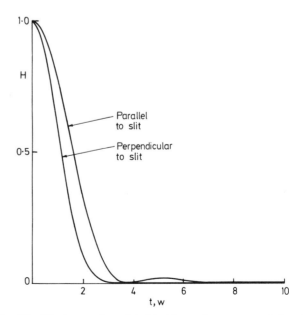

FIG. 22.   The image of a point object in a microscope consisting of a point source and an infinitely narrow slit detector. The image is shown in directions parallel and perpendicular to the slit.

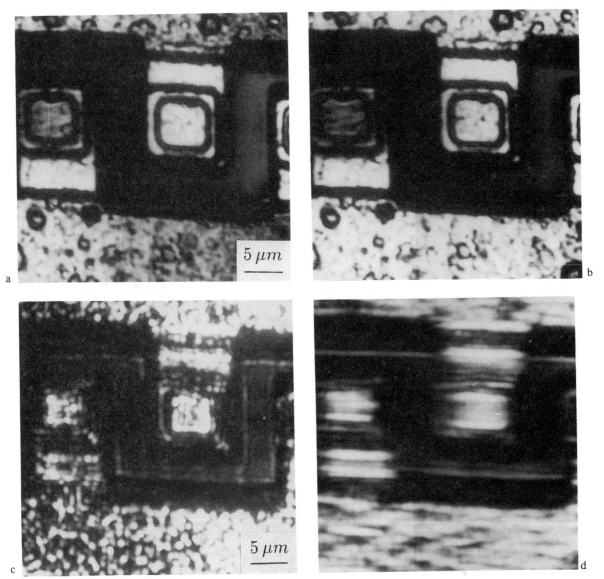

FIG. 23. Images of a portion of a microcircuit taken with microscopes using (a,c) point and (b,d) slit detector. The pairs of photographs (a,b) and (c,d) were taken in planes 6.0 μm apart. The slit was orientated in the horizontal direction.

sults from scattering within the object. The former, which is constant in either object or objective scanning microscopes, merely serves to reduce contrast and could, in principle, be measured and subtracted from the detected signal. In the case of beam scanning microscopes, however, this component is clearly not constant and will vary across the entire image field.

In an attempt to quantify these effects (Cox & Sheppard, 1986) we may consider a transmitted light system with no object but with a finite sized detector of radius, v_p. This permits us to write the detected signal as

$$I_{det} = \int \int \left(\frac{2J_1(V)}{V}\right)^2 D(x,y) \, dxdy \qquad (7)$$

where $D(x,y)$ represents the shape of the detector.

If we further assume that the intensity of the flare and scattered light is simply proportional to the area of the detector, we can also derive an expression for the signal-to-flare ratio as

a function of the size of the detector. In the case of a circular detector of radius V_p we can write

$$I_{det} = 1 - J_0^2(V_p) - J_1^2(V_p) \qquad (8)$$

We plot this function (A) in Figure 25 together with the signal-to-flare ratio (B) as a function of detector size. It is clear that the presence of any reasonably sized detector contributes greatly to the rejection of flare and hence to the production of higher quality images.

The case of the slit may be similarly modelled and the results are shown in Figure 26. In this case the slit width has been taken rather than the area in estimating the signal-to-flare ratio, which is seen not to fall off with increasing detector size as rapidly as in the circular case.

These considerations lead us to the very important conclusion that even if a particular detector geometry is used which does not give optimum optical sectioning, it may still allow

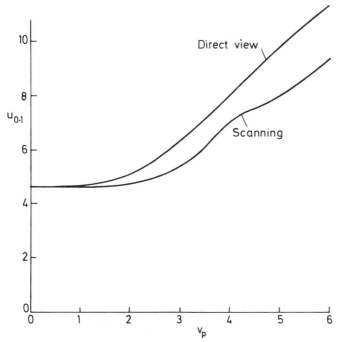

FIG. 24. The ten percent width of I_{plane} (u) curves as a function of detector aperture for the case of a laser scanning microscope and an incoherently illuminated tandem scanning (labelled Direct View) microscope.

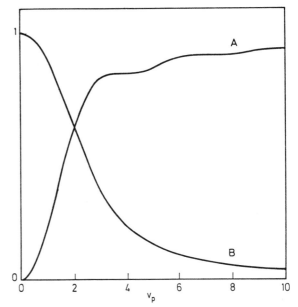

FIG. 25. Detected signal (A) and the detected signal to flare ratio (B) as a function of the normalised detector radius, v_p.

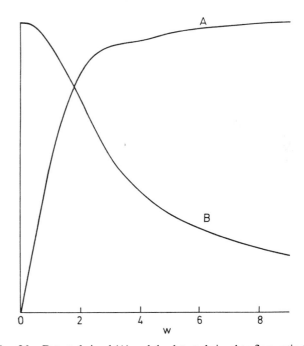

FIG. 26. Detected signal (A) and the detected signal to flare ratio (B) as a function of the normalised slit half-width w.

superior images to be obtained, in the sense of image clarity and lack of scattered light.

FLUORESCENCE IMAGING

It is probably fair to say that the ability to combine the three dimensional imaging capabilities of confocal microscopy with the fluorescent staining of biological specimens is one of the key reasons for the current surge of interest, both scientific and commercial, in confocal microscopy. All of our previous discussion has been concerned with what we might call bright-field confocal microscopy, in that our simple theory merely modelled our object as being affected by radiation and having a transmissivity or reflectivity, t. In the case of a perfect confocal microscope the imaging is purely coherent in the sense that we can write the image intensity as

$$I = |(h_1 h_2) \otimes t|^2 \qquad (9)$$

when $\otimes$ denotes the convolution operation and $h_{1,2}$ are the impulse responses (Fourier transform of the pupil function) of the two lenses. The situation in a fluorescent microscope is completely different. If the system employs an infinitely small detector then for a reflection system (Wilson & Sheppard, 1984)

$$I = |h_{eff}|^2 \otimes f \qquad (10)$$

where $\otimes$ denotes the spatial distribution of the fluorescence generation and h_{eff} is the product of the impulse response functions of the lens operating at the primary wavelength, λ_1, and the fluorescent wavelength, λ_2.

It is clear that the confocal fluorescent microscope behaves like an incoherent imaging system as opposed to the coherent imaging of the non-fluorescent confocal case. This difference is very important. It means that, although much of what we have already said about the role of the detector geometry in affecting the resolution in the non-confocal case is broadly true, none of it is directly applicable to the fluorescent case. We must, therefore, produce analogous design rules based on equation (10).

However before we launch into a discussion of detector geometries it will be useful to discuss the role of the fluorescent wavelength, λ_2. In order to have a metric of sectioning we consider, by analogy with a perfect reflector, the signal that we measure as we scan a uniform fluorescent object through focus,

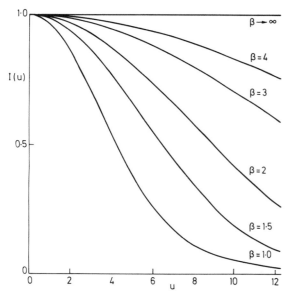

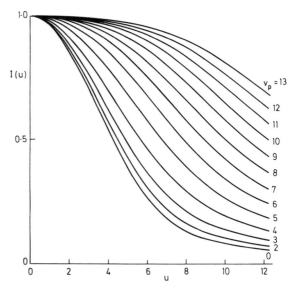

FIG. 27. The detected signal as a perfect planar fluorescent object is scanned axially through focus f or a variety of fluorescent wavelengths, b = (l2/l1). The axial distance, u, is normalised to the primary wavelength, l1. We note that if we measure the sectioning by the half-width of these curves, the strength of the sectioning is essentially proportional to b.

FIG. 29. (a) The detected signal as a perfect planar fluorescent object is scanned axially through focus for a variety of normalised detector radii, vp. The normalised parameters, u and vp, are normalised to the incident wavelength. The curves are drawn for the limiting case of b = 1.

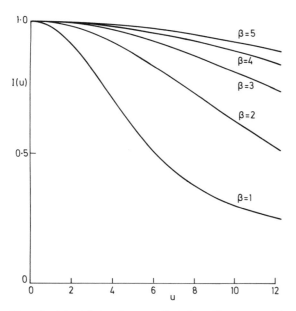

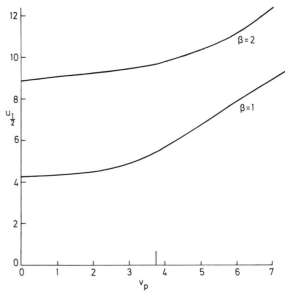

FIG. 28. The detected signal as a perfect planar fluorescent object is scanned through focus for a microscope employing an infinitely thin slit detector for a variety of fluorescent wavelengths, b. The axial distance is again normalised to the primary wavelength.

FIG. 29. (b) The half-width of the curves of 28a as a function of the normalised detector radius, vnp, for the cases of b = 1 and b = 2.

i.e. we set f$=1$. The results are shown in Figure 27 for various values of $\beta(=\lambda^2/\lambda_1)$. There are no zeroes in the response as there are in the non-fluorescent confocal case, and we see that the sectioning becomes coarse as the fluorescent wavelength increases. Indeed, in the limit as $\beta \rightarrow \infty$, the imaging resembles that of a conventional incoherent microscope, and the sectioning disappears altogether. We can also see that if we detect fluorescent radiation over a range of wavelengths, the final image will contain information from a variety of depths. However, in general, it is clear that to obtain optimum sectioning we should

try to operate as close to $\beta=1$ as possible. Similar conclusions are reached if, instead of the ideal point detector we use an infinitely thin slit detector, Figure 28.

It is now perfectly possible to calculate these responses for a specific value of β and finite sized detectors. We present the results of these calculations (Wilson, 1989) in Figures 29 and 30.

Finally, in this section, we compare the strength of sectioning which is available in fluorescent and non-fluorescent imaging, Figure 31. It is clear from this figure that, if we have a choice and want the strongest sectioning, a non-fluorescent method is the preferred choice. We should, in fairness, also say that practical requirements of signal level may well make the difference

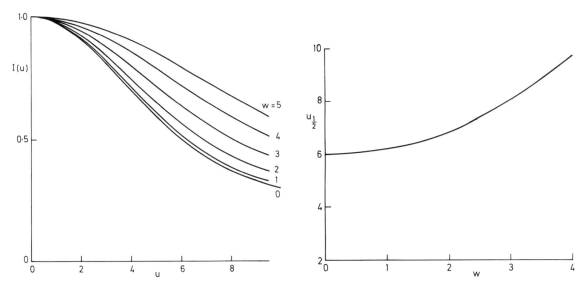

FIG. 30. (a) The detected signal as a perfect planar fluorescent object is scanned axially through focus for a variety of normalised slit widths, w. The normalised coordinates are all normalised to the incident wavelength. The curves are drawn for the limiting case of b = 1. (b) The half-width of the curves of (a) as a function of the normalised slit half-width, w.

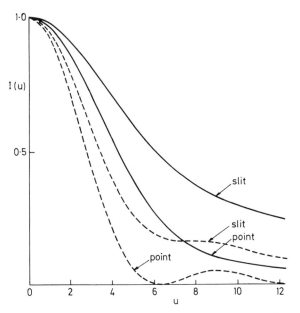

FIG. 31. The axial response to appropriate 'perfect planar reflectors' fluorescent (-) and non-fluorescent (---) microscope using both slit and central point detectors. The fluorescent curves correspond to the limiting case of b = 1.

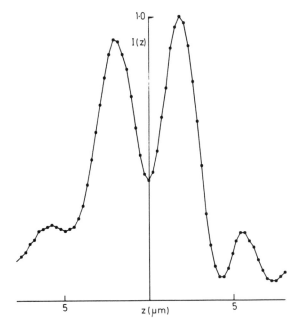

FIG. 32. Experimental signal detected when scanning a plane mirror through focus wiith detector offset. The conditions correspond crudely to dark field.

between the "point" detector response and the slit response less dramatic.

CONCLUSIONS

We have discussed the reduction in the strength of the optical sectioning that we can expect if we use a non-ideal detector. In many cases we have no choice but to use a large area detector because of signal to noise problems. The lateral position of the detector is also important and again the planar reflector proves to be a good test object because we can use it to align the system

laterally to get as sharp as response as possible. If the detector is laterally offset, the results can be quite dramatic, Figure 32, [Wilson and Carlini, 1988b]. However once the detector is properly aligned it should be possible to obtain acceptable images even when using detectors which are somewhat too large to give true confocal operation.

REFERENCES

Awamura, D., Ode, T. & Tonezawa, M. (1987) *Colour laser microscope.* SPIED, 765, 53–60.
Corle, T.R., Chou, C.H. & Kino, G.S. (1986) Depth response of confocal

optical microscopes. *Opt. Lett.* **11,** 770–772.

Cox, I.J., Sheppard, C.J.R. & Wilson, T. (1982) Super-resolution by confocal fluorescent microscopy. *Optik,* **60,** 391–396.

Cox, I.J. & Sheppard, C.J.R. (1986) Image Capacity and resolution in an optical system. *J. Opt. Soc. Am (A),,***3,**1152–1158.

Egger, M. D. & Petran,M.(1967) New reflected light microscope for viewing unstained brain and ganglian cells. *Science,* **157.** 305–308.

Hamilton, D.K., and Wilson, T. (1982a) Surface profile measurement using the confocal microscope. *J. Appl. Phys.* **53,** 5320–5322.

Hamilton, D.K., and Wilson, T. (1982b) Three dimensional surface measurement using the confocal scanning microscope. *Appl. Phys. B,* **27,** 211–213.

Koester, C.J., (1980) *Appl. Opt.* **19,** 1749.

Mathews, H.J., D. Phil Thesis, (1987) Oxford University.

Schutt, W. (1988) Proc. Conf. on Physical Characterisation of Biological Cells. Rostock GDR.

Sheppard, C.J.R. & Wilson T. (1981a) The theory of the direct-view confocal microscope. *J. Microsc.* **124,** 107–117.

Sheppard, C.J.R. & Wilson, T. (1981b) Effects of high angles of convergence on V(z) in the scanning acoustic microscope. *Appl. Phys. Lett.* **38,** 858–859.

Wilson, T. & Hamilton, D.K. (1982) Dynamic focussing in the scanning microscope. *J. Microsc.* **128,** 139–143.

Wilson, T. & Sheppard, C.J.R. (1984) *Theory and Practice of Scanning Optical Microscopy.* Academic Press, London.

Wilson, T. (1988) Depth response of scanning microscopes. *Optik* (in press).

Wilson, T. & Carlini, A.R. (1987) Size of the detector in confocal imaging systems. *Opt. Lett.* **12,** 227–229.

Wilson, T. & Carlini, A.R. (1988a) Three dimensional imaging in confocal imaging systems with finite sized detectors. *J. Microsc.* **149,** 51–66.

Wilson, T. (1989) Optical sectioning in confocal fluorescent microscopes. *J. Microsc.*

Van der Voort, H.T.M., Brakenhoff, G.J., Valkenburg, J.A.C., Nanninga, N. (1985) Design and use of a computer controlled confocal microscope. *Scanning,* **7,** 66–78.

Chapter 12

Photon Detectors for Confocal Microscopy

JONATHAN ART

Department of Pharmacological & Physiological Sciences, The University of Chicago, 947 East 58th Street, Chicago, IL 60637 USA

INTRODUCTION

The goal of confocal microscopy is to obtain better image quality than that achieved in conventional light microscopy by examining each point in an object plane in the absence of light scattered from neighboring points. In this respect confocal microscopy differs from conventional brightfield microscopy where the intent is to view an object under uniform field illumination. The detector in the disk-scanning confocal microscope of Petran, Hadravsky, Egger, & Galambos (1968), is the human eye, a highly sophisticated instrument that is simple to use. The eye is attractive as a detector in terms of its quantum efficiency, the number and size of detector elements, the high degree of parallelism, and the higher order processing that results in perception of an image. Any confocal microscope that projects points in the object plane coherently onto conjugate points in the image plane can employ this detector. If the scanning is rapid enough, a stable full-field image will be perceived. As a detector, however, the eye is less than perfect in reconstructing images if the scanning rate is too slow, or when the scanning is arranged so that all points in the object plane are sequentially projected back onto a single point in space. Nor is the eye able to implement averaging and filtering techniques to enhance the signal-to-noise ratio, SNR, in the image. It is also impossible to make precise temporal or kinetic measurements of fluorescence, nor is it easy to construct three-dimensional representations of an object. For these reasons and others, it is necessary to develop detection methods that at least approach, and in many respects surpass, the signal processing capabilities of the eye and that are amenable to further enhancement techniques. The task is important because, at present, the design goal of achieving the highest SNR in a confocal image for a given dose to the specimen is often degraded by elements in the detection system. When light levels are low (<20 photons/pixel) significant improvements in SNR can often be made by employing direct photon-counting techniques rather than traditional analog measurement schemes. (See Fig. 9 and also Chapter 2)

In this chapter we will consider the quantal nature of light and the interaction of photons with materials. We will compare a number of possible detectors in terms of their quantum efficiency, responsivity, spectral response, inherent noise, response time and linearity. We will then consider the design constraints in terms of the front-end circuitry that digitizes the data. The figures of merit for detection are usually that the estimate of the signal is limited either by the noise within the signal or by the background radiation. No physical detector can improve on these limits, and the response is always suboptimal. Finally, we will consider problems arising in available instruments and suggest future directions toward a more perfect detector with signal processing capabilities limited only by the stochastic nature of the signal. We will begin by considering the kinetic energy of photons.

THE QUANTAL NATURE OF LIGHT

At very low light levels, two aspects of the quantal nature of light can be demonstrated. First, each particle, or photon, has an associated kinetic energy. An incident photon stream transfers kinetic energy to a material and gives rise to the variety of effects used in light detection. Second, at low light levels it is apparent that even with perfect detection, the estimate of the intensity of a source is limited by the statistics of photon arrival at the detector. The statistical nature of photon flux will be considered in a later section.

Consider first the kinetic energy of a photon incident on a detector. The classical frequency of electromagnetic radiation, ν (s^{-1}), is related to the quantum mechanical kinetic energy, E (J), of an individual photon, by $E = h\nu$, where h is Planck's constant (6.626×10^{-34} in Js). The relation between the frequency, ν, and the wavelength, λ(in m), is given by: $\nu = c/\lambda$, where c is the velocity of light (2.997×10^8 ms^{-1}). Each photon in monochromatic green light, $\lambda = 550$ nm, has a kinetic energy of 3.58×10^{-19} joules, or 2.25 electron volts (eV). The human eye is sensitive to light with wavelengths between 400 and 700 nm. In confocal microscopy, the range of molecular probes used in biological experiments will most likely fluoresce at wavelengths that range from the ultraviolet to the near infrared, from say, 300 nm to 1200 nm. The associated photons will have kinetic energies between 4.16 and 1.03 eV. These modest energy levels will necessarily restrict the types of materials and the techniques that can be used for photon detection.

INTERACTION OF PHOTONS WITH MATERIALS

When metals or semiconductors are illuminated, the photons may be either reflected or absorbed. If they are absorbed, the kinetic energy, KE, of the photon is imparted to the structure. This energy may be transformed into a random motion as heat, or it may have a direct effect that changes the arrangement of charges in the crystal lattice of the material (Kittel, 1986). These direct effects are the bases of a number of *internal* and *external* techniques of photon detection.

Thermal effects do not depend on the photon nature of light and the response of the material depends on the radiant power, not the spectral content of the radiation. Thermal effects are characterized by changes in properties of a material arising from an increase in temperature due to the absorption of radiation.

Heating and cooling of a macroscopic detector is slower than techniques in which photons interact directly with electrons in the material. Roughly speaking, thermal effects are on a millisecond timescale, and photon effects are on microsecond or nanosecond timescales. In confocal microscopy, the slow response and lower sensitivity of thermal detectors as compared to direct photodetectors would restrict their use as primary detectors. They could, however, be used to calibrate the system because their response is independent of the radiation wavelength. The performance of thermopiles, Golay cells, bolometers and pyroelectric thermal detectors have been reviewed by Putley (1977) and will not be considered further here.

In direct photodetection, the photons interact directly with electrons in the material. These electrons can either be free or they can be bound to lattice or impurity atoms. For reasons of speed and sensitivity, the detectors used in confocal microscopy will generally be of the photon detection class. In metals and semiconductors, electrons are bound to their atoms within the material by electrostatic force. The average strength of this force is described by the material's ionization energy, or work function. An electron with energy greater than this can escape from the atom. The smallest ionization energy for any elemental solid is ~2.1 eV of metallic Cs. If an electron in solid Cs absorbs a photon with a KE ≥ 2.1 eV, a direct photoeffect can occur. The ionization energies of a number of materials are given in Table 1. Given the low KE of photons in the visible range, the materials employed for direct photodetection will almost always be semiconductors.

TABLE 1. WORK FUNCTIONS AND FORBIDDEN ENERGY GAPS FOR COMMON MATERIALS USED IN DIRECT PHOTODETECTORS

Metals	Work Function, emission from bulk material, eV.	Semi-conductors	Forbidden energy gaps, eV.
Be	3.67	CdS	2.40
Mg	3.66	CdSe	1.80
Ca	2.71	CdTe	1.50
Sr	2.24	GaP	2.24
Li	2.49	GaAs	1.35
Ba	2.38	Si	1.12
Na	2.29	Ge	0.67
K	2.24		
Rb	2.16		
Cs	2.14		

Direct photon effects can be divided into two classes, internal and external. Internal effects are those in which the electrons or holes stay within the material. Internal effects can be further subdivided in three ways: those in which the incident photon interacts with a bound electron; those in which the photon interacts with carriers that are already free; and those in which the photon produces a localized excitation of an electron into a higher energy state within the atom. The external photoeffect, or photoemissive effect, is one in which the photon causes emission of an electron from the surface of the absorbing material known as the photocathode. External devices often charge-multiply this free electron, producing gain. Of all the possible direct detection methods, the most often used are the photoconductive, photovoltaic, and photoemissive.

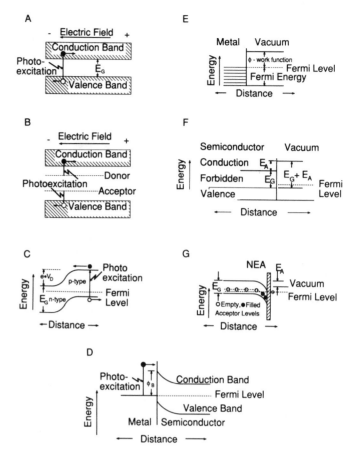

FIG. 1.   Direct photodetector energy-band models (energy vs distance). A. Energy profile of intrinsic photoconductivity producing an electron (filled circle) and a hole (open circle). B. Energy profile of extrinsic photoconductivity producing either a free electron or a free hole. C. Field induced separation of charge in the photovoltaic effect. D. Energy profile at the metal semiconductor interface of a Shottky diode. E. Energy profile for emission from classic photocathode material. F. Energy profile for emission from semiconductor photocathodes. G. Energy profile for emission from Negative Electron Affinity photocathodes.

Photoconductivity

In photodetectors exploiting the phenomena of photoconductivity, a photon effect is manifested by an increase in the free electron or hole concentration that causes an increase in the electrical conductivity of a material. Intrinsic photoconductivity occurs if the photon has enough kinetic energy to produce an electron/hole pair (Fig. 1a). Extrinsic photoconductivity occurs when an incident photon produces excitation at an impurity center in the form of either a free electron / bound hole, or a free hole / bound electron (Fig. 1b). In general, photoconductivity is a majority carrier phenomena, which corresponds to an increase in the number of electrons in an n-type semiconductor, or an increase in the number of holes in a p-type material. The minority carriers will also contribute, but with shorter lifetimes, their contributions are less. A circuit to detect the photoconductive effect is shown in Fig. 2a.

Photovoltaic

Unlike the photoconductive effect, the photovoltaic effect requires an internal potential barrier and field that separate the photoexcited hole-electron pair. This occurs at a simple p-n junction, but can be observed in p-i-n diodes, Schottky barrier diodes, and avalanche diodes as well. The field-induced charge

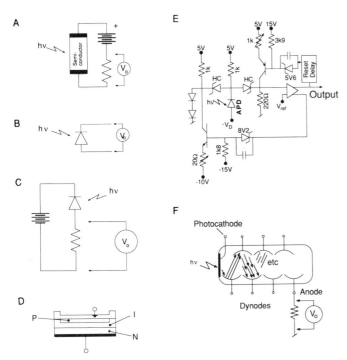

FIG. 2.   Direct photodetection circuits. A. Photoconductivity measurement using a bias voltage and measuring the voltage drop across the series resistor. B. Photovoltaic effect measures the potential difference generated across a simple p–n junction. C. Measurement of the voltage drop across a series resistor produced by the photocurrent through a reverse biased photodiode. D. Geometry of p-i-n photodiode with narrow intrinsic region between the p and n regions. E. Active quenching circuit for an avalanche photodiode (Brown, Jones, Rarity & Ridley, 1987). F. Charge multiplication as photoelectrons are accelerated along dynode chain by high potential between cathode and anode. Charge is converted to a potential difference across the load resistor at the anode.

Avalanche occurs in p-n diodes of moderate doping under reverse bias. Photoexcited or thermally excited electrons or holes are accelerated in the high field region of the junction. As they are accelerated, they collide with the structure and free more electrons. Thus, as the name implies, an avalanche of electrons occurs in the high field region. The advantage of the avalanche photodiode over other types of photodiodes is that it has internal gain. Under identical conditions, the response of such a diode is larger than that of the p-n diode. This internal gain cannot increase the SNR inherent in the detector, but it reduces the stringency of the noise and gain requirements of following stages. The high amplitude of the output and the speed of the response make avalanche diodes attractive for confocal microscopy, but the avalanche multiplication factor varies with the position of the initial photon absorption so the signal must be discriminated to remain a true measure of photon number. Additional difficulties with implementing avalanche diodes focus on the design of active drive circuits (Fig. 2e) that rapidly quench the avalanche response (Brown, Ridley & Rarity, 1986; Brown, Jones, Rarity & Ridley, 1987). Because of their inherent speed and gain, avalanche diodes are often used in extremely rapid kinetic measurements performed at low repetition rates. Low repetition is necessary since the response to an incident photon must be quenched before the arrival of a subsequent one.

Charge Coupled Devices

Photoconductive or photovoltaic effects can be used to produce free carriers which can then be injected into the transport structure of charge coupled devices (Boyle & Smith, 1970). Metal-insulator-semiconductor and metal-oxide-semiconductor capacitors in these devices can be used to store photogenerated electrons (Fig. 3a). Appropriate doping of the semiconductor substrate can be used to match the device to the wavelength of interest, and quantum efficiencies of greater than 85% can be achieved with commercially available devices when back-illuminated through the substrate (Fairchild, 1987). Generally these devices are packaged as either linear (Coutures & Boucharlat, 1988) or 2D arrays (Hier, Zheng, Beaver, McIlwain, & Schmidt, 1988, Mackay, 1988, McMullan, 1988), and are not available as simple elemental detectors. Since these devices have such high apparent quantum efficiency, they should be naturally suited to the low-light requirements of confocal microscopy. First, however, it should be noted that by their design (Fig. 3b), the 2D arrays will not have an available detector over the entire surface of the array. A percentage of the substrate will be occupied by the transport electronics, and will be unavailable for primary imaging. Consequently, though the material may naturally have high quantum efficiency, a large fraction of the surface area of the device may be unavailable for photon capture. Secondly, since the difference in the number of electrons in each potential well represents the spatial variation of light incident on the detector, it is crucial that this variation be preserved as packets of charge are transferred along the CCD to the output (Fig. 3b2). Incomplete transfer of charge packets, and the inability to transfer charge down the CCD structure in the absence of bias-, thermal-, or photon-generated electrons in all the wells presently limits the utility of these devices in applications where there may be large expanses of the field that are dark (Coutures & Boucharlat, 1988).

separation accompanying photoexcitation is shown in Fig. 1c. By definition the photovoltaic effect is obtained at zero bias voltage, i.e., the open circuit voltage (Fig. 2b). However, these detectors are frequently operated under reverse bias, so that the observed signal is a photocurrent (see, for example, the following avalanche diode section) rather than a photovoltage (Fig. 2c). In contrast to photoconductive phenomena, the photovoltaic effect is dependent on the minority carrier lifetime because the presence of both the majority and minority carriers is necessary for the intrinsic effect to be observed. Consequently, since the lifetimes of the minority carriers are less than those of majority carriers, the frequency response of photovoltaic detectors is higher than that of photoconductive devices.

P-i-n diodes differ from p-n diodes in that a region of intrinsic material is incorporated between the two doped regions (Fig. 2d). Absorption of incident radiation in the intrinsic region produces electron/hole pairs. Because of the high collection voltage and the small distance across the intrinsic material, the electron/hole pairs will drift rapidly through this region. As a consequence, the frequency response of a p-i-n diode will be higher than a comparable p-n diode (Mathur, McIntyre, & Webb, 1970).

The Schottky diode is formed at a metal-semiconductor interface (Fig. 1d). Such an interface forms a potential barrier that causes separation of electrons and holes. These devices are especially useful at ultra-high frequencies, and are often used as optical receivers operating in the GHz range (Sharpless, 1970).

A

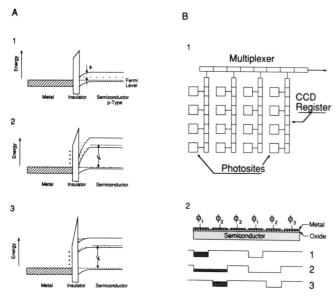

B

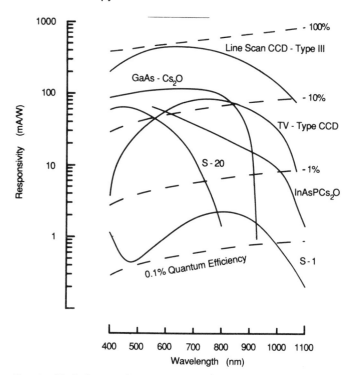

FIG. 3. Charge coupled devices used in photodetection. A. Energy vs distance profile in metal-insulator-semiconductor n-channel structure. The initial bands (1) are changed after application of a gate voltage V_G (2) and charge builds up at the insulator-semiconductor interface until equilibrium is approached (3). B. (1) Two dimensional devices can be built from an array of discrete photosites and CCD arrays arranged to sequentially shift out and read the charge packets collected at each photosite. (2) Method of transfer of charge packet along MIS CCD structure. Overlapping clocks transfer charge between neighboring electrodes.

FIG. 4. Typical spectral-response curves for internal and external direct photodetector materials.

Photoemissive

The third direct photon detection technique is photoemissive, also known as the external photoeffect. The incident radiation causes the emission of an electron from the surface of the absorbing material (Einstein, 1905), the photocathode, into the surrounding space (Fig. 1e,f,g), from whence it is collected by an anode. Photoemissive effects are used in simple vacuum phototubes, composed of a simple cathode and anode. They are very fast. They are also found in devices that interpose gain, such as gas-filled phototubes that rely on the avalanche effect of photoelectrons striking the gas within the tube. In the familiar photomultiplier tube, PMT, the primary photoelectron strikes a series of emissive surfaces interposed between the photocathode and the anode. At each surface the number of electrons emitted is multiplied, until at the anode millions of electrons may be collected for each photoelectron originally emitted from the photocathode (Fig. 2f).

Two special forms of photoemissive device should be mentioned, the image dissector and the microchannel plate. In addition to the fast response, wide spectral sensitivity, and photon counting capabilities of the usual types of PMTs, these devices have position sensitivity and can be used as full-field detectors.

Image dissector

A novel approach that combines the aperture and detection problems in confocal microscopy is the use of the image dissector tube (Goldstein, 1989). The image dissector consists of the usual photocathode and photomultiplier dynode chain. Between the two, in an image plane for the photoelectrons, a small aperture is centered in the field. Deflection coils sweep the image across the aperture, and only those electrons passing through the aperture undergo multiplication. All others are discarded. This type of field detector differs from normal vidicon tubes and CCD arrays in that integration does not take place in the detector between scans. Rather it functions as a movable point detector, and in this capacity can be used to electronically track the illuminated spot in a confocal microscope.

Microchannel plate

The microchannel plate photomultiplier, MCP-PMT, differs from the usual PMT by replacing the chain of discrete dynodes with a channel of continuous photomultiplication. The MCPs are secondary multipliers consisting of an array of capillary tubes, or channels, fused together to form a plate. The tube diameter can be as small as a few μm, and the interior of each is coated with a photoemissive compound. A high-voltage electric field is imposed along the length of the tube. Photons entering one end of the tube at an angle strike the channel wall with sufficient energy to generate secondary electrons. These electrons are accelerated and in turn strike the wall farther down the tube, and the process is repeated. Gains of 10^4 to 10^6 can result from this series of collisions (Kume, Koyama, Nakatsuga, & Fatlowitz, 1988). The MCP can thus serve as an intermediate gain stage in front of lower sensitivity detectors.

Detectors vary widely in their response properties. A comparison of the quantum efficiency, responsivity, spectral response, response time, and linearity of direct photodetectors is given in Table 2. Unlike thermal detectors, the response of direct photodetectors depends on the photon nature of light. Therefore, the response of the detector varies with the wavelength of radiation. The direct detectors differ widely in their maximum sensitivity and quantum efficiency. Graphs of the spectral response for examples of direct detectors are given in

TABLE 2.   RESPONSE PROPERTIES OF SAMPLE DIRECT PHOTODETECTORS

Type of Detector	Quantum Efficiency	Radiant Sensitivity (A/W)	Spectral Range	Response (nm) Peak	Response (seconds)	Range	Type
Silicon		0.4	190–1000	720	5×10^{-7}	10^{-11}–10^{-3}W	Hamanatsu S 1227
Photodiode	80.0%	0.5	190–1100	920	2×10^{-7}	10^{-11}–10^{-3}W	Hamamatsu S 1337
PIN Silicon Photodiode	83.0%	0.6	190–1060	900	3×10^{-9}	10^{-11}–10^{-2}W	Hamamatsu S 1721
GaAsP	—	0.18	190–680	610	1×10^{-6}	10^{-13}–10^{-3}W	Hamamatsu S 1025
Photodiode (Schottky)		0.22	190–760	710	0.8×10^{-6}	10^{-13}–10^{-3}W	Hamamatsu S 1745
Avalanche Photodiode	70.0%	—	350–1050	830	0.2×10^{-9}	2×10^6 cts/s	Hamamatsu S 2381
PMTs							
S-1	0.5%	2.5×10^{-3}	300–1100	800	15ns (FWHM)	5×10^7 cts/s	Thorn-EMI-9684
S-20	23.0%	64.0×10^{-3}	300–850	420	25ns (FWHM)	3.3×10^7 cts/s	Thorn-EMI-9890
GaAs:Cs-O	17.0%	120.0×10^{-3}	200–950	850			RCA–Type 60 ER
CCD linear	85.0%	4.5V/mJ cm^{-2}	330–950	680	50ns/pixel readout	7500:1	Fairchild CCD–134
CCD Areal 488 × 380 elements	15.0%	0.08V/mW cm^{-2}	500–1000	800	@ 60 Hz field rate	1000:1	Fairchild CCD–222

Fig. 4. PMTs with classic photocathode materials have greatest sensitivity in the blue to UV (QE ≤ 35%). The short wavelength limits are functions of the envelope materials rather than the photocathode materials and can be extended by using quartz and fluorite faceplates. Semiconductors are attractive photoemissive materials since they have high quantum efficiency at longer wavelengths and can be designed with ionization energies or work functions that match the wavelength of interest. As such they will be useful in the future either as negative electron affinity, NEA, emissive materials for cathodes and dynodes in PMTs or as solid-state detectors (QE ≤ 85%).

NOISE INTERNAL TO DETECTORS

An ideal detector would be one in which detection is limited by the noise or background of the radiant source, and no additional noise is added by the detector or subsequent amplification and conversion electronics. With present techniques, it is possible to design amplification and conversion stages with noise below that of the zero-signal output of the detector (Siliconix, 1986). Therefore, the detection scheme will generally be limited by the noise of the detector stage itself. We will consider the noise inherent in both internal and external devices in turn. Formal expression of each noise contribution is given in Table 3 as the noise power obtained by summing the contributions of the independent noise sources in quadrature (Schwartz, 1970).

Internal detection with semiconductor devices is associated with two general classes of noise. The first is measurable in the absence of an applied bias voltage. It arises from the thermal motion of charge carriers within a material and is known as Johnson, Nyquist, or thermal noise. The second category of noise sources is only measurable in the presence of a bias voltage, and is specific to the type of device and the variable meas-

ured in the photoconversion process. In photoconductors there also exists generation—recombination (g-r) noise, which is due to fluctuations in the rates of thermal generation and recombination of charge carriers, giving rise to a fluctuation in the average carrier concentration. This in turn is measured as a variation in average resistance. Complete analysis of g-r noise can be found in Van der Ziel (1959) and Burgess (1956). In diodes with an applied bias, shot noise is apparent. This noise is due to the quantal nature of current carriers and results in a statistical variation in the amplitude of the measured current. The final form of noise, which is not strictly amenable to analytic treatment, is 1/f noise, so named because the power varies more or less inversely with frequency.

For external photoemissive devices the limit to detection is given by the dark current. This current has three origins: ohmic leakage, thermionic emission from the cathode and dynodes, and regenerative effects. Ohmic leakage is a breakdown between active leads along the insulating material of the tube. It can be identified at low acceleration voltages by the linear relation between the voltage and the measured current. At higher voltages the thermionic component, formally equivalent to shot noise, becomes apparent because thermally generated electrons from the cathode (or first dynode) undergo the same multiplication as do photoelectrons. And the amplitude of this component will increase in parallel with the amplitude of the PMT response under low light conditions. This component of the noise is dependent on temperature and can be reduced by cooling the tube.

At higher voltages, regenerative effects can come in and can include the glow of the dynodes under electron bombardment. Glowing of the glass envelope also occurs as photoelectrons impact the tube wall if it is not at the cathode potential. This effect can be eliminated either by keeping the envelope at a negative potential, or by providing it with a shield at such a potential. After-pulses can also occur. One type is the result of

TABLE 3. NOISE CURRENTS IN DIRECT PHOTODETECTORS

All sources considered to be independent, and total noise current is the square root of the sum of the squares of the contributing currents. Abbreviations: B, bandwidth of measurement; C, shunt capacitance of anode lead; d, dynode gain; e, charge on an electron; f, frequency; g, shunt conductance of the anode lead; I, dark current; I_B, bias current; k, Boltzman's constant; K, multiplicative constant; M, charge multiplication or gain; N, number of electrons; P, number of holes R_L, load resistance; R_N, equivalent noise resistance of amplifier input; T, temperature in degrees kelvin; τ, carrier lifetime; ω, angular frequency. NEP calculations are rough estimates for each class of detectors. Noise effects due to the noise-in-signal and that resulting from converter Q.E. < 1 have not been included.

Type of Detector	Johnson Noise	Generation-Recombination Noise	Shot Noise	1/f Noise	Multiplication Noise	NEP (W/Hz$^{-1/2}$) Noise Equiv. Power
	$i_J=(4kTB/R_L)^{1/2}$ Peak Sensitivity (A/W) due to resistive components		$i_s=(2eIB)^{1/2}$ due to bias current	$i_F=(KI_B{\sim}^2B/f{\sim}^1)^{1/2}$ due to conjunctions with external conductors		Value at which SNR = 1
Extrinsic photo-detectors	same	$i_{grn}=2I_B(\tau B/N (1+\omega^2\tau^2))^{1/2}$	same	same	N.A.	
Intrinsic photo-detectors	same	$i_{grn}=(2I_B/N)(P\tau B/(1+\omega^2\tau^2))^{1/2}$	same	same	N.A.	
Avalanche photodiodes	same	N.A.	N.A.	same	$i_M=M(2eIBM)^{1/2}$	$\sim10^{-14}$
PMT alone	same	N.A.	N.A.	N.A.	$i_a=M(2eIB)^{1/2}(1+(1/(\zeta-1)))^{1/2}$	$\sim10^{-17}$
I-V converter Noise						
PMT & electronics	$(4kTgB(1+R_{Lg}+(4\pi^{2/3})(R_{N/g})B^2C^2))^{1/2}$	N.A.	N.A.	N.A.	same	N.A.

feedback from the dynodes to the photocathode (due to light given off from the dynode that impacts the photocathode and consequently gives off more electrons). This after-pulsing has a short delay (40–50 ns) after the initial pulse. A second type of after-pulse is due to the ionization of residual gases that are in the tube or are adsorbed in the envelope. Most prevalent are N_2^+ and H_2^+ ions that are accelerated back toward the negative cathode, giving rise to further electron emission. (The delay is somewhat longer, on the order of a few 100 ns.) Tubes run near a cooled helium environment will have troubles since the helium will permeate through the glass envelope and will remain within the tube (RCA, 1980).

Further sources of noise arise from radioactive elements within the glass, such as ^{40}K, or due to cosmic rays. Additional noise is often produced after exposure of the tube to blue or near-UV light. Normally this is due to fluorescent room lights, though it is likely to be an increasing problem in experiments where near UV light is used to stimulate the chromophores such as Fura-2 and Indo-1 indicators used in the study of $[Ca^{++}]_i$.

The statistics of the effects of these noise sources will be considered next, along with the necessary probabilistic effect of the finite quantum efficiency of the original production of photoelectrons at the photocathode.

Statistics of Photon Flux and Detectors

Several of the parameters of direct photodetector behavior were given in Table 2. Many of the noise contributions for each detector are summarized in Table 3. In practice, the utility of the various detectors will be determined not only by the speed of the response necessary to represent the unique values at each pixel, but also the absolute sensitivity of the device. In this section we will consider a figure of merit, the achievable signal-to-noise ratio, SNR, of the PMT, to demonstrate how the threshold sensitivity of a device is analyzed and predicted. This is not the only figure of merit that could be used for detectors. At the outset we suggested that confocal microscopy might examine light with wavelengths from the UV to the near IR. At the longer wavelengths the performance is limited by the background level of IR radiation. Comparisons of alternative figures of merit for detector function can be found in Seib & Aukerman, (1973). In general, noise sources will either be additive or multiplicative. Additive noise, for example, is the noise added by the process of photoemission at the photocathode to the noise already present in the original photon flux. We can perform a straightforward analysis of the behavior of a detector in terms of the degradation of the SNR (Robben, 1971).

The detection process is limited at the front end by the SNR of photon flux. If the average rate of emission of photons is I_p, then during the observation interval τ the average observation is $n_p = I_p\tau$, and the variance is given by $\sigma_p^2 = I_p\tau = n_p$. The SNR is given by: $SNR = n_p/\sigma_p = (I_p\tau)^{1/2} = (n_p)^{1/2}$.

For any photon incident on the photocathode, the quantum efficiency, η, is the product of three probabilities. The first is the probability that a photon will be absorbed rather than transmitted or reflected. The second is the probability that this photon will produce a free electron. The third stands for the probability that the free electron will actually reach the surface of the material and escape. Therefore, for all real materials, $\eta < 1$. Since the probability of release of a photoelectron per incident photon is related by the quantum efficiency, η, then $n_{pe} = \eta I_p \tau$. The variance of the number of photoelectrons, $\sigma_{pe}^2 = \eta I_p \tau$. Consequently, at the stage of emission of photoelectrons from the photocathode, we can reduce the signal-to-noise ratio to $SNR_{pe} = (\eta I_p \tau)^{1/2}$. The only way to improve on this SNR would be to use a material with the highest possible quantum efficiency, such as a NEA material.

During any recording period, τ, thermionic electrons will be emitted. The average number of these emissions is n_d, and their variance, $\sigma_{pe}^2 = n_d$. In all practical cases the SNR of photoemission is determined from the total emission, which is a combination of the terms due to photoelectrons and thermionic electrons. The number of photoevents, $n_{pe} = n_c - n_d = \eta I_p \tau$, where c and d indicate composite and dark terms respectively. Since the photoevents and the thermal ones are independent, the square of the variances add, $\sigma_{pe}^2 = \eta I \tau + n_d$. Thus, in the presence of dark noise the SNR of a realizable PMT is given by

$$SNR_{pe} = (\eta I_p \tau)/(\eta I_p \tau + n_d)^{1/2}.$$

Now consider what happens if we interpose j dynode stages all having identical gains, δ_j, and Poisson statistics of secondary emission. The gain seen at the anode will be $m = \delta_1 \cdot \delta_2 \ldots \delta_j$. The anode variance, $\sigma_a^2 = \eta n_p m^2 [\{1 + 1/(\delta-1)\} \cdot \{1 - (1/\delta_j)\}]$. If, for example, we use negative affinity materials and in each stage the gain, δ, is large, then term $1/\delta_j$ will be very small. Thus

$$\sigma_a^2 \simeq \eta n_p m^2 [1 + 1/(\delta-1)].$$

The corresponding SNR is given by

$$SNR \simeq [\eta n_p (\delta-1)/\delta]^{1/2}.$$

Which, if the gains are high, reduces to

$$SNR \simeq [\eta n_p]^{1/2}.$$

Thus, for any device with high gain at each stage the performance will be dominated by the quantum efficiency of the first stage, or perhaps by the photocathode and the statistics of the first dynode. In terms of current, the SNR_a at the anode for a PMT is given for two cases in Table 3. The first is for the current alone, and the second includes the noise contributed by the output circuit noise in the amplifier. A complete analysis using generating functions to predict the total noise of a detector system based on additive and multiplicative noise sources is given in (Jorgensen, 1984; Prescott, 1966).

Representing the Pixel Value

In the majority of confocal microscopes, the image is constructed sequentially from the output of a point detector. Ideally, the digitized value at each pixel should reflect the average detector response during the time the beam dwells on a point in the field. Two problems must be considered. First, can we define a suitable means of sampling the response of the detector over the period used to estimate a pixel value? Second, since the goal of confocal microscopy is to achieve the maximum resolution, how do we avoid degrading the image with spurious correlation between the sampled values at neighboring pixels? Ideally the measure of intensity would be an average of the detector response for the time of interest. For ease of manufacture and implementation, however, such a scheme is often approximated by the use of a capacitive integration (Fig. 5a). The time constant, τ, of such an integrator is often chosen to be 1/4 the pixel dwell time. Such an integrator has the advantage that, in some sense, it represents a running average of the detector output. Unfortunately, it can be shown (Jones, Oliver & Pike, 1971) that this form of integration results in a 2% correlation between neighboring pixels. (If the Nyquist bandwidth, as defined in Chapter 4 has been correctly chosen to be $1/2\pi\tau$, the signal will correlate between adjacent pixels by the same amount.) This correlation can be avoided by the use of true integration of the detector signal, whether this be in photon counting (Figs. 5b,c), or analog detection schemes (Fig. 5d). Other advantages of full integration will be considered specifically with photon counting and with analog detection.

At low light levels ($\leq 10^8$ photons/s), direct photon counting strategies have advantages over analog methods of light intensity estimation. The large gain inherent in most PMT designs is itself a distinct advantage in many photon counting techniques since these tubes produce large pulses that are well above other sources of noise in the tube or in the subsequent electronics. In PMTs designed and selected for photon counting, the pulses produced by single photon events are tightly distributed and widely separated from the amplitude of pulses produced by multiple photon events. It is possible with modest acceleration voltages to produce well-defined charge packets that develop mV pulses of ns duration across a 50Ω load. Further, removal of any variation in pulse amplitude at the load resistor can be accomplished by comparing the height of the pulse across the resistor with two well-defined thresholds. The lower threshold defines the minimum height of a pulse considered to be due to a single photoelectron emitted from the photocathode, multiplied along the dynode chain, and collected by the anode. The upper threshold is greater than the pulse height produced by a majority of single photoelectron events, and pulses exceeding this height are likely to represent multiple-photon events or other artifacts. The output of this two-stage detection scheme can be used to trigger a well-defined and tightly controlled pulse of known amplitude and duration. A minimum interval between pulses can be imposed to eliminate possible PMT artifacts such as those produced by correlated after-pulsing. Typically, pulses as short as 15 ns with a dead time between pulses of 5 ns can be used. Both Schottky TTL and ECL logic families are fast enough to count at the implied maximum rate of 50 MHz.

True integration of standard pulses can be accomplished as shown in Fig. 5b, c. In the analog method, pulses are directly integrated on a capacitor. Prior to integration the capacitor is shorted to ground by a switch. During the integration, the shorting switch is open. In response to a series of input pulses, the voltage measured across the capacitor rises in a staircase fashion, with the rise at each step determined by the size of the capacitor and the magnitude and duration of the input pulses. At the end of the integration period, the analog voltage is converted to a digital value using an ADC, and the capacitor is then reset. A duplicate capacitor and switch are arranged so that the capacitors integrate on alternate pixels, avoiding the loss of photon counts during ADC and capacitor resetting.

In the digital method, the pulses increment a TTL or ECL counter. At the end of the integration period, the count is latched in an output register. The counter is reset and begins

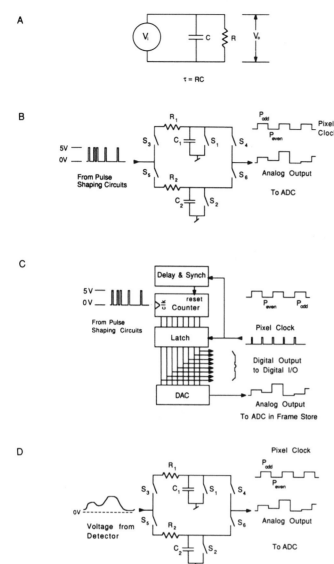

FIG. 5. Methods of photon quantification. A. RC integration. Charge or current from photodetector is changed into a voltage, and a running average is stored on a capacitor. Resistor in parallel should insure that the voltage across the capacitor decays with a time constant appropriate for the pixel dwell time but as this changes with scan zoom setting, the condition is not always met. B. Analog method of photon counting. During alternate pixels the upper and the lower half of the schematic circuit are used. During odd pixels charge pulses generated by detected photons are stored on C_1. At the end of the pixel S_3 is opened and the value on capacitor C_1 is converted to a digital word. This value is held for the duration of the pixel and then the capacitor is reset. While this conversion is taking place, the photon pulses for the next even pixel are accumulated on capacitor C_2, and the process is repeated. C. Digital method of photon counting. ECL or TTL logic is used to count the photon pulses and output is by way of digital word or DAC conversion back to a video voltage. D. Direct integration method used to store an analog output voltage. The circuit assumes that subsequent digital processing of the signal is used to normalize the response with respect to pixel dwell time.

accumulating counts for the next pixel. Additional logic can be configured to eliminate the loss of photon counts during output latching. The output of the digital latch can be used directly as input for the image buffer, or the value can be converted back into a standard video voltage with a digital-to-analog converter, DAC. One attraction of the digital technique is that once the

PMT pulses have been converted to logic levels, the process of integration with digital counters is immune to noise problems inherent in further analog processing. For either method of photon counting, with pixel dwell times on the order of a microsecond, we would expect at most a few tens of photons to be counted. The small number of distinct signal levels represented by these photons could easily be converted to the range of standard video between 0 and 0.75 Volts, and used as input to a typical 8-bit video ADC and frame grabber. Such a device would convert each voltage to a number between zero and 255.

For high light levels ($\geq 10^8$ photons/s) that might be typical of reflectance confocal microscopy as used in metallurgy or in the inspection of integrated circuits, the extreme measures needed to maximize the SNR under low light levels are unnecessary. A variety of different diode detectors with current-to-voltage converters can be used as, in these detectors, each photon absorbed deposits an identical amount of charge. In these instances, the output is continuous rather than discrete. Traditionally, low-pass filtering of the form of Fig. 5a ($\tau \simeq T/4$) is used to create a running average of the light intensity. The difficulty of pixel correlation remains whenever pixels are bigger than resels. It can be avoided by creating a technique similar to the analog method of integrating pulses in the photon detection scheme, Fig. 5d. With the exception of the fact that the input to the capacitors is a continuous voltage rather than a series of discrete pulses, the technique and the process is identical to the previous case in Fig. 5b though the results will be somewhat degraded by the fact that some photons contribute larger pulses to the total signal than others.

For either discrete or continuous estimates of luminance, the full integration technique is preferred over bandwidth limitation since it avoids the correlations inherent in using a running average. A second advantage is the ease with which different rates of confocal scanning can be implemented. With capacitive integration, the time constant of the integrator must be changed to match different rates of scan and pixel dwell-time and also to compensate for changes in the relative sizes of pixels and resels. With true integration, the match is automatic since the integration begins and ends at times defined by a pixel dwell-time. A third advantage of this technique is that the relative variance of the intensity estimate using full integration is half that obtained using capacitive integration with $\tau = T/4$ (Jones et al, 1971). Consequently, for any desired level of precision, full integration will require fewer frames for an average. This fact is important both in speed of data acquisition and in minimizing photodamage to the sample.

CONVERSION TECHNIQUES

The resolution of the analog-to-digital conversion required for confocal microscopy is determined in part by the detector. For the photon counting example above, all possible pixel values could be described uniquely with an eight-bit binary word. In full-field microscopy, however, a converter would need the resolution of a 14-bit binary word to take advantage of the linearity and large dynamic range of slow-scan CCD arrays. In essence, an ADC needs to have sufficient resolution to avoid degrading the SNR inherent in the conversion of the signal up to that point. The choice of converter is further restricted by the rate at which conversion is required. In general, confocal microscopy is characterized by a relatively high degree of resolution and high rates of digitization.

A

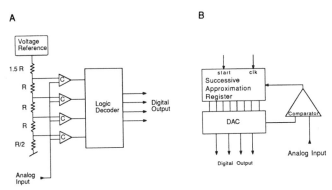

B

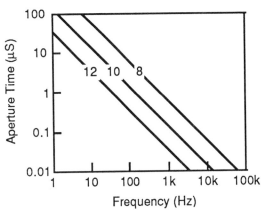

FIG. 7. Aperture time vs frequency of a full scale sinusoidal input for system accuracies to within one half of one least-significant bit error.

FIG. 6. Converter types. A. Parallel A/D converter in which the analog input is simultaneously compared with four reference levels. The delay through the system is determined by the logic delay, and conversion is very rapid. B. Successive approximation A/D converter. On each clock cycle the digital input to the DAC is toggled starting with the most significant bit. The output of the DAC is compared with the analog input and if the DAC voltage is too great, the test bit is set to zero. The next significant bit is then tested in turn until, for an n-bit conversion, after n cycles the closest n-bit approximation to the analog input is found. Since n clock cycles are used, the time used with this method of conversion may be relatively long.

Of the types of converters available, only flash and successive approximation converters (Fig. 6) will be considered. The flash converter uses multiple comparators and simultaneously compares the analog input with all analog code levels. The speed of conversion is limited only by comparator speed and the propagation delays through the logic. The successive approximation technique, on the other hand, operates on a feedback principle. The analog input and the output of a DAC are compared with a single comparator. The DAC is controlled by the output of a digital register whose bits are changed successively until the closest possible match is achieved between the DAC output and the analog input. This technique is relatively time consuming, and conversion often takes as much as a microsecond.

The rate of conversion and therefore the time window during which a conversion takes place is of prime importance when choosing the method and resolution of the converter. During the time that the conversion is taking place, it is critical that the input change by less than the amount coded by the least significant bit. If the input changes by more than this amount the conversion will be incorrect. This problem arises due to the uncertainty in the time aperture during which the conversion is performed. For the true integration schemes illustrated above, the problem does not arise since the output of the integrators is arranged to be constant for a large percentage of the pixel interval, and all that is required is that the conversion take place within this interval. For all the techniques that use a variant of the capacitive integration, the voltage will be changing during the period of conversion. In the capacitive integration we chose a τ equal to 1/4 the pixel dwell-time. For sampling periods of $1\mu s$, $\tau = 250$ ns, the integrator is equivalent to an RC filter with half-power band-width, or 3dB point, of roughly 640kHz. It is sobering to consider that to convert a sinusoidal voltage accurately at this frequency to 8-bit resolution the sampling aperture uncertainty would need to be shorter than one ns. The relationship between the desired resolution of the conversion, the frequency of a sinusoidal input, and the necessary aperture is given in Fig. 7.

To minimize problems created by the conversion aperture, either the converter must be extraordinarily fast or an additional component that samples and holds the input signal must be interposed between the detector and the converter. Such devices are similar to our integrator schemes in that they sample the analog input on a capacitor for a brief interval, and then the capacitor is disconnected from the input during the period that the conversion takes place. Consequently, the problems of rapidly sampling the input are transferred from the converter to the sampling-and-holding device. The ideal device for confocal microscopy must not only have a very short aperture uncertainty but must also obtain the input voltage on the sampling capacitor to the desired resolution within a small fraction of the pixel dwell-time.

Because the output of this conversion is only certain to within 1/2 of a least significant bit, the converter can be viewed as an additional source of uncertainty or noise. With an 8-bit converter this noise is relatively small compared to the sources mentioned previously. This is a necessary result of the finite resolution of the converter. In general, the dynamic range of the converter should be matched to the dynamic range of the detector. For example, if the SNR in the detector output is 1000, or 60dB, then the converter output should be at least 10 bits to permit an equivalent resolution. (See also Chapter 4.)

ASSESSMENT OF DEVICES

With a number of laser-scanning and disk-scanning confocal microscopes presently reduced to practice and available in the marketplace, it is convenient at this moment to consider aspects of practical instruments that can be examined to determine if the behavior of the implemented detection systems have been optimized. Of the possible detector schemes, we shall consider one for each type: the PMT for point detection, and the CCD for full-field detection.

Point Detection Optimization

Of current devices available for point detection, the PMT in photon-counting mode is the most suitable for low light tasks with fluxes of less than 10^8 photons/s and a λ shorter than 500 nm. Most present microscopes using PMTs convert the anode current into a voltage and use this output as a measure of the

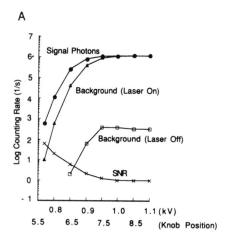

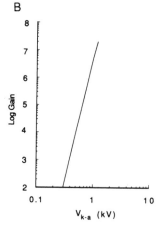

FIG. 8a. Behavior of BioRad PMT (Thorn 9828b) versus voltage. Confocal laser head mounted on a Zeiss UEM with a ×40, 0.75 NA water-immersion objective. A Thorn C604 head amplifier was used to generate and detect 1 mV pulses. The head amplifier output consisted of 15 ns ECL pulses with 5 ns deadtime. Responses were counted with the laser off, with the laser on and no object in the field, and with a FITC stained specimen. Fewer than 400 events were counted in the dark. The number of events versus PMT acceleration voltage increased without an object in the plane of focus when the laser was energized and the beam entered the confocal head. The number of counts increased again when a FITC stained object was in the plane of focus. The maximum SNR of near 60 was achieved at PMT voltages between 750 and 850 volts. On our BioRad head this corresponds to gain position between 5.5 and 6.5 but these exact readings may vary from instrument to instrument.
b. Gain versus acceleration voltage for PMT.

incident illumination. Gain can be achieved in such a system by varying the acceleration voltage along the dynode chain, thereby increasing the photoelectron multiplication within the tube (Fig. 8b). However, unfortunately, with progressively larger acceleration voltages, there is a tendency for the internal noise of the PMT to increase. This is particularly noticeable under low or absent light conditions when, with sufficient acceleration, the output of the headstage amplifier will display large-amplitude noise pulses. At lower voltages this noise will be seen to disappear. This is a simple demonstration in the analog mode that the PMTs have a preferred operating range, beyond which the noise of the device increases and the SNR decreases.

Most of the noise sources associated with anode current measurement can be avoided by using photon counting. In this mode SNR is maximized by finding and using the optimal setting for the acceleration voltage. Ideally, such operations are performed using a pulse height analyzer to characterize the amplitude of pulses at the anode both in the dark and under low light conditions. Though such analyzers are rarely part of a typical microscopy laboratory, an alternate strategy can be employed. For pulse counting, the threshold detectors are first fixed at some nominal value, say 1 mV for the lower detector. The output of the discriminator circuit can be counted digitally. Shown in Figure 8a is a comparison of the number of counts vs. acceleration voltage, acquired under no-light and two low-light conditions for the BioRad MRC 500. In the dark, with the laser off, the count rate rises gradually and then plateaus over an extended range (open boxes). Even at acceleration voltages in excess of 1 kV, there are fewer than 400 events detected by a Thorn C604 amplifier/descriminator. Under low light conditions, with the laser on and without neutral density filters attenuating the beam, the count rate versus acceleration voltage was determined under two conditions. In the first case the count was taken without a specimen in the object plane (filled triangles). Ideally, in this case no light would be reflected back through the system and onto the PMT. Apparently, significant light is scattered back through the system and is detected even in the absence of a specimen. When a FITC stained specimen

was placed in the object plane of the microscope, the number of signal photons detected (filled circles) was always greater than the background count. Perhaps because of the scattered light, the SNR of detection was a maximum of 60 at relatively low acceleration voltages between 750 and 850 volts. The SNR dropped dramatically for higher accelerations near 1 kV. For most PMTs the curve under low light conditions is similar to the curve recorded in the dark, but displaced towards higher counts. Therefore, in general there is a particular voltage for each photomultiplier for which the separation between the signal and the background noise is the greatest. The tube should be operated this voltage. Operation at higher voltages will degrade the SNR and, in the BioRad 500, degradation of the SNR is compounded by the additional problem of scattered light within the confocal head. Figure 8b plots the gain versus the acceleration voltage.

Using a fixed, optimal PMT voltage will, however, produce a requirement for variable gain in the pre-ADC amplifier so that the signal output level matches the input of the ADC.

The output of the headstage PMT amplifier is often used as input to a video-rate frame-buffer running in a slow-scan mode. The transmission and digitization stage can often be another source of problems. In one commercial microscope, we noticed that in response to a step change from white to black the detector/digitization system produced a series of damped oscillations or secondary bright levels. The problem could be eliminated by insuring that the transmission cable terminates with a matching impedance at the input of the video board digitization stage.

As mentioned earlier, problems arise from using a capacitive integration technique and the consequent wide variation in output that occurs under certain conditions. Consider the difference in response that results when a photon is incident on the PMT at the beginning and at the end of a pixel dwell time. Under full integration, the output in either case would be the same, and the result would be proportional to a single photon. Under capacitive integration, however, the voltage resulting from the photon that arrived at the beginning of the pixel dwell period would have decayed to 2% of its value by the time that the pixel value was sampled. By comparison, the photon arriving just before the detector voltage was sampled would be at full amplitude. Consequently the output of such a detector/digitization scheme carries with it a random variation of the output dependent on the time of arrival of the incident photons during the integration period. This increase in noise will often prevent achieving a satisfactory SNR with an acceptable number of image scans (See also Chapter 2, Fig. 3b).

The behavior of the PMT amplifier and conversion system can be tested directly by connecting a constant-current pulse generator capable of producing low level steady currents and pulses comparable to those produced by the PMT with optimal acceleration voltage. If a series of pulses comparable to single photon events are produced at a constant rate near, but not equal to, the inverse of the pixel dwell time, then capturing an image frame will reveal the method used to integrate during the pixel. If true integration is used, then the response can be one of three levels, with each pixel having a value equivalent to zero, one, or two pulses. Often it is convenient to map these values to, say, 0, 127, 255 for an 8-bit frame grabber. On the other hand, if capacitive integration is used, the pixel values will assume all values between 0 and 255. Such a result would suggest that the detection and digitization scheme would converge more slowly towards an unbiased estimate of the luminance at the measured point than the full integration method.

Field Detection Optimization

The disk-scanning confocal microscopes require a full-field detection system rather than a point detector. As mentioned in the introduction, the eye is often a suitable device, but suffers under very low light conditions. Alternatively, one could use the normal types of field detectors currently used in video microscopy. A recent review of the field is available (Inoué, 1986). Many of the present-generation imaging devices are inappropriate due to the speed of the response. In addition, in many of the most sensitive tubes there is significant lag or carry-over between the image recorded during one frame scan and the next. Alternatively, a cooled CCD camera could be used as the detector, given its large dynamic range and extraordinarily high quantum efficiency. As noted above, the difficulty that arises with CCD devices is the generation of a noise-equivalent photoelectron signal due to thermal generation during the integration time, to variations in the charge-coupled transfer efficiency, or to random variations in the conversion at the output. To be sure, this noise can be minimized and, for some CCD chips with slow scan readout, the noise can be reduced to 10–20 photon equivalents (rms). However, this still yields peak noise (5σ), readings of nearly 60 photon equivalents in the dark. Such a figure is not ideal under low light conditions. A further problem stems from difficulties in transferring the signal through the charge-coupled process when one of the detection sites contains too few photoelectrons. In this case, transfer along the device may be interrupted until sufficient charge accumulates from adjacent pixels in the row to permit transfer. This problem is likely to be exacerbated for fluorescent images in which there are likely to be large numbers of pixels without any photon hits during the integration period.

Since the distance between detector elements in 2D CCDs is on the order of 10 μm, it is be possible in principle to add a gain stage by interposing a microchannel plate (such as the

Hamamatsu HPK R2809, built with 6μm elements) in front of the CCD (Kume et al, 1988). A modest gain of 100 would bring us clearly above the noise floor of the CCD. Since these CCDs can store as many as 5×10^5 electrons in a well, we would still be able to detect 5000 photoevents before saturating the detector. Unfortunately, since the MCP is manufactured with S1, multi-alkali and bi-alkali photocathodes, we can expect the quantum efficiency of the composite device to be less than that of the CCD. In addition, because of statistical variations in MCP gain, all photons will no longer deposit identical charge in the sensor. However, a benefit of such a strategy is that the MCP can be gated on and off and perhaps phased-locked to periods following an illuminating pulse. In this manner, the kinetics of the response to illumination could be followed on a ns time scale. The response to such an experiment could be integrated simultaneously over the entire field, and after sufficient repetitions the value could be digitized in the usual fashion.

DETECTORS PRESENT AND FUTURE

In conclusion, we will consider two general topics. The first is the means of optimizing the performance of this first generation of confocal microscopes. The second is the specification of the qualities of the ideal detector to use in confocal microscopy. Our goal is to produce images with the least possible illumination of the specimen. In terms of constructing an image, this requires that the average be formed limited only by the uncertainties of photon flux. From the analysis of the contributions of noise sources, the SNR is degraded at each step in the conversion process. As was shown in the section on the statistics of the photon flux and the detector, the first point of departure from the ideal when using a PMT as the detector is the fact that the quantum efficiency of realizable PMTs is less than unity. Consequently, the emission of the photoelectron is itself a second probabilistic event in the cascade, and the SNR is reduced by $(\eta)^{1/2}$, where η is the quantum efficiency. SNR could be enhanced simply by increasing the QE of the photocathode and the first dynode in the multiplication chain and, towards this goal, it is common (but sadly not universal) to place a zener diode between these electrodes so that the gain of this step is high regardless of the total PMT voltage used.

The SNR in PMTs could be enhanced further by cooling the tubes to reduce the effects of thermionic emission, by running the cathode at near ground potential to reduce regenerative effects due to collisions between electrons and the tube wall, by reducing the effective cathode area and focusing of the photoelectron beam, and, finally, by reducing the number of stages in the dynode chain and increasing the gain at each stage. All of these argue for the use of more efficient negative affinity materials, a feature that would also move us towards the use of the less-damaging longer wavelengths. These maneuvers would also decrease the dispersion in the time of fight of the photoelectron cloud produced by a single incident photon. This would increase the temporal resolution of the detector, a feature that would serve us well in attempting kinetic studies of the rates at which compounds fluoresce.

Many present confocal microscopes use rather crude techniques to create a running average of the photon flux. Perhaps the two most straightforward improvements of the devices for use in biological or low-light measurements would be the fol-

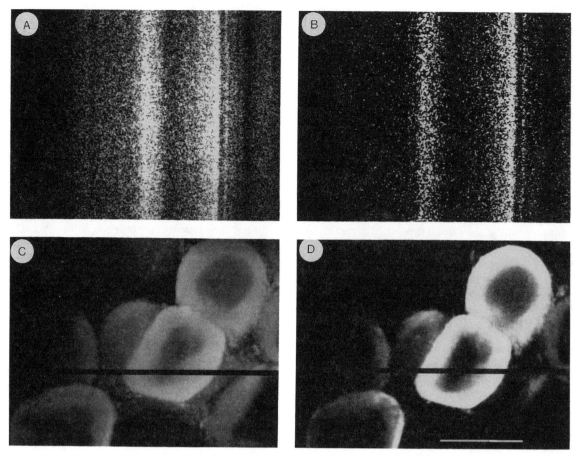

FIG. 9.   Comparison of the use of Bio-Rad MRC 500 confocal microscope in anode current measurement and photon counting modes at low light levels. Pedal ganglion of *Aplysia* stained with antibody raised to pedal peptide (Pep) conjugated with FITC. A. Background noise using anode current measurement apparent in the 512 scans of the single line indicated in part C. Successive scans displaced vertically. B. Output of photon counting circuit for the field line highlight in part D demonstrating relatively noise-free operation. C. Average of 512 fields using anode current measurement technique. Display restricted to values between 160 and 255 and expanded to the full dynamic range of the monitor before photographing. D. Average of 128 fields, at 1/10th the light level of part C, using photon counting. Sixteen quantal levels expanded to the full dynamic range of the monitor before photographing. Scale bar 100 μm.

lowing. First, one should eliminate the use of anode current measurements and the associated capacitive integration methods of pixel intensity estimation. Second, one should avoid the inappropriate use of the dynode acceleration voltage as a means of increasing the intensity of the image. The degradation of the SNR using these methods is too severe to warrant these techniques. The alternative to using the gain in this way is to increase the incident light levels or to use digital or electronic gain. As other authors in this volume point out, this can often result in severe photodamage to the specimen and bleaching of the photoprobe, again resulting in an inability to create a meaningful image in a minimum number of successive scans.

A convenient solution both to the problems of pixel convolution and to problems inherent in PMT operation can be implemented simply by using photon counting. The dark counts of photon counting tubes are often below 100 photoelectrons/s, and in an image that has perhaps 4×10^5 pixels/s, this contribution is negligible. Thus integrating over the pixel interval, the SNR will be limited by the photon statistics and the QE of the cathode material. The spurious noise due to regenerative effects and breakdown within the tube when run at high acceleration voltages can be eliminated. These effects can be demonstrated by comparing the average images collected under ex-

tremely low light conditions using the anode current measurement provided with the confocal microscope to a technique of direct photon counting (Fig. 9). Parts a and b of the figure demonstrate the SNR problem viewed as a measurement task after the primary detector. In Fig. 9a the signal is presumably buried somewhere within the extraordinary broadband noise in the trace. Since this is the input to the ADC stage, the signal will be sampled at the end of each pixel as an estimate of the pixel value. The result of averaging 512 frames acquired using this technique is shown in Fig. 9c. By comparison, the 16 levels from the photon counting circuit are shown in Fig. 9b. The result of averaging 128 images acquired under illumination reduced by a factor of ten are shown in Fig. 9d. From the viewpoint of capturing a useful image, photon counting is to be preferred. Furthermore, since in this photon counting unit the detection circuitry saturates at 10^7 photoelectrons/s (or 4×10^7 photons/s), the likelihood of bleaching the fluorescent probe has been minimized.

In the future, we should consider enhancing the quantum efficiency of the detectors. PMTs are presently limited in quantum efficiency to levels near 35% for blue light but may be less than 3% for rhodamine. An alternative approach would be to examine further the feasibility of using the solid-state detectors normally used in CCD arrays as the primary detector. The QE of the present generation CCD devices approach 80% well into the near infared, and this fact alone suggests that the solid-state direct photodetectors will ultimately come closest to achieving a SNR in the detected signal that is limited by the statistics of the photon flux. Presently, the sources of noise in realized devices are those due to thermal generation both in transfer along the readout registers and in resetting the readout capacitor. The problem of the minimum number of electrons is not insurmountable if the detector is arranged so that it always has the required minimum number of electrons in the well. Of course, the precise number will be a random variable and therefore will constitute a noise source to the detector that cannot be eliminated entirely. The second source of uncertainty is due to the readout noise. Since the readout of the voltage due to a packet of electrons can be made nondestructively, it is possible to shift each packet down a normal charge-coupled shift register and to make multiple readings along the register as the packet passes by. In this way, estimates of the pixel value would increase in precision with the square root of the number of estimates performed for each packet and with no apparent cost.

REFERENCES

Brown, R. G. W. , Jones, R., Rarity, J. G. & Ridley, K. D. (1987): Characterization of Silicon Avalanche Photodiodes for Photon Correlation Measurements. 2: Active Quenching. Applied Optics, **26–2**, 2383–2389.

Brown, R. G. W. , Ridley, K. D. & Rarity, J. G. (1986): Characterization of Silicon Avalanche Photodiodes for Photon Correlation Measurements. 1. Passive Quenching. Applied Optics, **25–22**, 4122–4126.

Boyle, W. S. & Smith, G. E. (1970): Charge Coupled Semiconductor Devices. Bell System Technical Journal **49**, 587–593.

Burgess, R. E. (1956): The Statistics of Charge Carrier Fluctuations in Semiconductors. Proceedings of the Physical Society, **B69**, 1020–1027.

Coutures, J. L. & Boucharlat, G. (1988): A 2 × 2048 Pixel Bilinear CCD Array for Spectroscopy (TH 7832 CDZ). Advances in Electronics and Electron Physics, **74**, 173–179.

Einstein, A. (1905): Über einen die Erzeugung und Verwandlung des Lichtes betreffenden heuristischen Gesichtspunkt. Annalen der Physik, **17**, 132–148.

Fairchild. (1987): CCD Imaging and Signal Processing Catalog and Applications Handbook. Fairchild Weston Systems Inc. CCD Imaging Division, Sunnyvale, CA.

Goldstein, S. (1989): A No-Moving-Parts Video Rate Laser Beam Scanning Type 2 Confocal Reflected/Transmission Microscope. Journal of Microscopy, **153–2**, RP1–RP2.

Hier, R. G. , Zheng, W. , Beaver, E. A. , McIlwain, C. E. & Schmidt, G. W. (1988): Development of a CCD-Digicon Detector System. Advances in Electronics and Electron Physics, **74**, 55–67.

Inoué, S. (1986): Video Microscopy. Plenum Press, New York & London. pp 584.

Jones, R., Oliver, C. J. & Pike, E. R. (1971): Experimental and Theoretical Comparison of Photon-counting and Current Measurements of Light Intensity. Applied Optics, **10**, 1673–1680.

Jorgensen, T. Jr. (1948): On Probability Generating Functions. American Journal of Physics, **16**, 285–289.

Kittel, C. (1986): Introduction to Solid State Physics, 6th ed. John Wiley & Sons, New York. pp 646.

Kume, H. , Koyama, K. , Nakatsugawa, K. , Suzuki, S. & Fatlowitz, D. (1986): Ultrafast Microchannel Plate Photomultipliers. Applied Optics, **27–6**, 1170—1178.

Lacaita, A. , Cova, S. & Ghioni, M. (1988): Four-hundred-picosecond Single-photon Timing with Commercially Available Avalanche Photodiodes. Review of Scientific Instruments, **59–7**, 1115–1121.

Mackay, C. D. (1988): Cooled CCD Systems for Biomedical and Other Applications. Advances in Electronics and Electron Physics, **74**, 129–133.

McMullan, D. (1988): Image Recording in Electron Microscopy. Advances in Electronics and Electron Physics, **74**, 147–156.

Mathur, D. P. , McIntyre, R. J. & Webb P. P. (1970): A New Geranium Photodiode with Extended Long-Wavelength Response. Applied Optics, **9–8**, 1842–1847.

Petran, M., Hadravsky, M., Egger, M. D. & Galambos, R. (1968): Journal of the Optical Society of America, **58**, 661–664.

Prescott, J. R. (1966): A Statistical Model for Photomultiplier Single-electron Statistics. Nuclear Instruments and Methods, **39**, 173 179.

Putley, E. H. (1977): Thermal Detectors. In Topics in Applied Physics, **19**: Optical and Infrared Detectors. Ed: R. J. Keyes. Springer-Verlag, Berlin. pp 71–100.

RCA. (1980): Photomultiplier Handbook. RCA Solid State Division. Lancaster, PA.

Robben, F. (1971): Noise in the Measurement of Light with Photomultipliers. Applied Optics, **10–4**, 776–796.

Schwartz, M. (1970): Information Transmission, Modulation, and Noise, 2nd ed. McGraw-Hill, New York. pp 672.

Seib, D. H. & Aukerman L. W. (1973): Photodetectors for the 0.1 to 1.0 mm Spectral Region. Advances in Electronics and Electron Physics, **34**, 95–221.

Siliconix. (1986): Small-signal FET Data Book. Siliconix Inc. Santa Clara, CA.

Sharpless, W. M. (1970): Evaluation of a Specially Designed GaAs Schottky-Barrier Photodiode Using 6328-ü Radiation Modulated at 4 GHz. Applied Optics, **9–2**, 489–494.

Sommer, A. H. (1968): Photoemissive Materials. John Wiley & Sons, New York. pp 255.

Van der Ziel, A. (1959): Fluctuation Phenomena in Semi-conductors. Academic Press, New York.

Chapter 13

Manipulation, Display, and Analysis of Three-Dimensional Biological Images

HANS CHEN, JOHN W. SEDAT AND DAVID A. AGARD

Department of Biochemistry and The Howard Hughes Medical Institute
University of California at San Francisco, San Francisco, Ca. 94143–0448

INTRODUCTION

Due to dramatic advances in optical microscope technology, it is now possible to examine biological specimens in three-dimensions with either electron microscopy or light microscopy. Although the algorithms used for generating the three-dimensional reconstructions are well known, much work remains on developing methods for the display and analysis of the resultant complicated three-dimensional data. After brief discussion of a rational file format designed for storing three-dimensional image data and its properties (e.g. pixel spacing, orientation, size etc), we will go on to discuss two major aspects of three-dimensional image data handling. The first covers image processing schemes for enhancing features in the data and some computational methods for manipulating three-dimensional data sets. In the second part, we will discuss the image display system in the context of software design and hardware requirements, which must be considered for convenient data visualization and measurement. Much effort has been spent on developing a generalized display system that can also be used for model building and analysis. By model building we mean the interactive tracking of features in three-dimensional volumetric images. Throughout this chapter we will make a distinction between display methods that directly utilize three-dimensional image data stored as a contiguous set of pixels (also called volumetric data, or voxel data) and those that convert the data into a set of polygon vertices that define a single-level contour surface. Although this latter approach contains much less information than volumetric approaches, it can make stunning pictures. Figure 1 shows a typical procedure for handling three-dimensional data involving image enhancement, data manipulation, data display and analysis.

STORAGE OF THREE-DIMENSIONAL IMAGE DATA

Three dimensional data can be obtained from a variety of microscopic sources. From light microscopy, three-dimensional data can be obtained as a series of two-dimensional images taken at different focus positions from either confocal microscopes or from conventional optical microscopes equipped with digitizing video cameras or cooled, scientific grade CCD detectors. Data from electron microscopy can be in the form of digitized images of physical thin sections or the result of tomographic analysis of thick sections. In all of these cases a three dimensional data set can contain an enormous amount of information. In our own work, we often have files of over 100 Mbytes in size for a single data set. There is thus a pressing

need for a convenient way of managing this data. Several years ago at the MRC labs in Cambridge, England a unified file format for storing and manipulating two- and three-dimensional pixel data was developed for handling x-ray density maps and images. It is absolutely essential that there be a single header (Table 1) that describes the geometric and physical contents of the file that is a part of the same file as the data. Furthermore, it is imperative that each set of three-dimensional data be stored in a single file. Random access capability then allows the rapid access to any single image section or part of a section. In this way, all of the sections of a three-dimensional image can be managed as a single unit. The file design that was chosen consisted of a 1024 byte header immediately followed by the image data. A mode flag in the header indicated the format of the data. Each pixel could be represented numerically either by a single byte (allowing numbers from 0–255 to be stored), by a two-byte integer (values from -32768 to 32767), a four-byte real number ($\pm 10^{\pm 33}$), or by pairs of either integer*2 or real data to represent the complex values from a 2D or 3D Fast Fourier Transform (FFT). In addition to containing information on the size of the image, the pixel spacings, mode, three-dimensional origin and orientation of the image, symmetry operators and unit cell parameters for the x-ray maps, the header also contain space for 10 text labels each 80 characters long. This is very convenient as each program that manipulates the

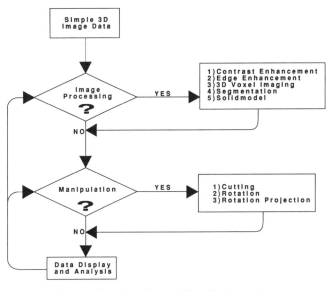

FIG. 1. Procedure for handling 3D image data.

TABLE 1

TABLE 1

MRC	Image File Header	data structure
1–3	NXYZ	# of columns, rows, sections
4	MODE	data type: I*1,I*2,R*4,Complex I*2,Complex R*4
5–7	NXYZSTART	number of first Column,Row,Section in map (default = 0)
8–10	MXYZ	number of intervals along X,Y,Z
11–13	XYZLENGTH	cell dimensions (cell/mxyz = pixel spacing)
14–16	ALP,BET,GAM	cell angle(Degrees)
17–19	MAPCRS	which axis corresponds to Columns,Rows,Sections
20	AMIN	minimum density value
21	AMAX	maximum density value
22	AMEAN	mean density value
23	ISPG	space group number
24	NSYMBT	number of bytes used for storing symmetry operators
25–40	EXTRA	user defined storage space
41	IDTYPE	type of data set, section, projection, etc
42	DV	data value 1, info related to data type
43	DV2	data value 2, more info for data type
44–49	Tilts	2 tilt sets (original and Tilts 2 tilt sets (original and current)
50–52	Waves	multiple wave length information
53–55	XYZORIGIN	x,y,z origin of image
56	NLABL	number of labels being used
57–256	LABEL(20,10)	ten 80 character text labels

file can add a label record allowing the processing history of the file to be clearly kept. A comprehensive set of subroutines has been developed to allow convenient manipulation of the image header as well as the image data itself. On disk, the data is stored in fixed length records to improve access and IO performance, however, all of this is completely transparent to the user who only needs to be concerned about images.

The convention chosen to specify the orientation of any image file is defined by the following equation.

$$[XYZ] = [M]^{-1} [IXYZ \times \Delta XYZ + OXYZ]$$

Where matrix M is the same rotation matrix used for rotating the original data file and creating this new file. In simple section image files, OXYZ is the coordinate of the first data point in this file with respect to the rotated coordinate system, Δ OXYZ is the pixel spacing. For a projection image file (see below), OXYZ is the coordinates of the center of the entire projecting volume. By making this information available to the image display system, it will be able to relate data from different types of image files.

IMAGE ENHANCEMENT

Once a three-dimensional data set has been obtained, it is often necessary to correct for systematic errors in the data. Such errors can be due to the lower resolution along the focus direction that occurs with either confocal data or conventional optical section data, or the missing data that occurs in electron microscopic tomography due to practical limitations on tilt angle. Further, confocal microscopy, especially laser scan methods, can suffer from scan irregularity and various geometric distortions occurring off the central axis. Three-dimensional data recorded on CCD cameras must be corrected for variations

in gain and offset for each pixel (Hiraoka et al, 1987). All of these artifacts can and should be corrected before proceeding to visualization or quantitative analysis. We have previously described methods for image restoration that dramatically improve the three-dimensional resolution obtainable with conventional optical sectioning microscopy (Agard et al, 1989). These methods are just as applicable to confocal data.

After suitably corrected image data have been obtained, there are several image enhancement schemes that can be used to enhance the visual appearance of an image (e.g. edge structure). As we shall consider it here, image processing (as distinct from image restoration) does not try to add or improve the information content of the three-dimensional images, but only serves to improve the clarity of presentation. The field of image processing methods is well developed and the reader is directed towards such classic texts as Castleman (1979) or Pratt (1978). Very often data that represent the part of the structure which is of interest falls within a small portion of the overall dynamic range. When this type of image is displayed without enhancement, the data range of interest will be translated into only a few intensity levels in the display, suppressing desired detail in the resultant image. Contrast stretching and histogram normalization are two standard approaches. Here we will concentrate on other methods that we have found to be particularly useful for three-dimensional microscope data. Most of these schemes work by remapping the image data according to a specific type of function. By choosing proper functions and parameters the desired enhancement can be accomplished. Because image quality is often a subjective criteria, it is generally necessary to try a few methods with a few sets of parameters.

Linear Filters

The use of various linear filters is a common and productive way to manipulate image data. Confocal microscope data is often quite noisy and it is useful to apply a smoothing filter. Enhancement can be achieved through the use of high-pass or bandpass filters. These can be applied to two- or three-dimensional data either as convolution operations in real space or as multiplication operations in Fourier space. In general, it is common to use filters that are circularly or spherically symmetric because there is little reason to distinguish particular directions within the image (although this can be simply done). We typically apply filters in Fourier space and prefer the use of gaussian filters to avoid the introduction of ripples and contrast inversions that can otherwise be generated. Low pass, smoothing filters are generated using a gaussian function ($\exp(-r^2/2\sigma^2)$) or for enhancement we often use a Fourier filter of the form (1-$\exp(-r^2/2\sigma^2)$). These can be combined, using different values of σ in each part, to give a bandpass filter.

Median Filters

These are a class of non-linear filters that have the property of smoothing data while maintaining edges. The general scheme is to choose an NxN or NxNxN box (N is odd) surrounding a particular pixel in either two- or three-dimensional space and to calculate the median intensity within the box. Recall, that the median intensity is that intensity value which is half way up the histogram. This can be quite distinct from the mean density within the box. Note that the median is rather insensitive to the absolute intensity of a point. The central value in the box is then replaced by either the median value (Median filter) or by the actual value minus the median (Median enhancement). The position of the box is then incremented by one pixel and the process repeated. The median filter has the property that objects smaller than about one half of the box size tend to be removed. With the median enhancement methods, broad backgrounds are effectively removed, and small features remain. This is a very powerful method, but can be quite time consuming. Several authors have described fast algorithms for computing these filters (Hung, T.S., 1979; Narendra, P.M., 1981).

Local Contrast Enhancement

Surprisingly, the local contrast enhancement method can often perform as well or better than the Median Enhancement method, above, and can generally be computed more rapidly. This scheme defines its mapping function based on the local mean and local contrast in the neighborhood of a particular pixel. As with the Median filter, the local neighborhood is defined in terms of an NxN or NxNxN box (N is odd) surrounding a particular pixel. The local mean is defined as the average of all the data values within the box, while the local contrast is defined as the difference between the central data value and the local mean. Once the local mean and local contrast values are calculated, the contrast and mean are separately re-mapped according to a pair of lookup tables (LUTs) and then summed to give the final value which is placed in the central pixel. Again, the position of the box is incremented by one pixel, and the process is repeated. This approach enhances an image by reducing the overall dynamic range of the data and by boosting the local contrast in a potentially nonlinear fashion. This approach is especially useful for microscope data as it allows background to be suppressed without the artificiality and error

caused by thresholding as in conventional contrast stretching. The use of separate LUTs to permit independant manipulation of the mean and contrast levels allows contrast in the important areas to be increased while maintaining a good overall sense of the image. The key to success with this method is the appropriate definition of the lookup tables. These can be designed to take into account the psychophysics of image perception. An example of this approach is shown in Figure 2. Clearly, significant detail is seen in image B (after 2D filtering of the final projection images) that is present, but not obvious, in A.

Gradient Method

This method is designed mainly for edge enhancement which is helpful in trying to determine connectedness in a complicated data structure or as a preparation for solid modeling (see below). This type of enhancement has been used extensively by the group at PIXAR (San Rafael, California) (Dreibin et al), and we find it to be extremely useful. The idea is to form a new three-dimensional image that is made by multiplying the value of every pixel by the two- or three-dimensional gradient in the neighborhood of that pixel. Although the gradients may be high in the background regions, the image values are small, thus noise seems to be effectively suppressed. Before calculating the gradient, it is often useful to remap the image by a sigmoidal function to further suppress background. The density mapping function used in this method is defined as below:

$$X_{out} = X_{in} \times (K + (1 - K) \times grad(F(X_{in}))) \quad 0 < K < 1$$

where grad is the modulus of the three dimensional gradient:

$$sqrt(g(x)^2 + g(y)^2 + g(z)^2)$$

Where the function F can be either unity or an ArcTangent (a convenient way to generate a sigmoidal function). K controls

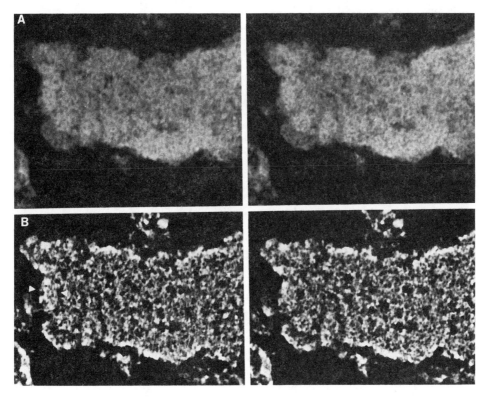

FIG. 2.   (A) and (R) show the difference between before and after LCE. Data shown is Epon sections of metaphase-arrested Kc chromosomes.

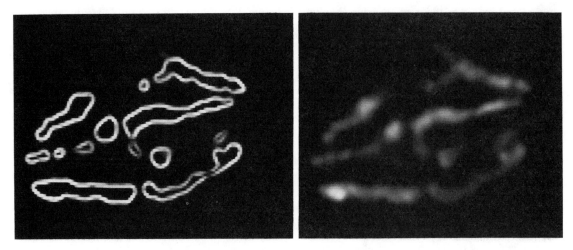

FIG. 3. The left picture is the result of gradient method with K = 1 and the right picture is the original image. Data shown is a Formaldehyde-fixed, devitalinized and DAPI-stained anaphase chromosome from a Drosophila early embryo.

the mix of image and image × gradient. Figure 3 shows both the original and an edge-enhanced image. A three dimensional automatic data segmentation scheme is being developed at UCSF which uses both three dimensional gradient and data value information to optimally define structures.

PROCESSING METHODS FOR DISPLAYING 3D DATA

Presenting three-dimensional data in a form where the vast amount of information present can be readily appreciated and analyzed is a challenging problem. Ideally, one would like to be able to wander around within a three-dimensional hologram under computer control to allow zooming in on particular regions or zooming out to see the entire data. Although one day this will undoubtedly be possible (there has been much progress in the computer generation of holograms), the present goals are to try to approach this immediacy of interaction with the data using considerably more mundane approaches. In order to visualize three-dimensional data, it must be converted in some manner to one or more two-dimensional images for display on a raster computer graphics system.

After 3D microscope data has been collected, reconstructed, processed, etc. it is generally thought of as a set of two-dimensional images. Each of which represents a slice through the data cube representing the three-dimensional specimen. A very simple way of displaying this data is to allow the user to examine each section individually, and when he is done to go on to another section. This can even be done in rapid succession, creating a movie. Unfortunately, although such approaches are ideal for examining the details of a single slice, they do little to provide a sense of the three dimensionality of the data as a whole because nothing has been done to integrate information into an image that appears to be distributed throughout three-dimensional space.

Three methods which we have found to be especially useful in visualizing the 3D aspects of these data sets are 1) simple display of stereo image pairs, 2) serial displays of mono or stereo projections of sequential rotations of the entire three-dimensional data cube, being displayed rapidly enough to achieve a movie effect and 3), simultaneous viewing of the same point in the data from multiple directions using two or more two-dimensional image sections derived from the three-dimensional data set at various rotations (e.g. orthogonal views).

Stereo Images

Stereo pairs can be calculated from a three-dimensional data set in either of two ways. The most accurate is to rotate the full three-dimensional data set by anywhere from ±3° to ±10° and then to project each of these rotate three-dimensional data sets onto a two dimensional plane (see also ROTPROJ, below). Another approach which is less accurate, but is less expensive computationally is the stacking method. Instead of actually rotating the three-dimensional image data, the required projection images are approximated by summing a series of section images with an appropriate pixel shift between the adjacent sections. The left eye part of the stereo pair is made by sequentially shifting each image to the left as one progresses from the farthest to the nearest plane. The number of the pixels to be shifted is dependent upon the actual pixel size and the distance between sections. In principle the angle resulting from the shift operation should fall between 3.0° and 7° for each image. To see the stereo effect on the computer monitor, the images can be displayed side by side and the viewer can wear simple 3D glasses which will fuse left and right images by properly adjusting angle between two reflecting mirrors in the glasses (very nice viewers are available from nu 3D vu Co, Eugene, Or.). A more convenient (and more expensive) system electronically alternates the display of the left eye and right eye right images on the monitor. The user can either wear a pair of mechanical or electro optical shutters, or a liquid crystal screen can be placed in front of the monitor that switches between left and right circular polarization in synchrony with the monitor. To assure that each image only reaches the appropriate eye, the user wears a pair of left-right circularly polarized "sunglasses" (available from Stereographics, San Rafael, Ca., or Tektronix, Beaverton, Or.). For more discussion see (Agard,et al 1989).

3D Rotations

With either display approach, computational methods are needed for generating new three-dimensional data sets in a different format or orientation. Two software programs have been developed at the Biochemistry Department at UCSF for computationally rotating three-dimensional data sets and either projecting entire data set onto an assigned imaginary image plane or reslicing the data cube along the rotated axis. ROT3D is a FORTRAN program for rotating three-dimensional images. The approach taken in this program is following:

- Determine the size of the new rotated image data set
- Calculate the inverse rotation matrix
- Loop through every point in the output image and determine the coordinate of data point within the original image by pre-multiplying the new coordinate by the inverse matrix
- Determine the data value by interpolating between adjacent points in the original data file.

Rotated Projections

The second program ROTPROJ is for calculating a series of projection images of any three-dimensional image data set calculated at different tilt angles. To speed up the process for calculating the rotated projection images, the rotation and projection operations are performed simultaneously; the result being a substantial saving in computer time (Agard et al 1989). Consider a two-dimensional slice of the three-dimensional image taken perpendicular to the desired rotation axis: for example the X-Z plane for tilts about the Y axis. Then the desired coordinate transformation is given by:

$$x' = (x-x_c)\cos\theta - (z-z_c)\sin\theta + x_c$$
$$z' = (x-x_c)\sin\theta + (z-z_c)\cos\theta + z_c$$

Where x_c, z_c are the centers of rotation and θ is the rotation angle. Instead of rotating all the data and then projecting it down the z' axis, we loop through the desired x' range and the original z solving for x as we go.

$$x = [(x'-x_c) + (z-z_c)\sin\theta] / \cos\theta + x_c$$

the value to be added into the projection vector at x' is then given by one-dimensional interpolation:

- loop on x' in the output projection vector
- loop on z in image
- calculate x in image that corresponds to the current x', z
- linearly interpolate in the input image to get value and add to value in projection vector at x'

By saving one loop, this approach can speed calculations by as much as 30 fold. For $|\theta| > 45$, because of the $\cos\theta$ in the denominator, it is advisable to loop on x',x and solve for z. Rotation about other axes can likewise be efficiently accomplished.

Simultaneously with forming the rotated projections, one can either alter the contributions of density values arising from the back of the image or add in the property of opacity to the sample. Opacity is especially useful, as often simply projected images tend to have an transparent quality to them that makes them hard to interpret. As each point is summed into the projected image, it is first multiplied by a weight that is kept for each pixel in the projected image. The initial value for the weight is 1.0, as each new point is added in, the weight for each pixel is multiplied by exp(-α*val /mean). This acts to make the higher values more opaque. For speed, a lookup table containing exponential factors is precalculated. Varying α, varies how opaque the object seems.

Pixar Displays

It is often particularly useful to combine this ROTPROJ method with the PIXAR edge enhancement approach (Driebin et al, 1988). When opacity is added, the net effect is very similar to the surface rendering methods described below. Another variation also developed by PIXAR, is instead of combing the overall three-dimensional gradient information when multiplying by the image, is to separately rotate the x,y,z components of the image gradient data and to then take the dot product with respect to a light source direction. This final value is the summed with opacity to produce a very nice and extremely rapid surface rendering that is rather insensitive to choice of contour level.

Contour Surface Representation

In this approach, a contour surface is defined by a single threshold level in a three-dimensional data set. Displaying this surface is done by finding a set of three-dimensional triangles which approximate the surface. The face of each triangle is colored with a constant value that is derived from the dot product between the direction of an imaginary light source and the triangle normal. Alternatively, it can be shaded by smoothly interpolating between intensity values calculated for each triangle vertex. These intensity values are determined in a similar manner by taking the dot product between the light source and vertex normal. The triangle or vertex normals are chosen to point away from the structure. An example of this type of surface representation is shown in Figure 4. Since the structure geometry is assumed to be completely random, finding a scheme which will automatically search for all these triangles is difficult. One scheme developed at UCSF, defines the location of each triangle and its normal by considering all of the possible ways that a three-dimensional surface can be enclosed by a unit box. Depending on how the intersections occur, triangles can be defined easily to approximate the enclosed surface. By looping through all the unit boxes in the sampling space, we can cover the whole surface of the structure. The approach seems to work best on simple data such as would be expected from stained axons or for data that has been processed using the Gradient method, above.

GRAPHIC SYSTEM FOR 3D IMAGE DISPLAY AND ANALYSIS

Programs such as FRODO (T. A. Jones, 1982) which utilize advanced computer graphics techniques to display x-ray data, are widely used by scientists in the field of protein structure research. Unfortunately, the cage contour representation of the three-dimensional data adopted in such programs is not suitable for microscopy data. This is mainly due to the greater level of structure irregularity, higher noise and nonisotropic data resolution. At the Howard Hughes Structural Biology Unit at UCSF an interactive computer graphics display system PRISM has been designed and built to serve the purpose of three-dimensional microscopy data display and analysis. It displays data as a gray level image on an computer raster graphics CRT

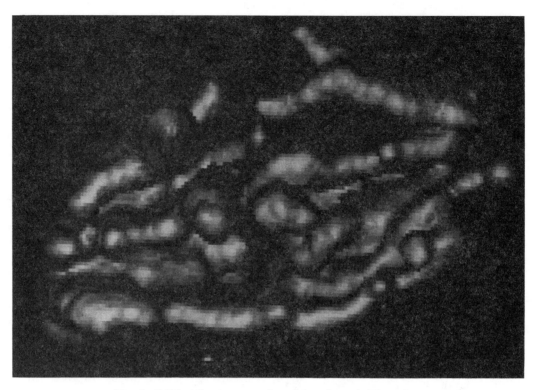

FIG. 4. Solid surface representation of data shown in Figure 3.

screen (1024 × 1280), the pixel brightness on the screen reflects the data density level. Since human eyes can only detect about 128 gray levels at most, an eight bit graphic device (256 gray levels) is quite suitable for the display. By properly scaling image data, the image recorded in the microscope can be easily reproduced on the screen.

Details of PRISM's Design and Implementation

The main goal of PRISM is providing the capability of three-dimensional image data analysis, especially model building, through data visualization. The design began with building the foundation of a flexible and versatile display functionality and then adding data analysis functions such as path tracing, density analysis, distance measurements, and point marking. The following is a list of design principals of PRISM.

i)   Being able to handle multiple image displays and allowing each display to be manipulated (e.g., zoom, pan, update etc) independently. Comparison between several images is probably the most common practice in data analysis. Especially when working with three-dimensional data sets, it is often necessary to simultaneously examine a region of the data from multiple angles of view in order to resolve and interpret complicated structures. Thus a windowing capability (allowing multiple, independent images to be simultaneously displayed and manipulated) is a definite must.

ii) The capability to rapidly and sequentially display a set of images. As discussed in the previous section, one of the best ways to perceive a 3D structure is by looking at a set of sequentially rotated projection images displayed in movie mode.

iii) Accommodate images up to 1024 by 1024 pixels. Most digital microscopy data is no larger than 1024 by 1024 in one section. The system should be able to display the whole data section when desired.

iv) Providing an on-screen cursor for interacting with data displayed on the screen. Since PRISM is the system for both data visualization and analysis, the ability to interact with the scene on the screen is very important. A mouse-driven cursor can give the user a convenient way to either select data on the display screen or input program commands.

v)   Functionality for tracing and building a model of a complicated biological structure from 3D microscope data. This is also the ultimate goal for PRISM.

vi) Model display. It can be difficult to appreciate the spatial aspects of the structure by looking at gray level images. Being able to display a simplified model in stereo with the capability to rotate the display gives the user an easy way to visualize the important aspects of a complex structure.

The Window System

The software solution for the independent manipulation of multiple images on the screen is known as windows. A window is a viewport in which an image can be displayed and manipulated. Every image on the screen has a window structure associated with it. Displaying an image requires that the image be copied from a storage area in the display memory (the image buffer) to a pre-defined location on the area of memory that can be displayed (the viewport buffer). To create a new display on the screen requires adding a new window to the window system. Since PRISM is designed for both data display and analysis, the functionality of this window system not only defines the mapping relationship between the image buffer and viewport buffer, but it also creates a geometrical link between a two-dimensional screen coordinate system and a real space three-dimensional coordinate system. Therefore, it is possible to determine the location in real space for data displayed on the screen. This is essential for doing three-dimensional model building and data analysis. This link is accomplished by tracking the source data file of every image loaded to the window system, its location in the data file, the screen coordinate of each window, and the geometrical information stored in the image data file header. (As discussed in the previous section, in doing three-dimensional analysis it is often necessary to examine the data stack from various angles. Since most computer systems are not capable of doing on-line three-dimensional volumetric rotations, these are often pre-computed and stored in several image data files. Each one represents some geometric transformation of the data. It is necessary that all of the relevant orientation information be stored in the file header, so that images from different files can unambiguously be related to one another.) Every window has its own set of attributes, which completely determines the on-screen display contents. The following is a list of window attributes defined in PRISM:

- Image source. This is the data file associated with this particular window. Different windows can link to the same file, but each window can have only one associated file. Every image file has a header attached to it, which contains the relevant information such as size, pixel spacing, data type (e.g., projection image vs section image), orientation and origin in three-space.
- Allocation of space in the image buffer for preloading images from the associated image file. As mentioned earlier, images need to be pre-loaded into the image buffer to allow rapid updates. Every window has an array which contains the location of each image stored in the image buffer.
- Region of the image that has been loaded into the image buffer.
- Window size and its location in the viewport buffer.
- Zoom Factor
- Display priority. The window system maintains a priority stack to determine the display order for overlapping windows. In the current system there are up to 8 windows. The window on top of the stack is called the active window. Only its content will be affected by the user input commands. Selecting the active window is done by raising the target window's display priority to the top of the stack and pushing the priority of all the other windows one level down. In the case where none of the existing windows are set to be on top (done by setting top entry to be 0), all the windows become active. This means that the same command will apply to all the windows. For instance if the command is ZOOMUP every window's zoom factor attribute will be incremented and the whole screen will be repainted with the new zoom factor. This gives users the ability to perform parallel operations among the windows. Using two windows to generate a stereo movie is one example of this. Images are manipulated on the screen by changing the value in the corresponding attribute and repainting the screen.

Since each window has its own set of attributes, images can be manipulated in a completely independent fashion. One aspect that should be emphasized here is zooming. The ability to have different zoom factors on a single screen gives great flexibility in data visualization. The traditional zoom is performed by display hardware and applies a single zoom factor throughout the whole screen. Whenever the zoom factor changes the size of the viewport area also changes. Because of this, it is difficult to maintain image layout on the screen. Furthermore, menu items that are displayed on the screen will also be zoomed up and down. This can be very inconvenient. For these reasons we have adopted the use of software zooms instead of hardware zooms. This is most easily done by pixel replication while copying the image from the image buffer to the viewport buffer. The bigger the zoom factor, the smaller the area of data that will be mapped onto display window. Zooming is set up to take place with respect to the image center instead of a screen corner.

Digital Movies

The hardware must be capable of accomplishing both the desired movie mode and the windowing functionality. To achieve the movie effect, it is necessary that images to be updated at the rate of 6 to 10 frames per second. Image display generally involves reading data in from disk, scaling between 0 255, and loading the result into the viewport buffer of the graphic imaging device. To obtain the desired speeds, extremely high speed, parallel transfer disks, and a fast host CPU with a high speed data bus between system memory and its graphic subsystem are required. In practice, extra CPU speed is needed for rotating the three-dimensional data set and calculating projection image. Except for a very few high-end graphics work stations, most of the computer systems that are readily available to the biologist do not have the hardware to meet this requirement. An alternative is to precalculate images and to load the images onto an image buffer in the imaging device itself, provided it has enough memory for all the images. Then, updating an image is done by sequentially copying the new image from image buffer onto the same location in the viewport buffer. Most inexpensive imaging devices take less than one tenth of a second to copy an image, providing the necessary speed. For this reason, having a large image buffer in which to store the pre-computed views becomes an important criterion in selecting graphic and image display hardware.

Choice of Display Hardware

Based on the above discussions, there are two major criteria for selecting display hardware. The first is that the display device must have a large image buffer for storing images. The second is that it must be able to perform an image copy operation with pixel replication. This function must be fast enough to allow smooth transitions in the movie mode (at least 5–10 frames-/sec). After a careful study of most of the imaging graphic devices commercially available, we picked the Parallax 1280 (Sunnyvale, CA) as the display device for the following reasons:

- It uses a high resolution, 1280 by 1024 pixel, 60 Hz, non-interlaced display. This provides sufficient space for displaying 1024 × 1024 images with room on the right side for menus. The 60 Hz non-interlaced ability results in flicker-free viewing even under fluorescent lights.
- It has 12M bytes of display memory which can be used either as three sets of eight bit pseudo color images or as a twenty

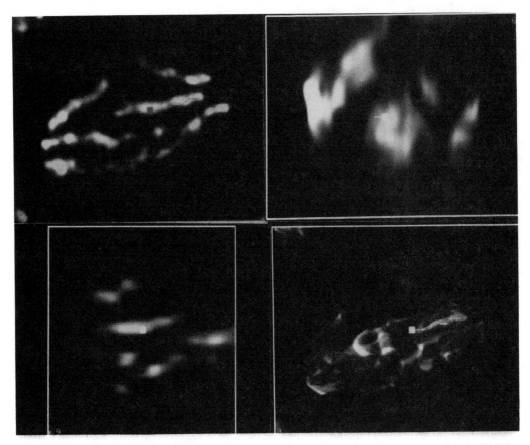

FIG. 5.   Shows various views of a 3D Anaphase chromosome data set. Top-left is the XY section image. Top-right is the XZ section image. Low-left is the YZ section image. Low-right is the computed projection image by using Pixar method. The square label marks the common spot in 3D data space where these XY, XZ and YZ planes intersect.

four bit true color system. The memory is organized as 2048 × 2048 with only 1280 × 1024 visible at any one time. Although pseudo color is more than enough for displaying gray scale images the true color mode is very useful for transparently overlapping images without losing any intensity information. This is obviously very important for examining multiply-labeled data sets.

- The Parallax 1280 processor is able to perform pixel replication and BLIT (Block Image Transfer) simultaneously at the speed of 12Mpixel/sec which is fast enough to support the movie function on the entire 1024 by 1024 display area.
- It supports a specialized macro instruction set. By loading the proper macro program, the Parallax is able to track the movement of a pointer device (such as a mouse) and represent it as an on-screen cursor completely independent of the host computer. The mouse can be programmed so that when the status of any button changes, a host interrupt will be generated, and the current screen position and button status will then be sent to the host.

Developments in hardware of this type are constantly being made, however, and interesting systems are currently offered by Indec Systems (Sunnyvale, Ca), Vital Images (Fairfield, Ia), ISG Technologies Inc. (Toronto, Canada) and others.

Model Building in PRISM

A model is defined as a stick figure representation of the path of a structure in three-dimensional space. It can be considered as a collection of separate objects. Each object is defined as a set of connected nodes which represent a single branch in the structure. A tree data structure is used to store the connectivity of all these nodes, and a position array is used to store the coordinates of every node in real space. To increase the generality of this data structure, the tree structure does not impose a limitation on the depth of the tree or on the number of entries at any level. The only limitation derives from total available memory space. For model display, each object has its own set of display attributes which PRISM uses to determine its visibility and color. On the node level, PRISM allows users to attach any of six predefined marks to a node. Thus when it is displayed, the attached mark will be shown at the same location and in the same color as the object to which it belongs. While building the model, PRISM maintains a data pointer within the tree structure. It determines the location in the tree structure where model command action takes place and the node pointed to by the mouse is called the active node. There are four basic commands for updating a model. They are ADD, DELETE, BRANCH and MODIFY. ADD will add a node right after the active node, and make the new node active. DELETE will remove the active node from the structure, and make the previous node active. BRANCH will create a new branch substructure at the active node, and set the first node in the new branch as the active node. MODIFY will not affect the tree structure, it simply alters the coordinates of the current active node. Besides these basic building commands, PRISM also provides a set of

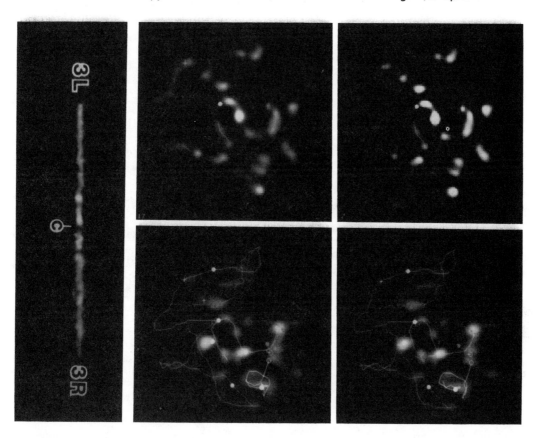

FIG. 6. Model building function in PRISM. The top-left square image is the deblurred image of a section, the top-right square image is the LCE image, and the two square images below are a projection stereo-pair of the 3D data set. The computer model is properly superimposed on each image. The vertical image on the left shows the result of applying the straightening procedure, described in the text, to unbend one of the chromosomes in this data set, revealing a banding pattern similar to that seen in a squash preparation. Data used are prophase chromosomes from a Drosophila embryo stained with a DNA-specific fluorescent dye.

commands for moving pointers within the tree structure so that any part of model can be retrieved easily.

Model Building

Building a model is accomplished by determining the locations of all the nodes. When displaying section images, a data point on the screen will correspond to a unique location in the data sampling space, as each image represents a slice in the sample. For such data, model building is accomplished by picking data points displayed on the screen. Stepping the section forward or backwards (which occurs rapidly because they have been preloaded) provides the third coordinate. As described in the previous section, the Parallax mouse will generate an interrupt whenever a mouse button is pushed, making it easy to send the screen coordinates to the host computer. Selecting nodes is also done by simply pointing to the data location on the screen with the cursor and pressing one of the mouse buttons.

When dealing with complicated objects, it is often necessary to be able to examine the data stack from multiple viewing angles. As described above, the program ROT3D can computationally reslice the data stack in any orientation. It is then

possible in PRISM to open several windows on the screen and have each of them display images of the same data, but sliced in a different orientation while building the model. PRISM will use the header information to keep track of the geometry of each window. Thus, in the model building function, PRISM will choose what (usually orthogonal) section to display in each window so that they all contain the same spot in three-dimensional space as defined by the cursor and the section number in the active window. This approach to window management and model building allows the PRISM user to simultaneously construct a model from multiple viewing angles (Figure 5). The models can only be updated when the cursor is in the active window which displays the section image. Modeling within multiple projections images (such as stereo pairs) can be performed but requires the use of a stereo cursor which has not yet been fully implemented. Nevertheless, a projection can be a very good reference window to check any mistakes made in the model as shown in Figure 6. In this regard, it is possible to allow the model to be corrected in the plane of the projection image in the active window. To aid in the identification of individual substructures, a computational method has been developed which extracts data within a defined radius perpendicular to the 3D line model and then linearizes the model and the surrounding extracted data as shown in Fig 6 (left).

Superimposing the Model on a Background Image

This is necessary for both model building and display. There are two types of background images: projection and section images. For projection images, the procedures for superimposing a model on the active window are:

- Transform all the model coordinates to the same orientation as the background image
- Project the 3D model onto the same imaginary projection plane as the background image
- Transform the projected 2D model to screen coordinates
- Clip the 2D model within the window boundary and display the model overlaid on an appropriate section or projection from the original 3D data set.

For section images, the procedures are the same except for the second step. Instead of doing the projection, the model will be clipped according to the boundary defined by the appropriate slice in the data stack. All the geometrical transformations are made possible because of the information stored in the image file header and the design of the window system. For the non-active windows, the procedures are the same except that in section windows, the background images need to be updated so that they contain the data point which is designated as the active node before overlaying the model.

Future Development and Discussion

The major drawback of PRISM is the need for precomputing all the images which are used for 3D data analysis. This is because the host microVAX computer is too slow to provide on-line calculations for generating these rotate-projected images. With today's high-end workstations which drastically increase the performance of both the CPU and its graphic subsystem, the existing problem can be eliminated. At UCSF we are currently designing a second generation image display system which will greatly improve both three dimensional image data display and analysis function in PRISM. The new system will be implemented on the Titan workstation (Ardent, Sunnyvale, California) using it as both a computing engine and graphics display device.

With this system we will be able to provide a display functionality which allows real time, random location and orientation of a 128 by 128 by 30 subregion of a larger three-dimensional data set. Manipulating the entire data set will be possible, but at slightly slower than real time. This will, for the first time, give the viewer complete freedom in visualizing complex three dimensional images of biological specimens.

A similar software system that permits rapid display of three-dimensional images without window or model building has been developed by Argiro (Van Zandt and Argiro, 1989) to run on Silicon Graphics workstations.

ACKNOWLEDGEMENTS

This work has been supported by funding from the Howard Hughes Medical Institute and by grants from the National Institute of Health to J.W.S. (GM-25101) and D.A.A. (GM-31627). D.A.A. is a National Science Foundation Presidential Young Investigator.

REFERENCES

Agard, D.A., Hiraoka, Y., Shaw, P. and Sedat, J.W. (1989). microscopy in three dimensions. "Methods in Cell Bilo. 30, p:353–377

Andrews, H. C., A. G. Tescher, and R. P. Kruger, 1972 "Image Processing by Digital Computer" IEEE Spectrum, 9, 1972, 20–32

Belmont, A. S., J. W. Sedat, and D. A. Agard, 1987 "A Three Dimensional Approach to Mitotic Chromosome Structure", J. Cell Biol. 105:77–92

Castleman, Kenneth R. "Digital Image Processing" 1979 Prentice-Hall, Inc., Englewood Cliffs, N.J.

Driebin, R. A., L. Carpenter, P. Hanranhan, 1988 "Volume Rendering," Computer Graphics Vol22 #4, 65–75

Huang, T.S., Yang, G.J., and Tang, G.Y. 1979. "A Fast Two-Dimensional Median Filtering Algorithm" IEEE Trans Acoust Speech and Sig Proc, 27:13–18.

Jones, T. A. 1982 "Computational Crystallography," D. Sayre, Ed. (Oxford Univ. Press, Oxford, 1982) p:303–317

Narendra, P.M. 1981. "A Separable Median Filter for Image Noise Smoothing." IEEE Trans Pat Anal and Mach Intelligence, 3:20–29.

Peii, T., and J. S. Lim, 1982. "Adaptive Filtering for image enhancement." Opt. Eng. 21:108–112

Pratt, William K. 1978 "Digital Image Processing," John Wiley & Sons, Inc. N.Y.

Van Zandt, W. and V. Argiro. 1989 A new "Inlook" of life, Unix Review, 7:52–57.

Chapter 14

Three-dimensional Imaging on Confocal and Wide-field Microscopes

WALTER A. CARRINGTON, KEVIN E. FOGARTY, LARRY LIFSCHITZ, FREDRIC S. FAY

Physiology Department, University of Massachusetts Medical School, 55 Lake Avenue North, Worcester, MA 01655, (508)856-6548, (508)856-2346, Supported by NSF Grant DIR-8720188

INTRODUCTION

The conventional (wide-field) light microscope accepts light from planes above and below the plane of focus. This lack of depth discrimination is the main limitation of the wide-field microscope for 3D imaging. The confocal microscope rejects this out-of-focus light with the confocal pinhole and provides greater resolution than the wide-field microscope. This depth discrimination of the confocal microscope makes it attractive for 3D optical sectioning microscopy. This advantage of the confocal microscope is balanced by inherent signal losses from the confocal pinhole (see also Chapter 2: Pinhole) and by the use of detectors in current commercial confocal microscopes that have substantially lower quantum efficiency than the cooled CCD cameras used in wide-field digital imaging microscopes. These additional losses of current commercial confocal instruments are especially important in 3D fluorescence imaging of single cells.

The light excluded by the confocal pinhole contains information that can be used by computer postprocessing techniques, called image restoration or deconvolution, to improve the quality of 3D images. These methods obtain 3D images from a wide-field microscope that are comparable in resolution and depth discrimination to images obtained from confocal microscopes. The disadvantage of these methods is that considerable computer processing time is required. The key question is how best to use the limited number of photons available from a fluorescent sample to answer the biological questions posed. We examine the question of which microscope, confocal, wide-field or wide-field with image restoration, is preferable in various situations.

A considerable part of the benefit of 3D digital imaging is achieved only if adequate computer software and hardware support is available. High resolution 3D digital images, however acquired, can be manipulated in a computer to provide views of a cell not possible by a direct view in a microscope. In a later section, we discuss 3D computer graphics. In addition to these computer graphics methods, as images increase in complexity, automated or semi-automated computer analysis becomes more important. Later, we discuss the different approaches to automated analysis, feature extraction and computer vision in 3D microscopy. Finally, we discuss the computer hardware requirements for operating with 3D data.

SIGNAL-TO-NOISE RATIO AND RESOLUTION

Fluorescently labelled, living single cells can emit a limited number of photons before the fluorescence is bleached away or

photodamage kills the cell. The choice a biologist must make is how best to use those photons to extract the most information from an experiment.

The confocal microscope gains its increased resolution and depth discrimination by excluding light with the confocal pinhole. The excluded light contains out-of-focus information that is not useful visually, but can be used effectively by image restoration (deconvolution). This procedure uses knowledge of the microscope's point spread function (image of a point source) to place that out-of-focus light in its proper place. This technique has been successfully applied to 3D optical-section images of fluorescently-labelled single cells of several types (smooth muscle, eosinophil, fibroblast) stained for a variety of molecular distributions, e.g., alpha actinin, actin, tubulin, calsequestrin, and mRNA. These images represent a general class of specific labellings usually yielding moderately sparse stainings. We have also applied image restoration to computer simulations of single isolated cells labelled for less sparse molecular distributions, such as fura-2 images of intracellular calcium with equally successful results (Fay et al, 1986; Carrington and Fogarty, 1987; Carrington et al, 1989; Agard, 1984).

The choice of whether to use a confocal microscope, a wide-field microscope, or a wide-field microscope with image restoration depends on the relative signal losses of the instruments and the nature of the object being imaged. We begin the analysis of the tradeoffs involved in making these choices in this section.

Signal Strength, Photo-damage and Photo-bleaching

Biological applications of microscopy frequently impose limitations on the light that may be collected from or delivered to the sample. Living cells can be damaged by too much light, or may move if the integration time is excessive. Fluorescent stains bleach with exposure to light. Indeed, the key question for weak signal fluorescence is how to most effectively use the limited amount of light that leaves the specimen before the fluorescence bleaches away or the cell dies. In 3D this is especially important because optical sectioning exposes the whole cell to approximately the same amount of light for each optical section. If 40 optical sections are taken with either a confocal or a conventional microscope, then the total light exposure of every part of the cell is 40 times the exposure for a single 2D image.

The confocal microscope achieves its improvement in resolution and depth discrimination by rejecting a portion of the light with the confocal pinhole. As the pinhole becomes smaller, approaching a point detector, less light reaches the detector, but transverse and axial resolution increase to a maximum of 1.4

TABLE 1. COLLECTION EFFICIENCY OF CONFOCAL MICROSCOPE WITH PHOTOMULTIPLIER TUBE DETECTOR VS. WIDE-FIELD MICROSCOPE WITH CCD DETECTOR AT EMISSION WAVELENGTHS OF 500μm–700μm

	Efficiency CF/WF
Confocal Pinhole	
No improvement in resolution (pinhole open)	100%
Significant improvement in axial resolution	50%
Significant improvement in transverse resolution	10%
Photomultiplier tube Quantum Efficiency vs. back-illuminated, thinned RCA CCD (80%)*	12%
Smaller pixels to make use of improved transverse resolution	50%
Summary: Relative efficiency for different final resolutions	
No improvement in resolution	12%
To improve axial resolution only	6%
To improve transverse resolution	0.6%

*For wavelengths near or below 400μm, the quantum efficiency of the photomultiplier tube may equal or exceed that of the CCD detector. The CCD detector has a higher fixed noise component (readout noise) than a high-quality, cooled photomultiplier tube. The high QE RCA sensor listed also has a high noise of ±40 photons/pixel while other devices may be as low as ±10 photons/pixel. This limit will ultimately determine the lowest useable absolute light level for the CCD.

times that of the wide-field microscope. (Wilson and Carlini, 1988; Shuman, 1988; Brakenhoff, 1989). For example, Wilson and Carlini (1988) state that the transverse resolution (in transmission mode) deteriorates with a pinhole radius greater than 0.5 (in normalized optical coordinates). By their eq. (6) this corresponds to a pinhole that passes 6% of the light a large pinhole passes. A pinhole with radius 2.5 has roughly half the improvement in transverse resolution over a wide-field microscope of a point detector, but theoretically has axial resolution and depth discrimination almost identical to a point detector. This 2.5 radius pinhole collects 74% of the light. Shuman (1988) obtains qualitatively similar but numerically different results: a pinhole that collects 50% of the light has 1.26 times the axial resolution and 1.2 times the transverse resolution of the wide-field microscope; collecting 10% of the light yields 1.39 times the axial resolution and 1.37 times the transverse resolution. Brakenhoff (1989) obtained similar results on resolution in fluoresence mode. Thus we see that to approach the full resolution of the confocal microscope, only 10% of the in-focus light will be collected. However, a much larger pinhole can still result in substantial improvement in axial resolution and rejection of out of focus light, collecting roughly 50% − 75% or more of the light from the in focus plane.

Current technology confocal microscopes use photomultiplier tubes. The best of these have quantum efficiencies that vary from 0.1 at 550 nm (typical of rhodamine dyes) up to 0.3 or 0.35 at 400 nm or shorter. The cooled CCD cameras used on wide-field microscopes can have quantum efficiencies as high as 0.8 at the longer wavelengths (500–600 nm) typical of many biological applications. CCD cameras, however, have a readout noise that is not present in PMTs. As shown in Table 1, PMTs are a good choice at short wavelengths (e.g. 400 nm) but require 1.5–4 times as many photons to produce a good signal to noise ratio at the longer wavelengths typical of the requirements of many applications of fluoresence microscopy to biology.

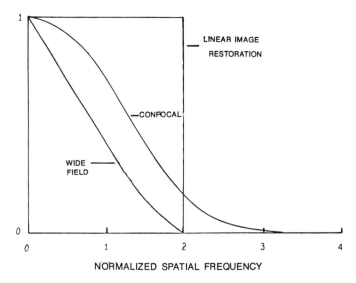

FIG. 1. Comparison of Incoherent Optical Tranfer Functions of Wide-field and Confocal microscopes, and Wide-field with image restoration (see Sheppard 1988).

Optical Transfer Function, Resolution and Noise

The optical transfer function (OTF) of a microscope measures the response of the optics to different spatial frequencies: higher spatial frequencies correspond to finer details. Fig. 1 presents the incoherent intensity optical transfer functions of wide-field and confocal microscopes using the same objective lens. Both OTFs have the same general characteristics. There is a cutoff frequency beyond which the optics pass no information; this cutoff frequency is higher for the confocal microscope than the wide-field microscope. Lower spatial frequencies are less attenuated than higher spatial frequencies; the fraction of light passed decreases until it becomes zero at the cutoff frequency.

We can now see the effect noise will have on the resulting image. When white noise is added to the image, we see that high frequency information is obscured by noise first because the signal contrast will be lower. This has the effect of decreasing the effective cutoff frequency, and decreasing the effective resolution. The higher the noise level, the lower the effective cutoff frequency becomes. It is now easy to see that there are cases where a wide-field microscope with cooled-CCD detector (without image restoration) can have greater effective resolution than a confocal microscope. This provides us with a crude way of comparing the various approaches on the basis of signal levels and spatial frequencies.

We can also see that the best an image restoration method can hope to do, without using additional information, is to eliminate the attenuation at higher spatial frequencies, so that the overall transfer function has a constant attenuation up to the cutoff frequency. We will see in the next section how simple additional information, such as the non-negativity of a fluorescent dye density or the finite spatial extent of a cell, can increase the power of image restoration.

THREE-DIMENSIONAL IMAGE RESTORATION AND CONFOCAL MICROSCOPY: A COMPARISON

A 3D image of an object is acquired as a series of optical sections in either a wide-field or a confocal microscope. Image

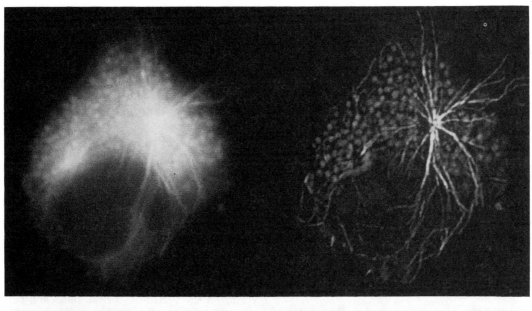

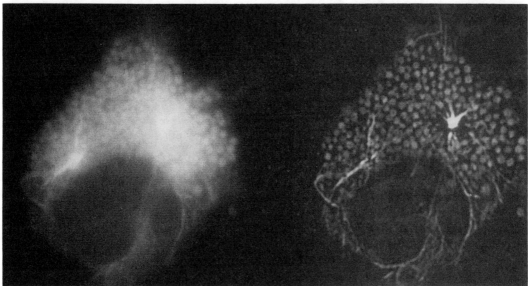

FIG. 2.   WIDE-FIELD MICROSCOPE: BEFORE (on left) AND AFTER (on right) IMAGE RESTORATION. Two optical sections 0.75 microns apart from a series of 46 optical sections at 0.25 micron increments of a Newt eosinophil with rhodamine labelled tubulin similar to the cell in Fig. 3, using a 63× 1.4NA lens on a Zeiss IM35 with Photometrics nitrogen-cooled CCD. Voxel size is 200×200×250nm. Note the detail revealed in the microtubule organizing that is obscured by out-of-focus flare in the original data on the left that is revealed in the image restoration on the right.

restoration, or deconvolution, combines this 3D data set with knowledge of the imaging process and other prior knowledge of the object imaged to invert the imaging process mathematically. The result is an image with better resolution, better contrast, and better accuracy for numerical measurements than the original data set (Carrington, 1989; Agard, 1984). Using a wide-field microscope and our image restoration method, we obtain 3D images of rhodamine-labelled cells with axial resolution, defined as the full-width at half-maximum intensity of a single microtubule, as good as the theoretical resolution of the un-processed confocal microscope (Figs. 2 and 3).

In computer simulations we obtain similar improvement in confocal images. In practice, the Bio-Rad MRC-500 confocal microscope provided images that had an unusably low S/N on the rhodamine-labeled cells we are studying.

Image Restoration Methodology

The 3D blurring of the microscope is described by $g = h * f$ where g is the blurred image, h is the instrument point spread function and f represents the object, e.g., a fluorescent dye density. In the frequency domain we can write this as $G = HF$ where capital letters denote Fourier Transforms. If we solve this for $F = G/H$, we obtain an estimate of f that is extremely sensitive to any noise present in the image. Some smoothing of the estimate is necessary, and this can usually be effectively performed by linear smoothing filters, (Castleman, 1979). These linear methods provide some improvement in the image and have an advantage in computation time over iterative methods. However, iterative methods that use the non-negativity of a fluorescent dye density provide significantly better results, especially when a substantial volume of the cell does not contain

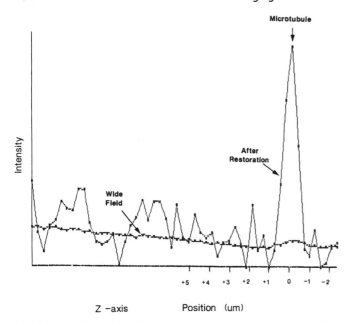

FIG. 3. Intensity profile along the optical axis through a rhodamine-labelled microtubule filament before and after image restoration. Actual filament cross-section dimension is about 28μm.

dye. We initially used a method due to Jansson (1970), and applied to 3D microscopy by Agard and Sedat, 1983, and Fay et al, 1986. This proved effective on images that consisted of small fluorescent bodies in a single cell, but was unreliable on other kinds of objects, such as the microtubules in Fig. 2 or cells loaded with Fura-2 because of the magnitude of the out-of-focus signal. We now use a regularization method (Carrington and Fogarty, 1987; Butler et al, 1981) that has proven effective on the whole range of fluorescent images. This method chooses for our estimate of the true dye density, the non-negative function, f, that minimizes:

$$\min ||g - h*f||^2 + a||f||_2^2 \qquad (1)$$

Where $||f||_2^2 = f^2$ and is the energy of f.

The first term measures how well the estimate fits the data. If there were no noise, we would let the parameter, a, equal zero and fit the data exactly. In the presence of noise, that would result in highly oscillatory solutions. More accurate estimates result if the parameter, a, is positive. Then the second term, which is the integral of the square of the function, f, enforces a certain amount of smoothness on the estimate. There are several mathematically sound ways of choosing this parameter (Butler et al, 1981; Carrington, 1982). A good numerical method has been developed for this minimization (Carrington and Fogarty, 1987; Carrington et al., 1989).

The advantages of this method over others are that it has a strong mathematical basis (Carrington, 1982; Butler et al., 1981) that provides guidance in applying it and ensures that it works reliably on the broad range of image types encountered in fluorescence microscopy, it is flexible in its use of data, and is computationally efficient. In practice, it has proven more reliable than other methods tested.

Requirements

The microscope point spread function must be either calculated or measured empirically. As our calculations of the

point spread function from optical theory have so far not proven accurate enough (Tellar, 1985), we use 0.1 or 0.2 micron fluorescently labelled polystyrene beads. Calculations of the point spread function from optical theory have so far not proven accurate enough (Tella, 1985). We use 0.2 micron polystyrene beads from Polyscience with free amino groups on the surface. Excess rhodamine isothiocyanate is reacted onto the beads at pH 9.0. The beads are then thoroughly washed with butanol to remove noncovalantly bound rhodamine. The beads are mixed with 2% gelatin at 40 degrees C in order to immobilize them and to simulate the index of refraction and scattering properties of protein-rich cytoplasm. A drop of suspension is placed on a glass slide which is allowed to cool, and an anti-bleach mounting medium was applied followed by a cover slip matching the indices of refraction of fixed cell preparations. Commercially available fluorescently-labelled beads (Fluorobrite beads, Polyscience) can be used. These beads offer the advantage of volume labelling, versus the surface labelling of our preparation, and thus are brighter. However, the fluorochromes in these beads will leach out when in a typical non-polar mounting medium, yielding a short shelf-life for the slides and potentially an incorrect point spread function measurement. These beads are useful for measuring the point spread function applicable to living cells in an aqueous environment and we have used them for such measurements.

Optical sections are taken at 0.2–0.5 micron intervals through the cell with pixel sizes of 0.2–0.25 microns. The cells we study are 5–15 microns thick; we generally take 20–50 optical sections but have used as few as 4 to remove out of focus flare from a single plane. Our algorithm allows the axial sampling to be non-uniform.

Geometric errors in the scanning mechanism can limit the geometrical accuracy of scanning microscopes for any quantitative measurement. Such errors can be corrected by postprocessing only if they can be measured accurately and do not vary from scan to scan. Image restoration procedures will degrade in performance if these errors remain significant after correction. Such errors are unimportant where the geometry is defined by a CCD detector.

Computer requirements depend on the required field of view, thickness of the cells and desired resolution. We currently use an array processor (Minimap. CSPI, Billevica Ma) with 16 megabytes of memory that performs about 3 million floating point operations per second attached to a VAX 11/750 (DEC, Maynard, MA). This performs the iterative restoration in 10–100 minutes for a $64\times64\times64$ image. We have just acquired a Silicon graphics 240 GTX (SGI, Mt. View, CA) that will perform a $128\times128\times64$ restoration in about the same time. Simulations show that resolution is currently limited by voxel size, which in turn is limited by the computer memory needed to hold the image.

Results

As expected from the nature of the *a priori* information, non-negativity that we use, results are best when most of the cell volume contains no fluorescence, or contains a background that can be measured and subtracted. When the fluorescence level is high in the whole cell volume, as it is with dyes such as Fura-2, our method improves the image, but not as much as in other cases (Fay et al, 1989).

The computer simulated images discussed in Table 2 are calculated using a theoretical point spread function for a $63\times$,

TABLE 2.   COMPARISON OF 3D POINT SPREAD FUNCTIONS, MEASURING FULL-WIDTH AT HALF-MAXIMUM INTENSITY OF PSF SAMPLED WITH 50 NM PIXELS SPACED 50 NM AXIALLY (EXCEPT WHERE NOTED)

	x	z	Integrated intensity in z plane
Wide-field	150 nm (185 nm)[1]	650 nm	infinite
Wide-field with Image Restoration	150 nm (122 nm)[2]	450 nm	250 nm
Wide-field with Image Restoration Noise added	150 nm (130 nm)[2]	450 nm	350 nm
Confocal	150 nm (135 nm)[1]	450 nm	550 nm
Confocal with Image Restoration	50 nm (71 nm)[2]	350 nm	250 nm

1. The numbers in parenthesis are taken from a theoretically calculated point spread function sampled at 5 nm transversely and 15 nm axially. All other results are in units of 50 nm voxels.
2. Interpolated linearly between 50 nm sample points.

1.4 NA, oil immersion lens at a 500nm wavelength (Tella, 1985). The simulations in Table 3 use the measured point spread of a Zeiss 63×, 1.4 NA planapo oil immersion ojective. The confocal microscope point spread function used in the simulations is the square of this theoretical point spread function. This assumes a point source and point detector (with no signal loss from this point pinhole) and equal excitation and emission wavelengths; this is an "ideal" confocal microscope. The point spread functions are scaled so that the total light from the 3D image is equal to the total gray level of the model object. Since the confocal microscope discriminates against out-of-focus light, this is equivalent to an assumption that the confocal sample emitted more total light. It would be more accurate to scale so that the total light from an in-focus plane is the same for both microscopes, then multiply by the light losses of each microscope.

When arbitrary signal levels are available, a wide-field microscope with image restoration provides greater resolution than our confocal microscope without image restoration on point sources. The best results are provided by image restoration combined with confocal microscopy. For a planar object imaged in 3D the result would be just the opposite; the wide-field microscope has no depth discrimination for planar objects (except for that due to changing magnification with axial position), so there is little axial information for the image restoration to extract.

Table 3 shows the results of computer simulations of a three compartment model of a cell, nucleus, cytoplasm, and sarcoplasmic reticulum. The cell is represented as a cylinder 7 microns in diameter, with the nucleus represented by a concentric cylinder 2.75 microns in diameter and the SR by a layer 0.5 microns thick on the cell surface; the relative dye densities in each compartment are 12,500 in the nucleus, 9,000 in the cytoplasm and 15,000 in the SR. The model is blurred with a point spread function corresponding to an objective lens of 1.4 numerical aperture in both a wide-field microscope and a confocal microscope. Pictures of the model and wide-field results are shown in Fay et al, 1989. Gaussian noise was added to each pixel; at these light levels, this is a reasonable approximation to the more accurate Poisson model. The standard deviation was empirically determined on a Dage/MTI SIT camera as a

TABLE 3.   PERCENTAGE ERROR IN ESTIMATED FLUORESCENCE INTENSITY

Compartment	Imaged Model	Restored Image	Confocal
Nucleus	8.6%	2.31%	2.44%
Cytoplasm	4.06%	1.51%	1.15%
Sarcoplasmic Reticulum	9.15%	4.6%	5.95%
Total Model	6.4%	2.90%	3.63%
Outside Model	3.0%	0.45%	0.92%

Values given are the square root of the sum of the squared residuals divided by the square root of the sum squares of the model pixel values for each compartment. The residuals are calculated from the model convolved with the 3D point spread function to simulate image formation for conventional microscope. Similar values are given for the imaged model after restoration by an iterative restoration method based on regularization theory also incorporating non-negativity according to Carrington and Fogarty (1987) and for a simulated confocal image formed by convolving confocal point spread function with the model. The errors outside the model are given as a percentage of the total square root of the sum of squares of the pixels within the bounds of the model cell (Fay et al, 1989).

TABLE 4.   COMPARISON OF POTENTIAL DOMAINS OF USE OF CONFOCAL MICROSCOPY AND IMAGE RESTORATION

3D Image Restoration and Wide-field
   Low signal
   High resolution single cell
   Fluorescence
   Localized fluorescence, small compartments, small discrete structures

3D
High resolution 2D by acquiring 3D optical sections to remove out-of-focus flare
When photobleaching or photodamage important.
Potential: Use of other *a priori* information
besides non-negativity—more resolution and better S/N.

Confocal
   Immediate images
   Thick tissue sections
   Bright images
   Uniform planar or volume images i.e., large membranes or large membrane-bound compartments
   2D imaging of 3D objects directly
   Photobleaching or photodamage less critical
   Potential: New designs using CCDs or multiple detectors may improve S/N and resolution and 3D image restoration can also be applied to confocal data.

function of number of counts, number of frames summed and gain setting. This is not the most appropriate noise model for either microscope, but was used to be consistent with results already calculated (Fay et al, 1989). The peak light intensities and signal to noise ratios for the 3D images were 12014 and 85:1 for the confocal microscope and 9281 and 71:1 for the wide-field microscope. The losses due to the confocal pinhole were not included in the model calculations. Surprisingly, image restoration of a wide-field 3D image provided numerical values slightly more accurate than the confocal microscope provided. Pictures calculated with this model are shown in Fay et al 1989.

In a comparison between two optical sections (out of a series of 46) obtained on a wide-field microscope and the same sections after our 3D image restoration procedure, out-of-focus flare is substantially eliminated, and axial resolution is substantially improved. Transverse resolution is limited by the size of our pixels (200 nm × 200 nm). Detail in the microtubule organizing center is revealed that is only hinted at in the original image. These microtubules are subresolution filaments; their axial half width in the restored image measures 850nm. This compares favorably with the 800nm axial half-width Brakenhoff, et al (1989) measure for confocal fluorescent imaging at similar wavelengths. In the data, the peak signal level is 14,705 photo-electrons with a mean of 669 photo-electrons. Near the microtubule organizing center in the unrestored data, individual microtubules are about 10% brighter than nearby pixels that appear to contain only out-of-focus haze.

One situation where confocal microscopy has the absolute advantage over image restoration of wide-field images is when imaging a uniform planar object of effectively infinite extent. In this case, the wide-field microscope provides almost no information on axial position (there is only the change in intensity as the magnification changes). In situations that approximate this we would expect the advantage to remain with confocal. This would include thick tissue sections with substantial fluorescence throughout the sample. For the advantage to be clearly with the confocal approach the thickness would have to be greater than the 5–15 micron thickness of the single cells to which we have applied image restoration (Table 4).

Multiple Detector Confocal Microscopes

The light discarded by the confocal pinhole contains information about the object. Multiple detectors can be used to sample the light distribution in the plane around the usual pinhole location (Chap. 2). Bertero, et al, (1987) and Sheppard, (1988) have proposed methods of using this information to improve resolution in 2D. Bertero, et al (1987), use an approach conceptually similar to the image restoration method presented in this chapter. They approximate the solution of the inverse problem of calculating the light at the scan position from the multiple detector data using a singular value decomposition. This approximation is simple enough to potentially be calculated in real time. They show that the resulting optical transfer function of this instrument has a spatial frequency cutoff double that of the wide-field microscope, or 1.414 times that of a conventional confocal microscope. Sheppard obtains the same resolution using a rather different method. Both methods are formulated in 2D, but in principle can be extended to 3D. Neither method incorporates *a priori* information such as non-negativity, so the ultimate resolution will be reached by combining these approaches with an image restoration technique such as that presented above.

Such multiple detector methods have the potential of collecting more light than the normal confocal microscope. In principle, they could detect most of the collected light, giving a major increase in signal levels over conventional confocal microscopes and at the same time retaining the Z-sectioning and the greater transverse resolution. If they prove practical, such methods could lead to superior microscopes for fluorescence microscopy.

Conclusions and Recommendations

For maximum 3D resolution on sparsely-stained fluorescent, single cell specimens, our simulation shows that image restoration of wide-field images is superior to the BioRad MRC-500 without restoration even when signal levels are high on both instruments and even when the cell is not flat but has significant axial depth (10μm).

When an image of only one plane is needed, using a confocal microscope is operationally easier than acquiring the series of optical sections that image restoration requires. However, while image restoration may require 10–40 optical sections on a wide-field microscope, the confocal microscope generally must rescan a single plane many times and average to obtain a usable image. The confocal microscope has the theoretical advantage on cells that have a substantial positive level of fluorescence everywhere. In cells that are intermediate in character between all white and all black, the theoretical choice is not clear, but clearly when only 10% of the light from a wide-field image represents contrast from the in-focus plane, there will be problems in extracting it. In practice, current technology confocal microscopes have substantially less collection efficiency than a wide-field microscope with cooled CCD since there are significant losses and inefficiencies besides the confocal pinhole. Until confocal instruments are available that, with the pinhole open, are as efficient as wide-field microscopes, the wide-field microscope with image restoration will remain our instrument of choice for the high resolution 3D fluorescence imaging of sparsely-stained single cells.

COMPUTER GRAPHICS 3D VISUALIZATION

A cell is inherently a 3D object, so 3D images are often needed to understand the cell's biology. Both confocal and wide-field microscopes can provide high quality 3D digital images by optical sectioning. Once a 3D digital image is acquired, it must be analyzed to answer the questions posed in the experiment. This requires the ability to view the cell in a variety of ways and to make measurements on selected regions (See Coggins, et al, 1986; van der Voort et al, 1989; Foley and van Dam, 1982, is the standard reference as are the adjoining Chapters).

The availability of true 3D digital data gives the biologist options in viewing the specimen that are not possible with microscopy alone. Structures may be selectively emphasized or eliminated. Multiwavelength or multimodal data of the specimen can be directly combined for viewing within a single image. An image can be generated of the specimen rotated to any angle, which may be impractical or impossible within the microscope. In fact the eye point can be placed anywhere, even inside the specimen. Unless computer software and hardware are available to perform these operations, a substantial part of the benefit of acquiring a 3D digital image is lost.

Display of 2D Slices of 3D Data

The first operation in analyzing 3D data is inspection. In the case of data resulting from optical sectioning, the simplest and fastest way is to display selected slices perpendicular to the three coordinate axes (X, Y and Z, Z corresponding to the microscope axial direction). These slices require no processing unless correction for geometric distortion is desired at this level of analysis. Ideally the microscope system itself should have software to display X-Z and Y-Z slices from digitized 3D data. Simple operations on each 2D image, such as thresholding or contrast stretching and simple measurements such as length or average intensity in a rectangle are useful and should be available.

Using a digital image display system with the capacity to internally store many 2D gray-level images (although only one can be viewed at a time), one can rapidly flip through a series of optical sections and attempt to quantify apparent spatial relationships. While simple to implement and comprehend, this approach loses its effectiveness as

- the complexity of the scene increases,
- as the amount of "noise" in the images increases such that individual structures become hard to identify in each 2D image,
- and as the amount of *a priori* information available about the structure to be identified diminishes.

In reconstructing a 3D structure from 2D slices, the investigator relies upon memory to build and validate the third dimension. While yielding a 3D impression that is otherwise not obtainable, all the available data is still not being brought to bear upon the analysis.

Volume Displays

Analyzing information from the high resolution 3D data sets produced by microscopy involves viewing and analyzing images consisting of as many as 512 x 512 × 128 voxels. One way of analyzing this enormous (32 million voxels) data set is to reduce it to a single image by projecting all or part of the volume onto a viewing plane, as if viewing the data through a window. This is called a ray-tracing volume display or a voxel-based display. The basic idea is to pass a "ray" through the data to the eye point, computing the observable "light" along the ray. Computing all the 3D translations, rotations, and scalings necessary to produce a single projection from an arbitrary eye position through a data set of this magnitude can involve over a billion calculations. Volume displays are useful for viewing sparse images, such as those produced when a dye is associated with specific organelles or filaments. By their nature, volume displays make no attempt to discriminate between useful data and digitizing noise, or between specific and non-specific staining.

Continuous dye density images such as those produced by ion concentration indicators (FURA-2, etc.) are difficult to display in a way that conveys meaningful information. The human visual system is not well suited to visualizing and understanding the 3D haze of these projected-density images. The display of density images is a difficult problem and the subject of current research (See Chapter 13).

Surface Model Displays

The amount of data that must be operated upon can be first reduced by spatially segmenting the image into "objects" representing regions of interest and ignoring the rest. A further reduction can be achieved by representing objects with surface descriptions instead of retaining all the pixels within object volumes. This approach involves rendering such segmented objects as "solid" model objects possessing physical attributes, such as length, width and orientation, extracted manually by interaction with a volume display or automatically by pattern recognition techniques. Because the dimensionality of the image has been reduced, less memory is required to store the image and faster display speeds are possible. Such images are also substantially easier for human comprehension. The trick is to ensure that the derived graphical surface portrays features of the data that have real significance.

3D Perception from 2D Displays

The use of solid modeling techniques offers many advantages. Perspective, shading, and reflectance cues produce the illusion of three dimensional information with a two dimensional computer display. Additional data attributes, such as densities or gradients, can be conveyed with the added dimensions of color, texture, translucency, etc. True stereo displays are useful for conveying 3D information, but are more effective on surface displays or sparse volume displays. The human visual system finds it difficult to see the stereo effect on blurred density images. (See Chapter 16)

User Interaction and Analysis

Ideally the experimenter needs to be able to interact with the graphics images in a variety of ways. We can move the "eye" position to any vantage point, even one that is apparently inside the cell. The ability to get extreme close-up views of specific regions within a cell from any arbitrary angle cannot be mimicked using conventional 2D microscopy.

We can extract quantitative information about structure beyond what can be inferred visually. One can quantify spatial relationships such as proximity and relative angle among any two or more objects by "pointing" to them (which is possible after objects have been given surface representations).

We can catalog relational information, breaking down complex structures into simpler ones, which can be displayed individually or visually differentiated from the whole using different color codings.

We can make movie loops to take advantage of the ability of the human visual system to extract 3D information from relative motion cues. The motions that are useful include cycling through the optical sections, rotating about an axis in space or flying the eyepoint through the cell, either interactively or along a predetermined path.

AUTOMATED IMAGE ANALYSIS: FEATURE EXTRACTION AND COMPUTER VISION

Analysis of 3D density images can be difficult and time consuming even when sophisticated computer graphics systems are available. A human observer can easily be overwhelmed by the information overload present in large complex 3D images. Computer based methods of simplifying the image, extracting the important features and suppressing extraneous details are necessary. Some measurements are difficult for an experimenter to make on 3D density images and computer assistance is necessary.

Thresholding

The most straight-forward methods of simplifying an image are intensity based, e.g., identifying objects of interest as any pixel with intensity between two fixed thresholds. An intensity based approach in this context means one which does not use any model of the object being searched for and uses only the most rudimentary of local spatial information during processing (e.g., if a voxel is surrounded by 26 voxels ([3×3×3]-1) of the same intensity, replace its intensity with that of its neighbors). The most common such approach finds objects by simple intensity thresholding (possibly followed by filling in small holes in large objects). This technique simply identifies as an object anything with an intensity above or below some threshold (which may be supplied or calculated automatically). These approaches, when they work, are usually fairly fast. They are also able to quantify parameters about the objects that have been identified and about their relative positions. Ideally this can be completely automated and allows massive amounts of data to be analyzed in fairly short order. The main drawback is that few interesting problems involve the analysis of objects having a geometry or an intensity profile simple enough to permit the application of this approach.

Certain image characteristics may invalidate an intensity-based approach. The object may not differ significantly in intensity from background. In fluorescence imaging, non-specifically stained objects may have the same intensity as the object of interest. Bleaching of fluorescence and non-uniform staining, illumination, or improper confocal scan rate may cause significant intensity changes across an image or between images, even when the stain is bound to the same substrate in all cases. If the signal-to-noise ratio is not high, then intensity may not be enough of a cue with which to find an object.

Human Interaction and Partial Automation

The next most complicated algorithm is interactive and partially automated. (Selfridge, 1987; Sobel, 1980). Since a human makes the decisions that are difficult for a fully automated system, this approach can work in diverse imaging situations. If the amount of data to be analyzed is not too large this is usually the method of choice. The utility of an interactive algorithm strongly depends upon the user interface, and most useful interfaces are graphical. Typically, the interface displays the image along with partial results; trouble spots may be highlighted in some manner. The human then assists the algorithm over the trouble spots (e.g., by drawing a line across a gap in an object boundary that the algorithm is unable to complete). With large 3D data sets, fast, well-designed, graphics display algorithms are essential. An interactive algorithm falters if the user must constantly struggle with the user interface. The major deficiency of this approach is that it can become too time consuming if the images are large or if the experiment requires results from many cells.

Fully Automated Analysis

The most complicated level of computer analysis is the completely automated one. This approach typically employs descriptions or mathematical models of the objects of interest. If the objects can be defined mathematically, detection and estimation theory can then be used to find them, thereby simplifying the problem. Of importance is the number of unknown parameters in the object model (e.g., position, orientation, size). The fewer unknown parameters, the easier the task becomes. Precise estimates of unknown parameters are also possible. Such a system, the Artificial Visual System, (AVS) has been developed for analyzing alpha-actinin dense bodies in 3D images of smooth muscle cells (Coggins, et al 1986 a, b,; Fay et al, 1989). This Artificial Visual System detects these dense bodies and measures their size, position and orientation. The measurement of orientation in particular is very difficult for a human exper-

imenter to perform at all. Analysis of a small section of a single cell by a human requires weeks of tedious work; the automatic system performs it in minutes with greater accuracy. The orientations can be estimated to within 5 degrees on this system, even though the dense bodies are very small and there is noise and distortion in the image. The user can then interact with a simplified display of the bodies to gain insight into the spatial relationships among them. The impressive performance of the AVS system is possible because the objects to be found are well-defined. We have constructed other artificial visual systems in 2D for locating colloidal gold particles and determining the length of smooth muscle cells (Abramson and Fay, 1989) and in 3D for locating and identifying cell receptors.

At the present state of technology, systems that perform identification and simple measurements on geometrically simple objects are easiest to implement. Successful systems are specific rather than general; they work on some very specific problem rather than a large general class of problems. Automation makes the most sense when there is a repetitive task , e.g., large numbers of similar measurements to make, or when the task is difficult for the human visual system to perform at all.

COMPUTER HARDWARE CONSIDERATIONS

The kinds of imaging tasks previously described place some imposing demands on the computer hardware and software needed to perform them. In particular, the availability of high resolution 3D data from confocal microscopes and from conventional microscopes coupled with image restoration places demands on data throughput and storage not easily met at the personal computer level. In addressing the requirements of the various systems functions (image acquisition, image restoration, image analysis and display, image archival storage, and computer networking) all computer subsystems come into play.

Image Acquisition

The major concerns in 3D image acquisition are speed and resolution. The two are necessarily linked as the required system bandwidth (speed) equals the number of pixels acquired (resolution) divided by the time to acquire those pixels. 3D image data sets are very large. A typical image of a single cell with a diameter of 50 microns and a thickness of 10 microns, taken with a transverse resolution of 200 nanometers/pixel and an axial resolution of 250 nanometers/pixel, requires at least 2.5 million pixels. Real-time (1/30s. or one standard video frame time) image acquisition of 512×512 optical slices with each pixel having two bytes (up to 16 bits) of information requires a sustained throughput of almost 16 million bytes/second. The Analog-to-digital (A/D) converters used to digitize images are capable of these rates. Most personal computers cannot process or store this much data this fast. In fact the limiting factor in acquisition throughput is usually data storage. Most computer disk systems transfer data at less than 5 million bytes/second. The software overhead in the computer's operating system will usually limit this to a few hundred thousand bytes/second of actual throughput. Thus, several seconds are usually required for 3D image acquisition. There are expensive solutions to this problem, such as real-time data disks ($30,000). New technologies, such as optical disks and high-speed digital signal processing (DSP) computer chips capable of real-time image compression/decompression, promise to solve both speed and resolution limitations in the near future.

Image Restoration

Image restoration is a computationally intensive operation. Our current algorithm requires 100 minutes to restore a $10 \times 10 \times 10$ micron volume at the resolution described above, using an array processor rated at 6 million floating point operations per second (6 MFLOPS). The algorithm requires ten megabytes (Mbytes) of memory, and the processor must have access to this amount of memory while maintaining its rated computational speed. Plug-in floating point accelerator cards for PCs, while rated as high as 20 MFLOPS, are usually inadequate as they must use the PCs limited memory for data storage, or access disk storage which is far too slow to keep the accelerator running at its rated speed. Rated speeds are often greater than that which can be achieved for a given application, especially when such large images are involved. The best rule of thumb is to try the application on the hardware being considered for the job. For our restoration algorithm we need the ability to perform $64 \times 64 \times 64$ fast Fourier transforms (FFT) in a maximum of five seconds. New RISC (reduced instruction set computer) based workstations are rated as high as 4 MFLOPS, can have more than 16 Mbytes of main memory, and are capable of performing image restoration without an attached array processor or floating point accelerator. These new workstations are available for as little as $20,000 and it is expected that the cost per MFLOP will continue to fall.

Image Analysis and Display

As already described, the process of 2D and 3D image analysis is visually interactive and thus graphically intensive. The generation and manipulation of volume displays is a large task, requiring lots of memory, fast computation, and fast image display. Most image acquisition systems provide more than 8 bits/pixel of gray level resolution. While the human visual system can only resolve about 60 gray levels (about 6 bits) at one instant, most image display systems provide 256 gray levels (8 bits) of output resolution. Even more bits/pixel are desirable for functions such as text and graphic overlays, image-image overlays (very useful for image registrations) and multicolor displays. Advanced display systems provide 24 bits/pixel for "true color" output (8 bits red, 8 bits green, 8 bits blue). As already discussed, a real-time system operating on a 512×512 pixel image requires a bandwidth of 10 million pixels/second. Therefore a display system should be able to update the image display at least this fast to provide smooth, real-time interactions such as 3D image rotation or through-focussing. If anything, 3D image processing requires more bandwidth on the output side than the input side, as images are acquired once but may be viewed many times in many ways.

Archival Storage

Three-D images are very large, containing millions of bytes. In the process of analyzing these images, many additional images may be produced. Sufficient cost-effective storage is necessary for serious 3D imaging. There are four basic alternatives for image storage and retrieval: magnetic disks, cartridge magnetic tapes, reel magnetic tapes, and optical disks.

Magnetic disks Floppy disks are impractical for either short or long term 3D image storage. A $512 \times 512 \times 50$ pixel image contains 25 Mbytes requiring 17 high-density floppy disks (1.44 Mbytes/floppy). Non-removable storage such as Winchester disks are useful for short term storage but they will quickly become full. Removable disks are fast and convenient, however the cost per megabyte of such storage ($>\$1$/Mbyte) is not competitive with other media.

Cartridge Magnetic Tape Cartridge tapes are a popular storage peripheral on personal computers and workstations. The initial hardware investment is reasonable ($1000-$5000). The capacity per tape varies between 40 Mbytes and 200 Mbytes and the cost per megabyte $0.20 to $0.50. Tape is a sequential-access medium and the storage and retrieval times are slow, measured often in minutes for a single image. The low capacity per tape means tape cartridges must be changed often, and the physical space and environment required for storing the tapes may be a concern.

Reel Magnetic Tape Half-inch reel-to-reel tape drives, as often found on larger minicomputers or mainframe computers, provide moderate storage capacity and speed but at a much larger initial cost ($10,000-$30,000). The upper-end tape systems provide 6250 bits per inch (BPI) tape densities and total tape capacity around 160 Mbytes. The time to retrieve a single image may be one-tenth of cartridge tapes; the cost per megabyte of storage is about the same. Reel tapes have the same physical requirements as cartridge tapes. The major advantage of reel tapes is for data exchange between computer sites and even between dissimilar computer operating systems. There are standardized formats for reel tapes and most formats are simple enough that decoding a non-standard one is usually possible.

Optical disk The optical disk is now a rapidly maturing technology. Write-once-read-many (WORM) disk systems have been available for several years. By their write-once nature, WORM disks provide a secure archival storage media. The initial cost of investment varies from $5000 for a single drive, 5-1/4 inch disk system storing more than 600 Mbytes per disk to more than $100,000 for a jukebox system holding more than 100 gigabytes at a time. The large single disk capacity (600 to 2000 Mbytes) means many weeks to months of 3D image data can be stored on a single volume and be available in seconds. The average access time to any file is less one-half second in current system, and while the data transfer rates are slower than magnetic disks, they are much faster than tape. The cost per megabyte of storage is currently about $0.20 for WORM disks and one cubic foot of space can hold more than 50 gigabytes. We have been using a 12 inch WORM system for four years with no more problems than we have experienced with any other storage peripherals. The major problem with optical disks is a lack of media format standards. Disks written on the system of one manufacturer probably cannot be read on that of any other manufacturer, even if the disk themselves are identical. Thus the disks are not universally useful for data exchange and the disks themselves probably will outlive the systems used to create them.

Networking

There may be no single computer system ideal for performing all aspects of 3D imaging. In our laboratories, we use

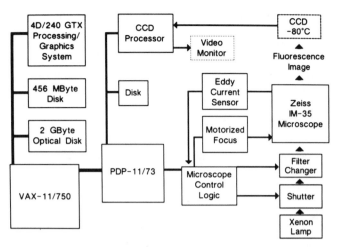

FIG. 4. Block diagram of the Digital Imaging Microscope used for acquiring and processing optical-section images. Image restoration and 3D image display and analysis are performed on the Silicon Graphics 4D/240GTX workstation (Mountain View, Ca.).

smaller, inexpensive microcomputers for image acquisition and real-time control of the microscope system, and larger, faster workstations optimized for image restoration, image analysis and image storage (Fig. 4). These computers are able to exchange images using a local area network (LAN).

MODEMs (1000 to 10,000 bytes/second) are too slow to exchange 3D image data on regular basis. The most common hardware system used in LANs is Ethernet, which is rated to carry 10 million bits/second. Ethernet uses a single cable to connect all computers in the LAN at a cost of $1-$2 per foot.

Each computer "taps" the cable; taps are approximately $200. Ethernet interfaces are available as plug-in options for most computer system and cost between $400 for a PC to $3000 for a minicomputer.

The choice of communication software used in an Ethernet LAN is independent of the hardware, and different software protocols can simultaneously communicate over the same cable. The UNIX operating system and its derivatives use the TCP/IP protocol. Digital Equipment Corp. uses DECNET for its line of VAX computers. Both are available for "IBM" PCs and clones are using the MS-DOS operating system but while DECNET and TCP/IP are able to operate over the same cable, they cannot exchange information.

While LANs allow the rapid exchange of image data between computer systems, the problem of total system integration remains. There are as yet no standard file formats for image data. Different computers, while connected by a network, may use different software for processing images. The images may need to be converted from one format to another before processing. Several general image processing packages have been or are being developed which include 3D image file formats as part of the package. These include "vsh" developed at the University of North Carolina, "qsh" developed at Columbia, and the ANALYZE package developed at the Mayo Foundation. An interesting project underway at University of Lowell in Massachusetts is the image kernel system (IKS), a proposed ANSI standard for creating hardware-independent image acquisition and image processing software. X-windows, developed at M.I.T. and placed in the public domain, represents an emerging standard for hardware-independent graphics software.

CONCLUSION

The confocal microscope is not automatically the instrument of choice. A wide-field microscope with an inexpensive video camera and computer will frequently provide adequate images and be more cost effective. A wide-field microscope with a cooled CCD camera has a substantial advantage over early commercial confocal microscopes in sensitivity. Light exposure of the cell by such a microscope can be orders of magnitude less than by a confocal microscope. Present commercial confocal microscopes are then the preferred instruments for 3D imaging of thick tissue samples or of single cells only when the staining is fairly dense and the signal levels are very strong so that photobleaching and photodamage are less important.

Image restoration applied to 3D optically sectioned images of sparsely stained single cells from a wide-field microscope provides 3D images with axial resolution as good as unprocessed images from a commercial confocal microscope. Our computer models show that transverse resolution, axial resolution, depth discrimination and numerical accuracy of images restored from 3D wide-field microscope data are comparable to those from confocal microscopes and that image restoration applied to confocal 3D images can provide a similar improvement.

Simple computer manipulations of 2D digital microscope images are very useful, but a 3D digital image provides the opportunity to view a cell in ways that are impossible in a simple microscope. The image of a cell can be viewed from any position, including from the inside, and measurements can be performed directly on the 3D image. This ability to manipulate 3D images substantially increases the information that can be gained from 3D images.

Three-dimensional cell images are very difficult and time consuming to analyze. Automated or semi-automated methods of analysis will become increasingly important.

The cost of computer equipment needed to perform 3D graphics and feature extraction efficiently is modest relative to the cost of any 3D digital imaging microscope, confocal or nonconfocal. Not having this capability essentially sacrifices a significant portion of the gain in 3D microscopic imaging. Computer hardware and software are increasingly integral components of a microscope.

REFERENCES

Agard, D.A. (1984) Ann. Rev. Biophys. Bioeng. 13:191–219.
Agard, D. and J. Sedat. (1983) Three-dimensional architecture of a polytene nucleus. Nature 302:676–681.
Bertero, M., P. Brianzi and E.R. Pike. (1987) Super-resolution in confocal scanning microscopy. Inverse Problems 3, 195–212.
Butler, J.P., J.A. Reeds and S.V. Dawson. (1981) Estimating solutions of first kind integral equations with non-negative constraints and optimal smoothing. SIAM, J. Numer. Anal. 19, No. 3, 381–397.
Carrington, W. (1982) Moment problems and ill-posed operator equations with convex constraints, Ph.D. Dissertation, Mathematics Dept. Washington U., St. Louis.
Carrington, W. and K.E. Fogarty. (1987) 3-D Molecular distribution in living cells by deconvolution of optical sections using light microscopy. In: Proc of the 13th Annual Northeast Bioengineering Conference, K. Foster, ed., IEEE, 108–111.
Carrington, W., K.E. Fogarty and F.S. Fay. (1989) Deconvolution and confocal microscopy in 3D. To appear, J. Microscopy.
Castleman, (1979) "Digital Image Processing", Prentice-Hall, Englewood Cliffs, New Jersey.
Coggins, J.M., F.S. Fay and K.E. Fogarty. (1986a) Development and

application of a three-dimensional artificial visual system. In Computer Methods and Programs in Biomedicine, Elsevier Science Publishers, 22. 69–77.

Coggins, J.M., K.E. Fogarty and F.S. Fay. (1986b) Interfacing image processing and computer graphics systems using an artificial visual system. Proceedings of IEEE Conferences on Graphics and Vision Interface.

Fay, F.S., W. Carrington and K.E. Fogarty. (1989) Three-dimensional molecular distribution in single cells analysed using the digital imaging microscope. J. Microsc. 153, pt 2, 133–149.

Fay, F.S., K.E. Fogarty and J.M. Coggins. (1986) Analysis of molecular distribution in single cells using a digital imaging microscope. In: Optical Methods in Cell Physiology, P. De Weer and B. Salzberg, eds., John Wiley & Sons, 51–62.

Jannson, P.A., R.H. Hunt and E.K. Plyler. (1970) Resolution enhancement of spectra. J. Opt. Soc. Am., Vol 60, No. 5, May, 596–599.

Kawata, S. and Y. Ichioka. (1980) J. Opt. Soc. Am. Vol. 70, 762–772.

Ortega, J.M. and W.C. Rheinboldt. (1970) Iterative solutions of nonlinear equations in several variables. Acad. Press, N.Y.

Sheppard, C.J.R. (1988) Super-resolution in confocal imaging. Optik Vol. 80 #2, 53–54.

Shuman, H. (1988) Contrast in confocal scanning microscopy with a finite detector. J. Microscopy 149:67–71.

Tella, L., (1985) The determination of a microscope's 3-dimensional point spread function for use in image restoration., MSc thesis, Worcester Polytechnic Institute, Worcester, MA.

Wilson, T. and A.R. Carlini. (1988) Three-dimensional imaging in confocal imaging systems with finite sized detectors. J. Microscopy 149:51–66.

Wilson, T. and C. Sheppard. (1984) Theory and practice of scanning optical microscopy. Academic Press, publishers: Harcourt Brace Jovanovich.

Chapter 15

Direct Recording of Stereoscopic Pairs Obtained From Disk-scanning Confocal Light Microscopes

ALAN BOYDE

University College London, Dept. of Anatomy and Developmental Biology

SUMMARY

The TSRLM is a practical tool for practical microscopy problems: it gives a real image in real time and real color, and the recording process is direct photomicrography. This chapter represents the advantages of the TSRLM in allowing stereo images to be acquired directly. Through-focussing during photography, repeated twice on inclined axes, provides the simplest direct means of obtaining stereoscopic views at the limit of resolution in light microscopy.

The method will be limited mainly by the characteristics of real objects and objective lenses. The translucency of the object will be impaired in proportion to the density of the light-scattering features which it is hoped to visualise. High resolving power objectives have a short free-working distance and collide with the specimen or its cover glass when one has focussed down through that distance.

INTRODUCTION

The usual simple and direct means of obtaining a stereoscopic view in a light microscope (LM) is to use two inclined, long-working-distance, low-aperture objectives which examine the same field in the object. If high-aperture lenses are used to secure high resolving power, the depth-of-field is so reduced that there is too little depth to perceive. Two such lenses cannot be used simultaneously because they are too bulky and too close to the sample at focus and it is therefore necessary to tilt the sample and record two separate images photographically. The depth of field is always a few times greater than the lateral resolution and useful information could be obtained from some 4 or 5 μm in Z, with a focus plane lateral resolution of 0.5 μm, but this would only work close to the line where the two tilted views intersect: away from this line, the microscope is focussed at different levels in the two images. This limit has led to the more general approach to direct stereoscopic imaging at higher magnifications using one objective, with split-field illumination (anaglyph or crossed polars for direct view, or a field stop for photography). However, such systems fall far short of providing an exact geometrical solution, and reduce the objective aperture by 50%. Wolf (1989) has described a system which is claimed to work at the full objective aperture, but this is also limited by the usual depth-of-field problems.

The lateral resolution in a light microscope (working with amplitude or phase contrast) is practically limited by the thickness of the sample because high contrast features present in out-of-focus layers obscure the in-focus components of the image.

To obtain the highest resolution, therefore, it is usual to use objects with a thickness close to both the wavelength of light and the resolving power of the objective, for example, the 0.5 μm plastic embedded sections used as optical overview controls in biological transmission electron microscopy. Since this use of a thin specimen has removed all the information from the other specimen layers, it is clear that the requirement for high resolution contradicts the demand for the preservation of 3D relationships, which is necessary for their appreciation.

This chapter deals with practical means for a general solution to the problem of producing high resolution stereo-pairs, and at the same time producing microscopical, stereo images with a much simpler geometry (parallel, as against perspective projection).

USE OF A CONFOCAL MICROSCOPE TO REDUCE THE DEPTH OF FIELD

All confocal scanning light microscopes (CSLMs) show high contrast in a very shallow focused-on plane. By scan-focusing in Z, while scanning in X and Y, it is possible to obtain signal intensity data for all the constituent sub-volumes in the volume to be analysed. For a solid specimen in the CSLM case, it is possible to produce a surface map or "range image" (Wilson and Sheppard, 1984) by digital image processing in which relative heights are displayed in grey level, pseudo-color coding, or as a contour map of a surface. For either solid or translucent specimens, the data can be processed to synthesize stereoscopic pair views of the sample from any mean vantage point and with any difference between the angles of view, as hypothesized by Brakenhoff (1979) and later demonstrated by Cox and Sheppard (1983); see also Wilson and Sheppard, (1984), Carlsson et al (1985), van der Voort et al (1985), Wijnaendts van Resandt et al (1985), Brakenhoff et al (1985) and Sugimoto and Ichioka (1985).

If a tandem scanning reflected light microscope (TSRLM: Petran et al, 1985; Xiao and Kino 1987) is used with objective lenses with an appropriate longitudinal chromatic aberration and a light source with a broad spectral coverage, at a single focus setting it will produce images of reflective specimen surfaces which are maps showing height level differences over a range of a few microns as contrasting colors (Boyde, 1985a). This is not the topic of the present chapter. In the present context, the advantage of the TSRLM or other disk-scanning confocal instruments is that they are the only CSLM to give an immediately viewable image without the intermediary of light-electronics-light conversion stages.

The TSM allows the formation of the image of a thin focal plane well below the surface of an intact block of translucent material or a high-contrast image of poorly reflective surface structures. No other reflected light microscope giving a real-time image can perform this function. In order to obtain three-dimensional information, it is necessary to examine sets of two-dimensional images corresponding to different focal planes. The operator looking down the microscope can have a strong psychological impression of 3D structure simply by focussing up and down rapidly. However, many three-dimensional structures are too complex to appreciate in this way. In addition, it is not possible to convey the 3D information to a third party and it is disappointing not to be able to record the 3D information by photographic means.

OPTICAL SECTIONING IN THE TSRLM

To study three-dimensional organization using the TSRLM, one can record images at regular focus intervals, reproduce these on photographic plates and make a stack of the plates to reconstruct the object; stereo-pair images can be generated from such a stack. Such images can alternatively be recorded in frame store, computer memory, video disc or tape and processed by computer, as was discussed in the preceding two chapters.

Stereo-pair images of the stack of photographs can be obtained either by shifting the stack in contact printing so that the rays of light which pass through the stack for each eye's view do so with differing, opposing obliquities, corresponding to left and right eye views through the stack; or by shearing the stack so that every optical section is shifted by a small amount relative to its neighbor: stack-shearing allows differing effective directions of view through the stack while viewing it from directly above. Two symmetrical and opposite sheared positions give a symmetric, mean normal incidence view of the stack. Alternatively, one normal and one sheared view can be employed to obtain a view at half that angular difference to the normal to the stack.

The disadvantages of employing stacked, recorded photographs of sections are that the specimen is sampled only at the intervals corresponding to the recorded images, and that the image densities for real features are so extreme (bright or dark) that overlapping them in one or the other or both directions of view through the stack means that the summed, stacked image may exceed the dynamic range of the final recording medium with the result that no local modulation of information is conveyed and no information about 3D position can be obtained. Consequently, although stereo-pair images can be generated from such a stack, the procedure is costly, time-consuming and not always satisfactory.

Direct Photographic Recording of the Stereo-pair

The information contained in such a stack can be contained in two images, which correspond to the two directions of view through the stack. Such images can be obtained directly by changing focus during the photographic exposure. The basis of the procedure is simply as follows: the operator selects the specimen volume to be reconstructed by direct view down the microscope. An image corresponding to one direction of view through this selected volume is recorded while changing the mechanical focus of the microscope. The image is therefore an

extended focus view in that direction. The same slice of tissue is then photographed in the same way through the same vertical interval, but along an axis inclined to the vertical, corresponding to a different view through the volume under study. The two photographs are viewed as a stereoscopic pair to give the three-dimensional effect.

Both members of the stereo-pair sample the same object depth. However, as with physical stack shearing, lateral shift need occur during only one of the exposures, the other axis of view being normal to the sampled slice volume. The more usual system would be to employ two equal and opposite lateral shifts (slews) so that the mean stereo viewing axis was normal to the plane of the slice within the object (Fig. 1).

Means for Stereo Imaging of a Layer Inside a Bulk

Any means for achieving the simultaneous combination of vertical (through-focussing = optical sectioning) movement and horizontal movement (equivalent to changing the direction of view through a real stack of photographically recorded images) may be employed. The simplest would be to employ two mechanical movement devices, both with their axes of movement nearly parallel with the usual (Z) focussing direction, but each tilted to correspond to the directions of stereo view through the "stacked" image. Several different mechanical means have been employed, and they are mentioned to encourage others to make preliminary experiments with this approach to stereo. The simplest devices were hand operated and did produce satisfactory results, but obviously there is a problem with vibrations introduced by an operator turning a mechanical focus control while recording a photograph. For routine application to high-resolution stereo imaging, the through-focusing needs to be done under high-precision remote control. The most precise systems are those operated by piezo-electric devices, which are also relatively simple to control by computer. The XZ movements can be applied either to the specimen or to the objective lens: the latter makes it simpler to use the microscope to examine specimens which are either bulky or which may move as a consequence of an experimental manipulation, e.g. because of a mechanical loading test.

Fixed Tilt Angle Difference: Hand-Operated Device

A mechanical stage was constructed with two identical standard LM fine-focussing mechanisms with an adjustable, pre-set fixed tilt angle difference to control two near-vertical movements. The focus was incremented at regular small intervals of 1, 2 or 4 um. The exposure duration was determined as the time taken for an exposure at one focus level using an (Olympus OM2 camera back) automatic exposure meter. The time interval was divided by the number of focus planes and an audio prompt given by a microcomputer.

DC-micromotor-controlled stage

A routine was developed to generate stereopairs using a (Sharp MZ80K) microcomputer to control a two-axis, DC micromotor-driven stage with optical encoder position readout (Oriel). This stage can be used with any TSRLM or, indeed, under any other confocal microscope. A very wide range of tilt angle differences and total height differences could be generated, and the arrangement proved to be particularly suitable for low magnification stereo work, i.e. in the range of scale which could otherwise be covered by 35 mm macrophotography and specimen tilting to generate stereo. The question will therefore be asked, why use anything as complex as TSRLM if a 35 mm camera will do? The answer lies with the advantage of the simple, parallel-projection geometry present in stereo images generated using a confocal microscope. This makes it easy to determine geometrical co-ordinates by stereophotogrammetry without the need to calibrate the camera system, as in conventional close range photogrammetry. We have worked with objective magnifications as low as $1.5\times$ and as high as $200\times$.

Piezo-electric Control of the Lens.

The Tracor Northern TSM has piezo-electric controllers giving a 50 μm range of movement in X and Z for the objective lens to a precision of one part in 4096. A (Tracor 8500) computer controls the objective lens movement. Again, the stereopairs are acquired completely automatically (Figs. 2 and 3). The operator needs to input, from the keyboard, the tilt angle difference to be stimulated, the depth of the volume to be reconstructed and the duration of each oblique through-focus pass. Both 35 mm and 70 mm format photography have been found satisfactory.

As an extension of this method, multiple photographs from different viewpoints at regular tilt angle difference increments can be processed into integrams (lenticular screen 3D displays or pseudo-holograms), which are very useful when attempting to analyze and appreciate complicated three-dimensional surfaces.

Alternatively, the images are acquired via a TV camera interface to the computer frame-store, using Kalman averaging as required and summing all the focal plane images to generate the two extended-focus views. In this case it is simple to display the maximum signal level at each pixel in the given line of sight, thus making it possible to obscure duller background objects which are overlain by brighter, more reflecting, foreground objects. The stereopairs may be displayed on the TV monitor, either as separate black-and-white images or as anaglyph (red and green) stereopairs displayed on the color display monitor, as soon as the second through-focus pass is completed.

Top or Bottom Overlap?

Each member of the stereo-pair contains information from a rhombohedron within the specimen. These rhombohedrons may be completely overlapped at the top or the bottom of the field of view, or outside the field altogether. The overlap plane is the level at which the fixed features in the images which constitute the two members of the pair have the same X shift and will appear to be in the plane of the screen. Any contribution(s) to the image(s) which do not derive from the real 3D distribution of features within the object will also be perceived as lying in this plane in the stereo view because such contributions are usually identical in both members of the pair and stem, for example, from dirt on lenses and the pattern of curved lines parallel with the scanning direction seen with imperfect disc design and/or manufacture. The author's preference is to project this "rubbish" information into the back of the stereo volume by overlapping the images at the deepest level of the reconstructed volume.

The sequence for recording the images is then to start focussed at the top of the desired volume, to record the first photo while focussing down into the specimen (with the required ratio of simultaneous movement in X), to stop the first photo, and start the second photo while focussing upwards with the same direction of movement in X. The common plane in the two images is then that at the end of the first photo and at the start of the second, both with the focus at its deepest level into the sample. If required, an additional increment of X movement in the same sense, applied at the bottom focus level will cause the overlap to lie beyond the deepest level in the reconstructed volume. Unwanted contributions to the image then appear to lie completely outside the 3D optical model.

STEREOPAIRS GENERATED FROM ONE THROUGH-FOCUS PASS

Given the availability of sufficient computer image framestore capacity, stereo-pairs can be generated from the set of images acquired in a single, vertical, through-focus pass recorded using a video or CCD camera. Using image subtraction routines, it is possible to provide a perfect background correction for the curved "scanning lines" caused by the imperfections in the manufacture of the Nipkow disc. The way in which we first generated stereoscopic pairs from a single through-focus set was as follows. To generate the left eye view, the (background corrected) images from each given focus plane were simply summed. The right eye view was generated by adding the images after a sideways shift of a defined number of pixels (to generate the stereoscopic angle). The advantage of this non-symmetrical approach was that one had an undistorted (left) image to compare with the pixel shifted (right) image: the former was always sharper because all confocal microscopes have greater resolution in the X-Y plane than they do in the Z direction. Stereopairs generated by this single-pass method show more blur than those acquired by the double-pass procedure described above. They also suffer from having a relatively small field of view: the principal limitation of any procedure using a TV camera is the resolution limit of the camera.

The photographic procedure has many advantages! It is capable of recording $100\times$ more pixels/image and, in addition, reciprocity failure in the film tends to suppress background stray light automatically.

Topographic Mapping

Given the precision computer-control of the TSRLM focus and image transfer to the computer, the XYZ co-ordinate of every point in the surface can be determined fully automatically by through-focussing and determining for every pixel the focus level for which the brightest signal level is recorded. This information is used to construct a derived image which is a topographic map of the surface. Having acquired such a full three-dimensional data set for a surface, this information can be re-displayed from any given projection. Thus, it is possible to generate stereopair images per computer from any desired angle of view and to use color depth coding and overlay grids to ease interpretation (see Chapter 11).

Color Coding Without a Computer

The thickness of the slice imaged in the two extended-focus projections which constitute the photographic stereo-pair is far

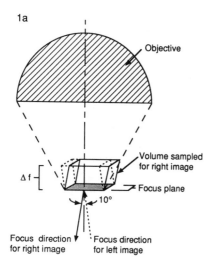

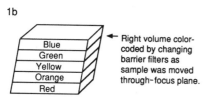

FIG. 1. Diagrams showing the means of recording stereo-pair images in the TSRLM. In Fig. 1(a) a conventional LM specimen is visualized as sandwiched between a slide and the coverslip. It is intended to make a stereo image of the volume of the sample indicated by the blank square. In Fig. 1(b) the volume to be reconstructed in a stereo image is figured as a series of optical slices through the required region. While recording the first image, the specimen is moved along one of the inclined vertical axes with the camera shutter open for the whole period. The color of the illuminating light could be changed at each of the levels shown (blue, green, yellow, orange, red). The camera shutter is then closed and a second exposure is commenced in which the specimen, is moved vertically, but along the alternate inclined vertical axis, through the same set of slices and with the same color changes. The two images will overlap at the top of the stereo image if the arrangement shown here is copied: however, they can be overlapped at the bottom, in the center of the 3D field of view or outside the field of view. This affects the perceived 3D level of the image of the curved scanning lines which are due to the (imperfect, 'Nipkow') aperture disc of the TSRLM (See Petran et al. 1985) for a detailed account of the microscope and Boyde (1985b) for an account of the stereo imaging procedure.)

greater than either the depth of field of any objective lens in conventional use or the depth of the field giving rise to color coding due to chromatic aberration in the TSRLM. However, artificial, photographic color coding for depth can be achieved by changing the color of the illuminating or recording light with a sequence of filters, so that the reflective features lying within different depth bands are imaged in contrasting colors (Boyde, 1987).

In a prototype arrangement, gelatin filters were arrayed in a sliding filter holder in the usual spectral (rainbow) sequence. Test exposures were made to determine the relative exposure necessary with each filter. Exposures determined with the automatic exposure meter of an Olympus 2 camera gave a good workable balance with Ektachrome 400 transparency film. From this data, fractional constants were apportioned for the proportion of the total exposure period which should be represented by each color.

In the combined color-coded-depth plus stereo procedure, the focus is changed at set (e.g. 1, 2 or 4 μm) intervals, using an additional shutter in the illumination channel to stop the

light while focusing to the next level when it is also necessary to change the color filter.

Using different colors to image different depths within the sample has implications for both lateral and depth resolution. Red-imaged areas might demonstrate lower resolution than blue-imaged levels according to the ratio of wavelengths, but this would only be a problem when trying to stretch this method to the limit. On the other hand, red light suffers less scattering and would therefore be expected to produce less hazy images at greater depths. As regards the definition of the depth at which a feature is imaged, the chromatic aberration of the objective has to be considered.

Considering the value of combining the methods of conveying the depth information: a mono-colored mono-image of a thick depth slice (e.g. one half of a stereo pair) taken by through-focusing while recording gives little clue as to the real 3D arrangement of structural features. A single color-coded image could be reasonably interpreted, given the information about the vertical separation corresponding to particular colors. A mono-colored stereo image would show the real distribution. However, the effects are additive: the color-coded-for-depth stereo images are easily interpreted even by those with limited experience in the interpretation of stereo images. The apparent vertical separation can often be so great that it is certainly helpful to be able to utilize both sets of cues. It is helpful to have the added information that all features in one color lie in one plane (and vice versa) since it is difficult to micro-inspect the stereoscopic optical model (concentrating in one part of the field and at one depth level) without losing something of the global impression of the distribution in the 3D volume. This is particularly true if the images are inspected without the aid of a lens or prism viewer. Color enhancement of stereo-depth information is also useful when dealing with shallower image fields of less-well-stratified structures. However, artificial color-coding has the disadvantage that it does away with one of the major advantages of the TSRLM: that it works in real color in both reflection and fluorescence.

Depth Limitation

A very robust limit to the depth to which one can image within a given object is set by the free working distance of the objective lens for a surface-reflecting object and by the light-scattering properties of a translucent object (it has to scatter some light or we see nothing!); however, there is another limit in simple photographic stereo recording of a deep, translucent object.

Consider the extreme cases of features which we may wish to analyze by stereoscopic microscopy. In one, there are randomly distributed, small, high-contrast features which could give rise to peak signal levels at any optical section level. In another, there are continuous sheet- or layer-like features running nearly parallel to the viewing axis which may give high or low signal values at specific section levels. If there are overlapping high-signal features of uniform intensity in a stack of images, then the maximum number of sections which could be accurately recorded would be the same as the number, n, of grey levels which can be appreciated by the unaided eye. In the recording process, each level should be given 1/n of the exposure level necessary just to record the peak level (black in a photographic negative, for bright features). The same will apply whether the stack is stepped or continuous. There must therefore be a limit to the depth of the total layer in an object which

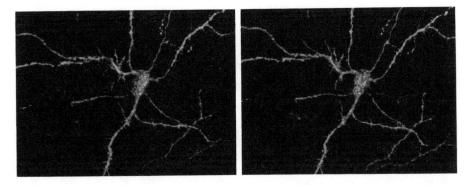

FIG. 2. (898–8–15) Stereo-pair showing the cell body and dendritic processses with dendritic spines of a pyramidal cell in hamster cortex (preparation made by Dr. Miguel Freire). The angular difference between the two views is 10 degrees, the depth of field is 40 μm. The originals were recorded on Kodak Kodachrome 64 film. The field height is 167 μm.

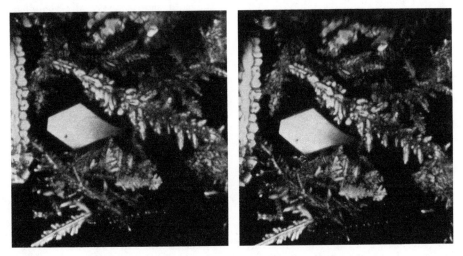

FIG. 3. A stereo view of silver crystals dried on a microscope slide and viewed with a Nikon 200x/.95 dry objective. The vertical range of the stereopair is 3μm. The tilt angle simulated between the two views is 14.4 degrees. Field width is 37 μm.

can be reconstructed equal to 1/n times the number of feature layers giving a high signal level which may overlap in projection in one or other member of the stereo pair (see also Chapter 4).

Particle Counting

Unbiased estimation of particle density can be conducted in the TSRLM by counting the number of particles that lie within a counting "brick" (or 3D counting frame), or which intersect one set of three of its six sides (Howard et al, 1985). The stereo images described in this chapter are just such bricks, and they could be used for retrospective particle counting in just this way.

Geometric Properties of the Stereo Images

Confocal microscope stereo images have the interesting property of parallel projection geometry: perspective is eliminated, because every imaged feature is recorded at the same scalar magnification regardless of where it is in the brick. This is an advantage because the theory for parallel projection stereo photogrammetry is much simpler. Familiarity with its usage stems from work with special stereophotogrammetric instruments for SEM stereo-pair images (Boyde et al 1986).

DISCUSSION: TSRLM or LSCM

Three-dimensional reconstruction of the nature proposed here could only be performed with a confocal scanning microscope. Since we have used the TSRLM, we should consider the alternative of using a laser confocal microscope. In the object-scanning type, only one point in the specimen is illuminated at one instant and the scanning to obtain the two-dimensional plane image is achieved by mechanically moving the specimen in relation to the optical beam. This type of microscope has the advantage that three-dimensional images of the nature proposed here can be achieved by further scanning the specimen in Z. However, in this type of microscope, image reconstruction is necessarily done by computer technology, and it is not possible to view the specimen to gain an impression as to whether an area of interest is significant before making the three-dimensional reconstruction. In object-scanning laser confocal microscopes it takes several seconds to form one frame of the image and successive focus levels can only be examined over a long period. Even in beam scanning LSCMs with moving mirrors, the fastest frame speed at full resolution is about one per second. (The new acousto-optic deflection LSCMs can function at full standard TV rate, however.) In spite of the advantages in image analysis of doing everything by computer, therefore,

I feel that the practical advantages of having a real-time image with which to search the specimen, in addition to the larger field-of-view, make reconstruction by optical/photographic techniques decidedly preferable as long as there is sufficient signal. A further significant advantage of the TSRLM is that it works with white light, so that "real" color effects can be retained. Although photography may be less "sophisticated" than computer technology, the information recording ability of the photographic emulsion still handsomely outstrips that of any affordable "framestore" or display CRT.

What the practicing biological microscopist means by recording an image is literally to record it—and that means by photographing it. The procedures for generating stereo-pairs from LSCM through-focus series are the equivalent of recording a stack of images, subsequently combined with some means of producing a stereo-pair from the stack. Being able to record the stereo pair directly from the TSRLM in the first instance (i.e., as an integral part of the procedure of photographing the field of view) is a major step forward, however simple the procedure seems. Getting a reconstruction back from a computer is not the same thing as photographing what you can see and know to be there—which is what happens in the procedure outlined here.

ACKNOWLEDGEMENTS

The TSRLM project was funded by the MRC and the SERC. I am very grateful for the excellent technical assistance of Roy Radcliffe and Elaine Maconnachie.

REFERENCES

Boyde, A. (1985a) The tandem scanning reflected light microscope. Part 2—Pre-Micro 84 applications at UCL. Proc Roy Microsc Soc 20, 131–139.

Boyde, A. (1985b) Stereoscopic images in confocal (tandem scanning) microscopy. Science 230, 1270-1272.

Boyde, A. (1987) Color-coded stereo images from the tandem scanning reflected light microscope (TSRLM). J. Microsc. 146, 137-142.

Boyde, A., Howell P.G.T., Franc F. (1986) A Simple SEM Stereophotogrammetric method for three dimensional evaluation of features on flat substrates, J. Micros 143: 257–264.

Brakenhoff, G.J., Van Der Voort, H.T.M., Van Spronsen, E.A., Linnemans, W.A.M., & Nanninga, N. (1985) Three-dimensional chromatin distribution in neuroblastoma nuclei shown by confocal scanning laser microscopy. Nature 317, 748–749.

Carlsson, K., Danielsson, P.E., Lenz, R., Liljeborg, A., Majloef, L. & Aslund, N. (1985) Three-dimensional microscopy using a confocal laser scanning microscope. Optics Letters 10, 53–55.

Cox, I.J. & Sheppard, C.J.R. (1983) Digital image processing of confocal images. Image and Vision Computing 1, 53.

Howard, V., Reid S.A., Baddeley, A. & Boyde A. (1985) Unbiased estimation of particle density in the tandem scanning reflected light microscope. J. Microsc. 138, 203–212.

Minsky, M. Microscopy Apparatus. United States Patent Office. Filed Nov. 7, 1957, granted Dec. 19, 1961. Patent No. 3,013,467.

Petran, M. and Hadravsky, M. (1968) Zpusob a zarizeni pro omezeni rozptylu svetla v mikroskopu pro osvetleni shora. Czechoslovak Patent No. 128936, application 5–7-66, granted 15–2-68, published 15–9-68.

Petran M., Hadravsky, M. & Boyde, A. (1985) The tandem scanning reflected light microscope. Scanning, 7, 97-108.

Sugimoto, S.A., & Ichioka, Y. (1985) Digital composition of images with increased depth of focus considering depth information. Applied Optics 24, 2076–2080.

Van der Voort, H.T.M., Brakenhoff, G.J., Valkenburg, J.A.C. & Nanninga, N. (1985) Design and use of a computer controlled confocal microscope for biological applications. Scanning 7, 66-78.

Wijnaendts Van Resandt, R.W., Marsman, H.J.B., Kaplan, R., Davoust, J., Stelzer, E.H.K. and Stricker, R. (1985) Optical fluorescence microscopy in three dimensions: microtomoscopy. J. Microsc. 138, 29–34.

Wilson, T. & Sheppard, C. (1984) Theory and practice of scanning optical microscopy. Academic Press—London 1984.

Wolf, R. (1989) A novel beam-splitting microscope tube for taking stereopairs with full resolution Nomarski optics: phase contrast; or epifluorescence. J Microsc. 153, 181–186.

Xiao, G.Q. & Kino, G.S. (1987) A real-time confocal scanning optical microscope, Proc. SPIE, Vol. 809, Scanning Imaging Technology, T. Wilson & L. Balk, Eds. 107-113 (1987)

Chapter 16

Fluorophores for Confocal Microscopy: Photophysics and Photochemistry

ROGER Y. TSIEN[1] AND ALAN WAGGONER[2]

[1]Department of Pharamacology M-036, School of Medicine, University of California, San Diego, CA 92093, [2]Department of Biological Sciences and Center for Fluorescence Research in the Biomedical Sciences Carnegie Mellon University, Pittsburgh, PA 15213

INTRODUCTION

Fluorescence is probably the most important optical readout mode in biological confocal microscopy, because it can be so much more sensitive and specific than absorbance or reflectance, and because it works so well with epi-illumination, which greatly simplifies scanner design. These advantages of fluorescence are critically dependent on the availability of suitable fluorophores that can either be tagged onto biological macromolecules to show their location, or whose optical properties are sensitive to the local environment. Despite the pivotal importance of good fluorophores, little is known about how to rationally design good ones. Whereas the concept of confocal microscopy is only a few decades old and nearly all the optical, electronic and computer components to support it have been developed or redesigned in the last few years, the most popular fluorophores were developed more than a century ago (in the case of fluoresceins or rhodamines) or several billion years ago (in the case of phycobiliproteins). Moreover, whereas competition between commercial makers of confocal microscopes stimulates ardent efforts to refine the instrumentation, relatively few companies or academic scientists are interested in improving fluorophores.

PHOTOPHYSICAL PROBLEMS RELATED TO HIGH INTENSITY EXCITATION

Singlet state saturation

The properties of current fluorescent probes relevant to conventional fluorescence microscopy have been reviewed recently (e.g. Waggoner et al, 1989; Tsien, 1989a,b; Chen & Scott, 1985) and are listed in Table 1. Absorption spectra of several representative fluorescent probes in relation to the common laser line wavelengths available for confocal laser scanning microscopes are presented in Figure 1. Confocal microscopy using multiple apertures scanned across an image plane, i.e. disk-scanning confocal microscopy, is essentially similar to conventional microscopy in its requirements on fluorophores. By contrast, laser-scanning microscopy subjects each fluorescent molecule to brief but extremely intense bursts of excitation as the focused laser beam sweeps past. If the laser-scanned image consists of n pixels (typically $n > 10^5$), any one pixel is illuminated for $1/n$ of the total time, or even somewhat less if some of the cycle time must be devoted to scan retrace; therefore the peak instantaneous intensity must equal or exceed n times the long-term average excitation intensity. Some idea of the quantitative

magnitude may be gathered from the following example, analogous to that discussed by White & Stryer (1987). If just 1 mW of power at the popular 488 nm line of the argon-ion laser is focused to a Gaussian spot whose radius w at $1/e^2$ intensity is 0.25 μm, as is achieved by a microscope objective of 1.25 numerical aperture (Schneider & Webb, 1981), the peak excitation intensity I at the center will be $10^{-3}W/[\pi \cdot (0.25 \times 10^{-4}cm)^2] = 5.1 \times 10^5$ W/cm², or about 1.25×10^{24} photons/(cm²-s). Such intensities are well able to excite fluorophores so rapidly that few molecules are left in the ground state and the population is emitting photons nearly as fast as the limit set by the excited-state lifetime. For example, if fluorescein is the fluorophore, its decadic extinction coefficient ϵ at 488 nm is about 80,000 liters·mole⁻¹cm⁻¹ at pH > 7. To convert this to the optical cross-section per molecule, one must multiply ϵ by $(1000 \text{ cm}^3/\text{liter}) \cdot (\ln 10)/(6.023 \times 10^{23} \text{ molecules/mole}) = 3.82 \times 10^{-21}$

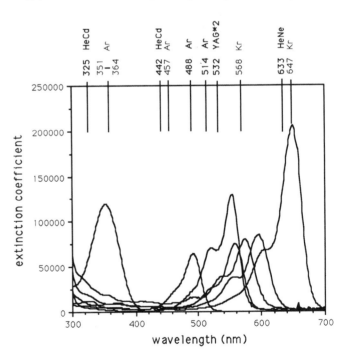

FIG. 1.   Absorption spectra from left to right of Hoechst 33342+DNA, and fluorescein, CY3, TRITC, Lissamine Rhodamine B, Texas Red, and CY5 conjugated to antibodies. Extinction coefficients are given on a per dye basis. Common laser emission wavelengths are presented at the top of the figure. Wavelengths in bold are for the lower power, less expensive lasers, which provide sufficient excitation intensity for most fluorochromes imaged with laser scanning microscopes with higher power objectives.

TABLE 1. SPECTROSCOPIC PROPERTIES OF SELECTED PROBES

Parameter	Probe (a)	Absorption Maximum (b)	Extinction Max. (c)	Emission Maximum (b)	Quantum Yield	Measurement Conditions	References (d)
Covalent labeling reagents	Fluorescein-ITC, DCT, IA, MAL (e)	490 494	67 76	520	0.71	pH7, PBS pH 9.2, 0.1M borate	[1], W, MP [21]
	FITC-Antibody	490	*	520	0.1-0.4 (f)	pH7, PBS	W
	TRITC-amines	554	85	573	0.28	pH7, PBS	[1], MP
	XRITC-amines	582	79	601	0.26	pH7, PBS	W
	XRITC-Antibody	580	*	604	0.08 (g)	pH7, PBS	W
	Texas Red®-amines	596	85	620	0.51	pH7, PBS	[3], W, MP
	Texas Red®—Antibody	596	*	620	0.01 (h)	pH7, PBS	W
	Lissamine Rhodamine Sulfonamide	570		590	med		MP
	CY5.8-ITC-amine	664	129	663	0.09	pH7, PBS	[4]
	CY7.8-ITC-amine	550	100	777		pH7, PBS	[4]
	CY5.4-IA-actin	652	140	672	0.15	pH7, PBS	[5]
	CY3.12-OSu-amine	556	130	574	0.05	pH7, PBS	[27]
	CY5.12-OSu-amine	650	200	674	0.13	pH7, PBS	[27]
	CY5.12-OSu-amine	755	200	784		pH7, PBS	[27]
	CY3.18-OSu-antibody	554	130	568	0.14 (f)	pH7, PBS	[28]
	CY5.18-OSu-antibody	652	200	672	0.18 (f)	pH7, PBS	[28]
	CY7.18-OSu-antibody	755	200	778	0.02 (f)	pH7, PBS	[28]
	Cascade Blue®	378, 399	26	423		water	MP
	NBD-amine	478	24.6	520-550	0.36/0.21	EtOH/MeOH	[6], [7], [8]
	NBD-S-CH2CH2OH	425	12.1	531	0.002 0.015	pH 7.5, 10% glycerol 80% glycerol	
	Dansyl-NH-CH3	340 (pH 7.4, 0.1M Tris)	3.4	578 539 508	0.068 0.5 0.41	water ethanol chloroform	MP, [9]
	Coumarin-phalloidin	387		470		water	[29]
	Phycoerythrin-R	480-565	1960	578	0.68	pH 7, PBS	[10]
	Allophycocyanine	650	700	660	0.68	pH7, PBS	[10]
DNA-RNA content (i)	Hoechst 33342	340	120	450	0.83	+DNA (excess)	W
	DAPI	350		470		+DNA (excess)	W
	Ethidium Bromide	510	3.2	595		+DNA (excess)	[11]
	Propidium Iodide	536	6.4	623	0.09	+DNA (excess)	W
	Acridine Orange	480 440-470		520 650		+DNA +RNA	[12], [13]
	Pyronine Y	549-561 560-562 497	67-84 70-90 42	567-574 565-574 563	0.04-0.26 0.05-0.21 LOW	+ds DNA (j) +ds RNA (j) + ss RNA	[14], [15]
	Thiazole Orange	453	26	480	0.08	RNA	[16]
Membrane potential	diO-Cn-(3)	485	149	505	0.05	MeOH	[17], W
	diI-Cn-(3)	548	126	567	0.07	MeOH	[17], W
	diI-Cn-(5)	646	200	668	0.4	MeOH	[17], W
	diI-Cn-(7)	740	240	770	0.28	EtOH	W, [18]
	diBA-Isopr-(3)	493	130	517	0.03	MeOH	[17], W
	diBA-C4-(5)	590	176	620		EtOH	W
	Tetramethylrhodamine ethylester	549	100	574		MeOH	MP, [31]
	Rhodamine 123	511	85	534	0.9	EtOH	EK, [19]
Lipid content and fluidity	Nile Red	485 530		525 605		Heptane Acetone	[20], [21]
	Diphenylhexatriene (DPH)	330, 351, 370	77 (351nm)	430		Hexane	MP
	diI-C18-(3)	546	126	565	0.07	MeOH	W
	Dansyl-PE	335	4.5				
	NBD phosphatidylethanolamine	450	24 (k)	530		Lipid	[22]
	Anthroyl stearate	361, 381	8.4, 7.5	446		MeOH	[23]
	Pyrene-sulfonamidoalkyls	350	30	380-400			MP
pH	BCECF	505 460		530		High pH Low pH	MP MP
	SNARF-1 (pKa = 7.5)	518 548 574		587 636		pH 5.5 pH 10.0	MP MP
	DCDHB (j)	340-360 340-360		500-580 420-440		High pH Low pH	[24], MP
Calcium (m)	Fura 2	335 360	33 27	512-518 505-510	0.23 0.49	Low Calcium High Calcium	[25]
	Indo 1	330 350	34 34	390-410 482-485	0.56 0.38	High Calcium Low Calcium	[25]
	Fluo-3	506 506	83 78	526 526	.183 .0051	High Calcium Low Calcium	[32], MP

TABLE 1.　SPECTROSCOPIC PROPERTIES OF SELECTED PROBES (continued)

Parameter	Probe (a)	Absorption Maximum (b)	Extinction Max. (c)	Emission Maximum (b)	Quantum Yield	Measurement Conditions	References (d)
Enzyme substrates	Rhodamine-di-arg-CBZ substr.	—	Low at 495nm	532	0.09	Hepes pH7.5 + 15% EtOH	[26]
	Product of rxn. (rhodamine)	495	67	523	0.91	Hepes pH7.5 + 15% EtOH	
	Coumarin-glucoside substr.	316	13	395		Acetate pH 5.5 + 1%Lubrol	W
	Product of rxn (hydroxy coumarin)	370	17	450		Glycine pH10 + 1%Lubrol	W

(a) Abbreviations: ITC=Isothiocyanato-; DCT=Dichlorotrizinyl-; IA=Iodoacetamido-; MAL=Maleimido-; BCECF=2',7'-bis-(2-carboxyethyl)-5(and 6)carboxyfluorescein DCDHB=dicyano-dihydroxybenzene.
(b) Measured in nanometers
(c) Multiply value listed by 1000 to get liters/mol.cm*, Suggest using value for amine adduct,
(d) EK, Eastman Kodak Chemical Catalog; MP, Molecular Probes, Inc catalog or personal communication; W, Waggoner laboratory determination; [1] Haugland, RP (1983) In "Excited States of Biopolymers." (Steiner, R.F., ed). pp 29–58. Plenum Press, New York; [2] Wilderspin, AF & Green, NM (1983) Anal Biochem, 132, 449–455; [3] Titus, JA, Haugland, RP, Sharrow, SA, Segal, DM. (1982) *J. Immunol. Meth.* 50, 93–93; [4] Mujumdar, RB, Ernst, LA, Mujumdar, SR, Waggoner, AS (1989) *Cytometry* 10, 3–10, 11–19; [5] Ernst, LA, Gupta, RK, Mujumdar, RB, Waggoner, AS (1989) *Cytometry* 10, 3–10; [6] Kenner, RA & Aboderin, AA (1971) *Biochemistry,* 10, 4433–4440; [7] Allen, G & Lowe, G (1973) *Biochem, J.,* 133, 679–686; [8] Bratcher, SC (1979) *Biochem. J.,* 183, 255–268; [9] Chen, RF (1968) *Anal. Biochem.,* 25, 412–416; [10] Oi, V, Glazer, AN & Stryer, L (1982) *J Cell Biol* 93, 981–986; [11] Pohl, FM et al. (1972) *Proc, Natl. Acad. Sci. USA* 69, 3805–3809; [12] Kapuscinski, J, Darzynkiewicz, Z & Melamed, M (1982) *Cytometry* 2, 201–211; [13] Shapiro, H (1985) *Cytometry* 2, 143–150; [14] Darzynkiewicz, Z et al. (1987) *Cytometry* 8, 138–145; [15] Kapuscinski, J & Darzynkiewicz, Z (1987) *Cytometry* 8, 129–137; [16] Lee, LG, Chen, C-H & Chiu, LA (1986) *Cytometry* 7, 508–517; [17] Sims, PJ et al. (1974) *Biochemistry* 13, 3315–3330; [18] Duggan, JX, DiCesare, J & Williams, JF (1983) In "New Directions in Molecular Luminescence". (D. Eastwood, ed.). pp. 112–126. ASTM Special Technical Publication 822; [19] Kubin, RF & Fletcher, AN (1983) *J. Luminescence*, 27, 455–462; [20] Greenspan, P & Fowler, SD (1985) *J. Lipid Res.* 26, 81–789; [21] Sackett, DL & Wolff, J (1987) *Anal. Biochem.* 167, 228–234; [22] Struck, DK, Hoekstra, D & Pagano, RE (1981) *Biochemistry* 20, 4093–4099; [23] Waggoner, AS & Sryer, L (1970) *Proc. Natl. Acad. Sci. USA,* 67, 579–589; [24] Valet, G et al. (1981) *Naturwiss* 68, 265–266; [25] Grynkiewcz, G, Poenie, M & Tsien, RY (1985) *J Biol Chem* 260, 3440–3450; [26] Leytus, SP, Patterson, WL & Mangel, WF (1983) *Biochem J* 215, 253–260; [27] Southwick, PL, Ernst, LA, Tauriello, EW, Parker, SR, Mujumdar, RB, Mujumdar, SR, Clever, HA, Waggoner, AS, Submitted; [28] Mujumdar, RB, Ernst, LA, Mujumdar, SR, Lewis, CJ, Chao, J, Wagner, M, Waggoner, AS. In preparation; [29] Small, JV, Zobeley, S, Rinnerthaler, G, Faulstich, H. (1988) *J. Cell Sci.* 89, 21–24; [30] Wolfbeis, OS, Furlinger, E, Kroneis, H, Massoner, H. (1983) *Fresenius Z. Anal. Chem.* 314, 119–124; [31] Eherenberg, B, Montana, V, Wei, M, Wuskell, JP, Loew, LM. (1988) *Biophys. J.* 53, 785–794; [32] Minata, A, Kao, JPY, Tsien, RY. (1989) *J. Biol. Chem.* 264, 8171–8178.
(e) Covalently bound to amino group (ITC, DCT) or sulfhydryl group (IA, MAL)
(f) Dye/antibody ratio of 2–5
(g) Dye/antibody ratio of 2.5
(h) Dye/antibody ratio of 1.2
(i) See Table III in Arndt-Jovin, DJ and T. Jovin, TM (1989) In *Meth. Cell Biol.* 30, 417–448 for additional DNA content probes.
(j) Base pair dependent
(k) Value for NBD-ethanolamine in MeOH which has an abs.max at 470 nm and an emission max at 550 nm. [Barak, LS, Yocum, RR, (1981) *Anal. Biochem.* 110, 31–38]
(m) See Tsien, RY (1989) In *Meth. Cell Biol.* 30, 127–156 for additional details and other ion indicators.

cm³·mole·liter⁻¹·molecule⁻¹, giving a cross-section σ of 3.06 × 10^{-16} cm²/molecule. In a beam of 1.25 × 10^{24} photons·cm⁻²s⁻¹, each ground state molecule will be excited with a rate constant $k_a = \sigma I$, or 3.8 × 10^8 s⁻¹ in this example. The excited state lifetime τ_f of fluorescein in free aqueous solution is known to be about 4.5 ns (Bailey & Rollefson, 1953), which means that molecules in the excited state return to the ground state with a rate constant k_f of 2.2 × 10^8 s⁻¹. Note that k_f is defined here as the composite rate constant for all means of depopulating the singlet excited state, the sum of the rate constants for fluorescence emission, radiationless internal conversion, intersystem crossing to the triplet, etc. Because of the Stokes shift between excitation and emission wavelengths, k_f is not significantly enhanced by stimulated emission effects. If x is the fraction of molecules in the excited state and $(1 - x)$ is the fraction in the ground state, at steady-state $k_f x = k_a(1 - x)$. significantly enhanced by stimulated emission effects. If x is the that in this example 63% of the fluorescein molecules would be in the excited state and only 37% in the ground state. Obviously the emission is nearly saturated, and further increase in excitation intensity could hardly increase the output. The actual in the excited state and only 37% in the ground state. Obviously where Q_e is the emission quantum efficiency, about 0.9 for free fluorescein dianion (but usually less for fluorescein bound to proteins, see IV.C. below). In this example each molecule would be emitting at an average rate of 1.3 × 10^8 photons/s, close to the absolute maximum of $Q_e k_f$ of about 2 × 10^8 photons/s. In current typical scanning confocal microscopes, the beam dwells on each pixel for 1–10 μs, so one would expect each molecule

to produce several hundred photons. However, only a minority enter the microscope objective, only a fraction of these manage to pass all the way through the scanner optics, and only 10–20% of these create photoelectrons in the photomultiplier cathode, so that each molecule probably contributes on the order of only one photoelectron per pixel per sweep. Because of fluorescence saturation, increasing the laser power will not significantly increase the signal amplitude. In reality, it is difficult to accurately predict the laser power at which a fluorophore will saturate. Accurate knowledge of the extinction coefficient at the wavelength of excitation and the excited state lifetime of the fluorophore is essential but not always easy to obtain. Coumarins, for example (Table 1), have extinction coefficients approximately 2–5 times smaller than the fluoresceins, rhodamines and cyanines, and would be expected on this basis alone to require a 2–5-fold increase in laser power before saturation. However, the emission lifetimes of coumarins are intrinsically longer than those of the fluoresceins, rhodamines, and cyanines, so that the factor of 2–5 is not realized in practice. To make calculations more difficult, the extinction coefficients and the excited state lifetimes of most probes depend on the environment of the fluorophore. For example, increasing the fluorochrome to protein ratio of a labeled antibody from 2 to 5 can reduce the average excited state lifetime of the bound fluorochromes several fold. For these reasons, the power saturation values for the probes listed in Table 1 are not given. However, as a general rule, fluorochromes with extinction coefficients and quantum efficiencies similar to fluorescein will also saturate under similar conditions.

Triplet state saturation

The above calculation considers only the ground state and lowest excited singlet state. Saturation of emission could occur at even lower excitation intensities if a significant population of fluorophores become trapped in a relatively long-lived triplet state. This would take place if a significant quantum yield exists for singlet-to-triplet conversion, or intersystem crossing. For example, if ground-state fluorescein molecules each absorb 3.8 $\times$ 10^8 photons·s^{-1}, have an excited singlet lifetime of 4.5 ns, cross to the triplet state with a quantum efficiency Q_{ISC} of 0.03 (Gandin et al, 1983), and reside in the triplet state for a mean time τ_T of 10^{-6} s, the triplet state would contain 81% of the fluorophore population at steady state, which would be attained so that the factor of 2–5 is not realized in practice. To make about 190 ns in this case. Only 12% and 7% would be left in the first excited singlet and ground states respectively at steady state, so that the fluorescence emission would be weakened about 5-fold compared to its initial value just after the illumination began but before significant triplet occupancy had built up. Therefore, if the dwell time per pixel is comparable to or greater than the triplet lifetime, then a severe reduction in output intensity may be expected beyond that due simply to the finite rate of emission from the singlet state.

In the above calculation, the most uncertain figure is that for the triplet lifetime τ_T; in very thoroughly deoxygenated solution, τ_T for the fluorescein dianion is 20 ms (Lindqvist, 1960), but oxygen is expected to shorten τ_T down to the 0.1 − 1 μs range. The rate at which different fluorophore environments in a sample quench triplet states and reduce τ_T will of course affect the extent of triplet-state saturation and the apparent brightness of each pixel at these high illumination levels. When τ_T is long, triplet-state saturation is easily attained even without laser illumination (Lewis et al, 1941).

Contaminating background signals

Rayleigh and Raman scattering

Meanwhile, there may be unwanted signals such as Rayleigh scattering, due either to excitation wavelengths leaking through the dichroic mirror and barrier filter, or to imperfect monochromaticity of the excitation source, for example if the laser is being run in multiline mode with only an interference filter to select one line. Even if all the wavelength filtering is perfect, Raman scattering will contribute a fluorescence-like signal, for example at a wavelength of [λ_{exc}^{-1} -3380cm^{-1}]$^{-1}$ due to the characteristic 3380 cm^{-1} Raman band of water. For an exciting wavelength λ_{exc} of 488 nm, the Raman peak would appear at 584 nm. At high concentrations of protein or embedding media, additional wavelengths closer to the excitation might appear. Both Rayleigh and Raman scattering are directly proportional to the laser power and will **not** saturate as the desired fluorescence does, so that excessive laser power diminishes the contrast between fluorescence and such scattering signals.

Autofluorescence from endogenous fluorophores

Another major source of unwanted background is autofluorescence from endogenous fluorophores. Flavins and flavoproteins absorb strongly at 488 nm and emit in the same spectral region as fluorescein. Reduced pyridine nucleotides (NADH, NADPH) and lipofuscin pigments absorb light from UV laser lines. These fluorophores usually have lower extinction coefficients or shorter fluorescence lifetimes than most exogenous fluorophores. For example, FMN (flavin mononucleotide) and FAD (flavin adenine dinucleotide) have the extinction coefficients of 1.1–1.2 $\times$ 10^4 M^{-1}cm^{-1} at 445–450 nm (Koziol, 197) and fluorescence lifetimes of about 4.7 and 2.3 ns respectively (Lakowicz, 1983), whereas NADH has an extinction coefficient of 6.2 $\times$ 10^3 M^{-1}cm^{-1} at its 340 nm peak (Kaplan, 1960) and a lifetime of about 0.4 ns (Lakowicz, 1983). Therefore autofluorescence from these molecules will be more difficult to saturate than the fluorescence from most of the common probes.

What is the optimal intensity?

The above discussion shows that if laser power is increased to nearly saturate the desired fluorophores, autofluorescence as well as Rayleigh and Raman scattering will increase background levels and decrease the overall S/N ratio. What is the optimal intensity? Assuming the system is limited by photon counting statistics, the irreducible noise level N is proportional to the square root of the background signal level B. Both B and the absorption rate constant k_a of the desired probe are directly proportional to the illumination intensity I and to each other. Therefore N is directly proportional to $k_a^{1/2}$. If triplet state saturation can be ignored, for example if the dwell time per pixel is short compared to the time for the triplet state to build up, then the desired signal is $Q_e k_f k_a/(k_a + k_f)$ as derived above, so that S/N is proportional to $k_a^{1/2}/(k_a + k_f)$. Regardless of the proportionality constant, this expression is maximal when $k_a = k_f$. This is a remarkably simple but important result, which we are grateful to Prof. R. Mathies (U of Calif. Berkeley) for pointing out.

At the other extreme, once the ground state and excited singlet and triplet have all come to an equilibrium steady state, the desired signal is readily calculated to be

$$Q_e k_a/[1 + k_a (k_f^{-1} + Q_{ISC}\tau_T)]$$

so that the S/N is proportional to

$$Q_e k_a^{1/2}/[1 + k_a (k_f^{-1} + Q_{ISC}\tau_T)].$$

This reaches its maximum when $k_a(\tau_f + Q_{ISC}\tau_T) = 1$, where $\tau_f = k_f^{-1}$ is the lifetime of the excited singlet. In this approximation, appropriate for slow scans in which the dwell time per pixel is long compared to the time for triplet state equilibration, the laser power P in photons/s should be optimal at about $\pi w^2/[(3.82 \times 10^{-21}\text{cm}^3\cdot\text{M})\epsilon(\tau_f + Q_{ISC}\tau_T)]$. For the present values of $w = 2.5 \times 10^{-5}$ cm, $\epsilon = 8 \times 10^4$ M^{-1}cm^{-1}, $\tau_f = 4.5 \times 10^{-9}$ s, $Q_{ISC} = 0.03$, and $\tau_T = 10^{-6}$ s, this expression gives an optimal P of 1.86×10^{14} photons/s, or about 76 μW at 488 nm. If triplet formation could be neglected, the optimal P would be 590 μW, slightly less than the 1 mW initially postulated to be the input.

PHOTODESTRUCTION OF FLUOROPHORES AND BIOLOGICAL SPECIMENS

One obvious way to increase the total signal is to integrate for a longer time, either by slowing the scan, or by averaging for many scans. Given that image processors are now relatively cheap, the latter alternative is likely to be the easier to implement, and it has at least two major advantages: repetitive scans give time for triplet states to decay between each scan, and the user can watch the signal-to-noise ratio gradually improve and choose when to stop accumulating. However, irreversible photochemical side effects such as bleaching of the fluorophore or damage to the specimen set limits on the useful duration of observation or total photon dose allowable. Photochemical damage is one of the most important yet least understood aspects of the use of fluorescence in biology; in this discussion we can do little more than define our ignorance.

At intensities of up to 3×10^{22} (Hirschfeld, 1976) or 4.4×10^{23} photons·cm^{-2}·s^{-1} (Mathies & Stryer, 1986), fluorescein is known to bleach with a quantum efficiency Q_b of about 3×10^{-5}. If this value continues to hold at the somewhat higher intensity of the above example, the molecules would be bleaching with a rate constant of $Q_b k_f k_a/(k_a + k_f)$, or about 4.2×10^3 s^{-1}. This would mean that $1/e$ or 37% of the molecules would be left after 240 μs of actual irradiation. The corresponding number of scans would be 240 μs divided by the dwell time that the beam actually spends on each pixel. The average number of photons emitted by a fluorophore before it bleaches is the ratio of emission quantum efficiency to bleaching quantum efficiency, or Q_e/Q_b; this is generally true regardless of whether the illumination is steady or pulsed. For fluorescein under ideal conditions, the above Q_e/Q_b works out to 30,000–40,000 photons ultimately emitted per dye molecule (Hirschfeld, 1976; Mathies & Stryer, 1986). The number of photons detected from each molecule will of course be considerably less.

Thus, in obtaining an image at a single plane by averaging say 16 scans, one would expect from 6–50% bleaching of a fluorescein signal (in the absence of antifade reagents), resulting from exp[-(16 sweeps)·(1–10 μs dwell time per sweep)/(240 μs lifetime)]. In an optical sectioning experiment, the cone of light illuminating the sample above and below each plane of data being acquired is causing photobleaching even though under confocal conditions no signal is being recorded from these regions. This means that if 16 optical sections are obtained with only one sweep each, the last image will have been bleached 10–50% by the preceding sweeps. If the signals are large, it may be possible for software to adjust the intensities of sequential images to compensate for bleaching. Of course, for quantitative fluorescence measurements it would be most desirable to use the most bleach-resistant fluorophores available.

Dependency on intensity or its time integral?

Theory

One major uncertainty is whether the bleaching quantum efficiency Q_b really does remain constant even at such high instantaneous excitation intensities. Theoretically, Q_b could rise at high intensities due to multiphoton absorptions. For example, the normal excited singlet or triplet state could itself absorb one or more additional photons to extra-high energy states, which will probably have picosecond lifetimes. If their main reaction pathway were back to the lowest excited state, then such higher-order states would be innocuous, but if bond dissociation competes with decay to the lowest excited state, then photodestruction will rise steeply as intensities reach levels that significantly deplete the ground state, (as in the previous example).

One can also imagine the opposite dependency: bleaching mechanisms whose quantum efficiency might decrease when the excitation was bunched into brief intense pulses. For example, suppose the dye is bleached by a 1:1 reaction of its excited state with a molecule of oxygen, and that the overall

dye concentration exceeds the oxygen concentration. Then within the zone of intense illumination, the first few excited dye molecules might react with all the locally available O_2, so that the rest of the excited molecules would be protected by the anoxic environment. Oxygen would be diffusing in from the surrounding non-illuminated environment, but the time required would be on the order of the spot radius squared divided by the diffusion constant, i.e. $(0.25 \times 10^{-4}\text{cm})^2/(3 \times 10^{-5}$ cm^{2}s^{-1} or 20 μs, i.e. considerably longer than the time for the beam to move to the next pixel. By contrast, with low intensity illumination, no local anoxia would develop, and each fluorophore would take its chances with the full ambient oxygen concentration. Such a mechanism would be the photochemical equivalent of predator-prey interactions in ecology, where it is often advantageous for the prey to school together or breed in synchrony in order to minimize losses to predation (Wilson, 1975).

Experiment

Theory is all well and good, but empirically how does the photodestruction quantum yield depend on intensity? White and Stryer (1987) tested R-phycoerythrin in a flow system and found that the rate of photodestruction was indeed directly proportional to laser power so that the quantum yield was constant. Unfortunately, the range of intensities tested only went up to about 10^{20} photons·cm^{-2}·s^{-1}, so that they were still 3 orders of magnitude below saturation of the phycoerythrin. Very recently Konan Peck, Lubert Stryer, and Richard Mathies (manuscript in preparation) have been examining B-phycoerythrin and find that photodestruction saturates with increasing input intensity in just the same way as fluorescence emission does, so that the photodestruction quantum yield is roughly constant even when the phycobiliproteins are heavily driven into saturation. However, there is some indirect evidence that simpler fluorophores may undergo a nonlinear acceleration of bleaching under such conditions. White, Amos and Fordham (1987) reported that bleaching by their scanning confocal microscope seemed to be greatest at the plane of focus. Since the plane of focus receives about the same time-averaged photon flux but much higher peak intensities than out-of-focus planes do, preferential bleaching at the plane of focus would imply that a given number of photons are more injurious when they are bunched, i.e. that the photodestruction quantum yield increases at high intensities. Obviously, further testing of this possibility and improvement in photon collection efficiency will be of great importance in confocal microscopy.

A number of workers have reported that damage to biological structures (as distinct from bleaching of the fluorophore) can sometimes be reduced if the given total number of photons is delivered with high intensities for short times rather than low intensities for long times. An early report of the advantage of pulsed illumination was by Sheetz and Koppel (1979) studying the crosslinkage of spectrin by illumination of fluoresceinated concanavalin A on erythrocyte membranes. Bloom and Webb (1984) found similar results for lysis of XRITC-labeled air-equilibrated erythrocytes, whereas well-deoxygenated cells were much more resistant but lysed after a constant total photon dose regardless of whether delivered quickly or slowly. Recently Vigers et al (1988) showed that increasing the illumination intensity up to about 10^3 W/cm^2 decreased the time required for fluorescein-labeled microtubules to dissolve, as one might expect. Surprisingly, intensities above this threshold actually stabilized the microtubules against dissolution, so that the dissolution time became a linearly *increasing* function of intensity. This paradoxical stabilization at high intensities was attributed to local heating based on the assumption that diffusion of heat was negligible. Because this assumption needs to be checked (see Axelrod, 1977; Bloom & Webb, 1984) and because microtubule stabilization and dissolution are not well-defined molecular events, the local heating hypothesis should be viewed with caution. Bonhoeffer and Staiger (1988) have reported that photodynamic damage to rat hippocampal cells was reduced if the light is delivered as 100 exposures each 200 ms long separated by 30 s dark periods rather than continuously for 20 s. They speculated that intermittent illumination was better because it allowed repair mechanisms to operate during the dark intervals. It should be noted that in all the above biological examples, the illumination intensity was well below that expected to be necessary to reach saturation of excited state dye populations.

Protective agents

As mentioned above, light-induced damage to both the fluorophore and to the biological specimen is often dependent on the presence of molecular oxygen, which reacts with the triplet excited states of many dyes to produce highly reactive singlet oxygen. Reduction of the partial pressure or concentration of oxygen often greatly increases the longevity of both the fluorophore and the specimen. In dead, fixed samples, it has become common to add antioxidants such as propyl gallate (Giloh & Sedat, 1982), hydroquinone, *p*-phenylenediamine, etc., to the mounting medium. The preservative effects of these agents may go beyond removing oxygen, since White and Stryer (1987) found propyl gallate to be more effective at protecting phycoerythrin *in vitro* than thorough deoxygenation was. One might speculate that polyphenols like propyl gallate might also quench dye triplet states and other free radicals, which would prevent other forms of photodegradation, not just singlet oxygen formation.

The problem of protecting living cells from oxygen-dependent photodynamic damage is more difficult. The above antioxidants would not be attractive, since they would be expected to have strong pharmacological effects at the high concentrations generally employed on fixed tissue. If the tissue can tolerate hypoxia or anoxia, one would probably prefer to remove O_2 by bubbling the medium with N_2 or Ar rather than using chemical reductants. Biological oxygen-scavenging systems such as submitochondrial particles or glucose oxidase + glucose are often helpful (Bloom & Webb, 1984).

If one cannot reduce the O_2 concentration, the next best tactic may be to use singlet oxygen quenchers. The most attractive here are those already chosen by natural selection, namely carotenoids. Their effectiveness is shown by classic experiments in which carotenoid biosynthesis was blocked by mutation; the resulting mutants were rapidly killed by normal illumination levels at which the wild type thrived (Matthews & Sistrom, 1959). A water soluble carotenoid would be easier to administer acutely than the usual extremely hydrophobic carotenoids such as carotene itself. The most accessible and promising candidate is crocetin, which is the chromophore that gives saffron its color, and which consists of seven conjugated C=C

units with a carboxylate at each end. Crocetin quenches aqueous singlet oxygen with a bimolecular rate constant of 5.5×10^9 $M^{-1}s^{-1}$, which is almost diffusion-controlled; of this rate, about 95% represents catalytic quenching and about 5% represents bleaching or consumption of the crocetin (Manitto et al, 1987; somewhat more pessimistic rate constants are reported by Matheson & Rodgers, 1982). Longer-chain carotenoids are supposed to be even more efficient at destroying singlet oxygen without damage to themselves, but have not yet been tested in aqueous media. There is some evidence that 50 μM of either crocetin or etretinate (a synthetic aromatic retinoid) can protect cultured cells (L cells and WI-38 fibroblasts) from hematoporphyrin-induced photodynamic damage (Reyftmann et al 1986). Other water-soluble agents that might be considered as sacrificial reactants with reactive oxygen metabolites include ascorbate (e.g. Vigers et al, 1988), imidazole, histidine, cysteamine, reduced glutathione (Sheetz and Koppel, 1979), uric acid and Trolox, a vitamin E analog (Glazer, 1988); these would have the advantage over carotenoids of being colorless and nonfluorescent, but would have to be used in much higher concentrations (probably many millimolar) since their bimolecular reaction rates with oxygen metabolites are not as high and they are consumed by the reaction rather than being catalytic. It should also be remembered that thorough deoxygenation may increase the triplet state lifetime τ_T and worsen the problem of excited-state saturation.

STRATEGIES FOR SIGNAL OPTIMIZATION IN THE FACE OF PHOTOBLEACHING

Light collection efficiency

The above discussion has shown that to increase signal amplitude and signal-to-noise ratio in laser scanning confocal microscopy, increasing laser power helps only until the onset of saturation, and increasing observation time is limited by photodestruction. What other measures can be tried? Obviously any increase in light-collection efficiency (i.e. higher numerical aperture of the objective), transmission efficiency through the scanner and wavelength filters, and quantum efficiency of photodetection is extremely valuable. Despite the importance of these factors, newcomers to low-light-level microscopy often use low N.A. objectives, excessively narrow emission bandpass filters, inefficient optic couplings, and photomultipliers of less-than-optimal quantum efficiencies. Nearly all the fluorophores that fluoresce strongly in aqueous solution with visible wavelengths of excitation are characterized by small Stokes shifts, or difference between absorption and emission peak wavelengths. It may then be difficult to find or fabricate filters and dichroic mirrors that efficiently separate the two wavelength bands. In that case, it would usually be preferable to displace the excitation wavelength to shorter wavelengths away from the peak of the excitation spectrum, so that the emission filters can accept as much of the entire output as possible. Although the excitation is less efficient, this can be made up by increased laser power as long as the photobleaching is reduced by the same factor. By contrast, if the excitation is at the peak wavelength and the emission acceptance band is pushed to longer wavelengths that exclude much of the emission spectrum, then emitted photons are being wasted. This is often a severe problem with rhodamine excited using the 512 nm line of the argon-ion laser.

Spatial resolution

Another tactic to increase signal is to increase the effective size of the confocal apertures, i.e. decrease the spatial resolution. If the illuminating and detecting aperture sizes are doubled, the pixel area quadruples and the volume sampled will increase eightfold; assuming the total laser power is increased to maintain the same intensity in photons·cm^{-1}·s^{-1} and that the fluorophore concentration is uniform in the increased volume (as might be true for an ion indicator distributed in the cytosol), the signal should increase eightfold, though at the price of degraded spatial resolution.

Fluorophore concentration

Increasing the concentration of fluorophore molecules will only increase the signal as long as they do not get too close together. When multiple fluorophores are attached within a few nm of each other on a macromolecule, they usually begin to quench each other. For example, the relatively high quantum yield for free fluorescein in aqueous solution at pH 7 is reduced to near 0.25 when an average of 5 fluorophores are bound to each IgG antibody (Waggoner, in preparation). Charge-transfer interactions with tryptophanes are yet another mechanism for quenching fluoresceins bound to a protein, for example anti-fluorescein antibody (Watt & Voss, 1977). Most rhodamines and certain cyanines also show a striking reduction in average quantum yield, which appears to arise from dye interactions on the protein surface. Absorption spectra of labeled antibodies clearly show evidence of dimers, and fluorescence excitation spectra demonstrate that these dimers are not fluorescent. The propensity of relatively nonpolar, planar rhodamines to interact with one another is not surprising. Even if the fluorophores do not form ground-state dimers, they can also rapidly transfer energy from one to another until a quencher such as O_2 is encountered. In other words, proximity-induced energy transfer between fluorophores multiplies the efficacy of quenchers. Perhaps fortunately it also shortens the excited-state lifetime, so that a higher intensity of laser excitation can be applied for a given degree of saturation (Hirschfeld, 1976). If such increased intensity is available, much of the emission intensity lost by fluorophore proximity can be regained, but at the cost of increased background signal from Rayleigh and Raman scattering and other non-saturated fluorophores.

Choice of fluorophore

Perhaps the most drastic alteration is to change to a different fluorophore altogether. Aside from the well-known labels such as fluorescein, rhodamine (including rigidized variants such as Texas Red), phycobiliproteins, and nitrobenzoxadiazole (NBD), and acridines, a few new tags are being developed, such as cyanines and borate-dipyrromethene ("Bodipy") complexes (Wories et al, 1985; Kang et al, 1988). There is much anecdotal lore about which chromophore gives better signals in various preparations, but most of the data are probably not generalizable, being heavily influenced by variations in the quality of the labeling reagent, in spectral match between excitation source and fluorophore, and the match between the emission and the spectral sensitivity of the detector. Ernst et al (in preparation) have shown that, at least in the case of cyanine dye labeling agents, appropriate placement of charged groups on the fluorophore can reduce dye interactions and increase the brightness of relatively heavily labeled antibodies. Particularly promising in this regard are the indopentamethinecyanines CY5 (excitation 630–650 nm, emission 670 nm) and indotrimethinecyanines CY3 (excitation 530–550 nm, emission 575 nm). Antibodies labeled with these dyes have a brightness comparable to fluorescein-labeled antibodies and have little tendency to precipitate from solution even when labeled with as many as ten dye molecules per antibody. CY5 is somewhat more photostable than fluorescein, and CY3 is significantly more stable. CY5 can be optimally excited with a helium-neon laser, whereas CY3 can be excited fairly efficiently with the 514 nm line and marginally well with the 488 nm line of the argon-ion laser. Thus these new reagents in combination with fluorescein or "bodipy" fluorophores should make it possible to do three color immunofluorescence with laser scanner microscopes equipped with an argon and a helium neon laser. However, it is essential to change laser lines and rescan to obtain the signals from all three fluorophores.

Phycobiliproteins (Oi et al, 1982) currently hold the record for the highest extinction coefficients and largest number of photons emitted before bleaching (Q_e/Q_b; Mathies & Stryer, 1986), partly because each macromolecule simply contains a large number of component fluorophores, partly because the proteins have been engineered by natural selection to protect the tetrapyrrole fluorophores from quenching processes (Glazer, 1989). Recently it has been shown that with suitable optimization of laser power, optics, flow rate, and detection, it is possible to detect fluorescence pulses from single phycobiliprotein molecules in flowing systems (Peck et al, 1989; see also Nguyen et al, 1987). Phycoerythrin (PE) in combination with fluorescein has been valuable for immunofluorescence determination of cell surface markers by single laser (488 nm excitation) flow cytometry. This approach can also be useful in confocal microscopy, provided that the emission signal is split into a 530 nm (fluorescein) and a 575 nm component (PE) and two photomultipliers are used for detection. This method is likely to prove less useful for intracellular antigens, because the size of a PE-antibody conjugate, around 410 kDaltons, restricts penetration into denser regions of fixed cells and tissues. Efforts to develop low molecular weight analogs of PE that have similarly large Stokes shifts and excitation wavelengths have not yet been successful, but work in this area continues. If fluorophores with large Stokes shifts could be found for both 488 nm and 633 nm excitation, a two laser microscope could obtain 4-color immunofluorescence images. Other probes are listed in Table I along with laser lines that are currently available.

FLUORESCENT INDICATORS FOR DYNAMIC INTRACELLULAR PARAMETERS

Membrane potentials

The use of confocal microscopy to measure dynamic properties of living cells such as membrane potentials (Gross & Loew, 1989) or ion concentrations (Tsien, 1988, 1989a,b) deserves some special comment. Preliminary attempts to use fast-responding, non-redistributive voltage-sensitive dyes in neuronal tissues were unsuccessful (Fine et al, 1988); the dye could be seen, but the signal-to-noise ratio was inadequate to observe voltage-dependent changes, which would have been at most only a few percent of the resting intensity. Lasers are inherently noisy light sources; even with optical negative feedback, their fluctuations are greater than the stabilized tungsten filament lamps conventionally used for fast voltage-sensitive dyes (Cohen & Lesher, 1986). "Slow" redistributive dyes, which accumulate in cells according to the Nernst equilibrium (Ehrenberg et al, 1988), would seem to be more suitable for present-day confocal microscopes, since their signals are much bigger, and their slowness of response is actually a better match to the rather slow scan times of the current instrumentation. Confocal optical sectioning should be quite beneficial for such accumulative dyes, since in principle one could directly compare the internal concentrations of dye accumulated without having to correct for the greater pathlength of a thicker cell or for extracellular dye above and below the plane of focus.

Ion concentrations

Wavelength ratioing

Some indicators of ion concentrations respond not just with changes in fluorescence amplitude but with wavelength shifts of excitation or emission spectrum or both. Such shifts permit ratioing between signals obtained at two or more wavelengths (Tsien, 1989 a,b). Ratioing is highly valuable because it cancels out differences in dye concentration and pathlength as well as fluctuations in overall intensity of illumination (Tsien & Poenie, 1986; Bright et al, 1987). Emission ratioing is the most valuable, since with a single excitation wavelength, the emission can be passed through a dichroic mirror to split it into two bands that can be monitored absolutely simultaneously. Such ratioing would give the best possible cancellation of laser noise or movement of the specimen as in motile cells. Emission ratioing is particularly easy to do with a laser-scanning system, since one can simply add a dichroic mirror and an extra photodetector after the scanning system. Whereas geometrical registration of all the corresponding pixels in two separate low-light-level video cameras is quite difficult (Jericevic et al, 1989), the registration problem is trivial in a laser-scanning system assuming the deflection is achromatic, which it must already have been in order to get excitation and even one emission in register. Disk-scanning confocal microscopes use low-light-level video cameras as detectors and lack this elegant compatibility with emission scanning.

Excitation ratioing of images requires sequential illumination with the two excitation wavelengths. Intensity fluctuations of the source and movement of the specimen are cancelled out only if they are much slower than the rate of alternation. Excitation ratioing would be most applicable to tandem-scanning systems, where conventional systems for alternating two grating monochromators or interference filters could be used, whereas alternating between laser lines may involve more construction work and is less flexible in choice of wavelength pairs.

pH indicators

Quite a number of ratiometric pH indicators are available (reviewed by Tsien, 1989b). The most popular excitation-ratioing indicator is probably the modified fluorescein BCECF, whose pH-sensitive and insensitive wavelengths are around 490 nm and 439 nm respectively. The former coincides with the major 488 nm line of an argon ion laser, so non-ratiometric

operation is possible on the BioRad confocal microscope (unpublished preliminary results of R. Tsien and J. White) though less accurate than ratioing. Several emission-shifting probes, 3,6-dihydroxyphthalonitrile (also known as 2,3-dicyanohydroquinone; Kurtz & Balaban, 1985), and various naphthofluorescein derivatives (SNAFs and SNARFs; Haugland, 1989) are also available.

Ca²⁺ indicators

Three currently available Ca^{2+} indicators have different sets of advantages and disadvantages for confocal microscopy (Tsien, 1988, 1989a,b). Fura-2, the dye most used in conventional microscopic imaging, shows a good excitation shift with Ca^{2+}, typically ratioed between 340–350 and 380–385 nm, but hardly any emission shift, so it would probably do best with a UV-enhanced tandem scanning instrument. Considerable enhancement would be necessary because current designs of tandem-scanning confocal microscope were designed mainly for reflectance rather than fluorescence. The beam-splitting pellicles used are inefficient because they are partially reflective but not dichroic; also, they are sometimes made from UV-blocking material in which the excitation has to pass through the pellicle whereas the emission would have to reflect off the pellicle. Even if the pellicle were replaced by a dichroic, this choice of beam geometry would be unfortunate, since it is much easier to make good broadband dichroics in which the shorter wavelength reflects and the longer wavelength transmits than vice versa. Disk systems in which the same area of the disk is used for both source and detector may be more flexible (see Chapter 10.)

Indo-1, the dye most used in laser flow cytometry, shows a fine emission shift from 485 to 405 nm with increasing Ca^{2+} and would be preferred for ratiometric laser-scanning. However, a UV laser, e.g. high-power argon-ion or krypton-ion system, is required for excitation in the 350–365 nm region. Also, indo-1 fluorescence has wavelengths similar to those of reduced pyridine nucleotides, so autofluorescence could be a problem, and indo-1 also bleaches much more quickly than fura-2.

Fluo-3 and its less-tested rhodamine analogs are the only Ca^{2+} indicators currently available with visible wavelengths suitable for low-power visible lasers (Minta et al, 1989; Kao et al, 1989). Therefore it has been the first to be exploited in confocal microscopy (e.g. Hernandez-Cruz et al, 1989), even though it lacks either an excitation or emission shift and is restricted to simple intensity measurements which are relatively difficult to calibrate in terms of absolute $[Ca^{2+}]_i$ units.

Of course, the ideal would be an indicator excitable at 488 nm with a large emission shift, high quantum efficiency, and strong resistance to bleaching, but this goal is a difficult challenge in molecular engineering. In general, strong fluorescence in aqueous media is much easier to obtain using shorter excitation wavelengths, because fluorescence demands planarity and molecular rigidity, which is obviously easier to assure in small molecules that absorb short wavelengths than in the larger molecules with longer chromophores. Most of the known chromophores that combine large size, long wavelengths, and rigidity are essentially insoluble in water. Even if solubilizing groups are added on the periphery, the huge expanse of hydrophobic surface still promotes formation of nonfluorescent aggregates. Finally, the quantum mechanics of absorption and fluorescence predict that the intrinsic radiative lifetime of a chromophore is proportional to the cube of the wavelength if other factors remain constant (Strickler & Berg, 1962). Short radiative lifetimes mean that fluorescence emission competes more successfully with nonproductive forms of deactivation and therefore correlate with high quantum yields of fluorescence.

Other forms of ratioing

Because ratioing is so desirable for quantitative measurements, but appropriate wavelength shifts are often unavailable, several alternatives to wavelength ratioing have been proposed. The easiest is simply to ratio poststimulus image intensities against a prestimulus image. An example is shown by Smith & Augustine (1988). This method has the advantage of minimal hardware requirements and high time resolution, though it only cancels out variations in dye loading and pathlength, not shape change or dye bleaching, and by itself cannot yield an absolute calibration of the analyte, e.g. $[Ca^{2+}]_i$. Another approach would be to covalently link the fluorescent indicator to a separate reference fluorophore. This approach would ideally gene rate a composite molecule in which the ratio of the indicator fluorescence to the reference fluorescence would signal the analyte concentration. Potential disadvantages would be the requirement for significant skill in organic synthesis, the likelihood that the conjugate would be too large for loading by ester hydrolysis, and the possibility that the two fluorophores would bleach at different rates, so that the operation of ratioing would fail to correct for bleaching. Yet a third mode of ratioing could be based on temporal dissection of excited-state lifetimes, as first shown for quin-2 by Wages et al (1987). If the free and bound forms of the indicator have sufficiently different fluorescence lifetimes, their relative contributions to the (ideally) biexponential decay might be separated by nanosecond or high frequency modulation techniques. However, even if the instrumentation challenge of combining lifetime kinetics with imaging can be solved, the problem remains that probes like fura-2 and indo-1, which are fairly strongly fluorescent both when free and when bound to Ca $^{2+}$, have almost the same lifetimes in those two states. For example, fura-2 with and without Ca^{2+} has lifetimes of 1.8 and 1.3 ns respectively at 25°; for indo-1 the corresponding numbers are 1.7 and 1.3 ns at 20° (Wages, et al 1987). In order to get a big difference in lifetimes between Ca^{2+}-bound and free indicator, as in quin-2 (10.1 and 1.3 ns respectively at 25°), one of the species has to be much more dimly fluorescent than the other. As a result the weaker and faster component will be hard to measure accurately and to distinguish from autofluorescence background.

Ratiometric measurements can also be applied to other parameters such as probe polarization and local viscosity (Axelrod, 1989; Dix & Verkman, 1989; Tinoco, et al 1987), proximity between macromolecules by fluorescence energy transfer (Herman, 1989; Uster & Pagano, 1986), and even water permeability (Kuwahara & Verkman, 1988; Kuwahara et al, 1988).

FUTURE DEVELOPMENTS?

Speculation on future directions in fluorophore designs is difficult, because the small number of laboratories working on fluorophore chemistry means that progress is a much noisier function of time than advances in instrumentation or computers. One thought prompted by preparation of this review is that, for present purposes, the triplet excited state of the fluorophore is a major villain without any redeeming virtues. It is responsible for a pernicious form of output saturation, for singlet oxygen production, and for nearly all covalent photochemistry such as bleaching. Similar problems have been encountered in laser dyes; a proposed solution (Schäfer, 1983; Liphardt et al, 1982, 1983) is to attach triplet-state quenchers to each fluorophore. Such a construction is reminiscent of the way that evolution has assembled photosynthetic complexes and may be an area where biology can repay its debt to synthetic chemistry.

ACKNOWLEDGMENTS

We wish to thank Profs. Richard Mathies and Alex Glazer for helpful discussions and criticisms of the manuscript and permission to cite their unpublished data. This work was supported by NSF Grant BBS-8714246 and NIH Grant GM 31004, EY 04372, and NS 27177 to RYT and MSN 19353 and GM 34639 to AW.

REFERENCES

Axelrod D (1977) Cell surface heating during fluorescence photobleaching recovery experiments. Biophys. J. 18, 129–131.

Axelrod D (1989) Fluorescence polarization microscopy. Meth. Cell Biol. 30, 333–352.

Bailey EA jr, Rollefson GK (1953) The determination of the fluorescence lifetimes of dissolved substances by a phase shift method. J. Chem. Phys. 21, 1315–1322.

Bloom JA, Webb WW (1984) Photodamage to intact erythrocyte membranes at high laser intensities: methods of assay and suppression. J. Histochem. Cytochem. 32, 608–616.

Bonhoeffer T, Staiger V (1988) Optical recording with single cell resolution from monolayered slice cultures of rat hippocampus. Neurosci. Lett. 92, 259–264.

Bright GR, Fisher GW, Rogowska J, Taylor DL (1987) Fluorescence ratio imaging microscopy: Temporal and spatial measurements of cytoplasmic pH. J. Cell Biol. 104: 1019–1033.

Chen RF, Scott CH (1985) Atlas of fluorescence spectra and lifetimes of dyes attached to protein. Analyt. Lett. 18, 393–421.

Cohen LB, Lesher S (1986) Optical monitoring of membrane potential: methods of multisite optical measurement. In Optical Methods in Cell Physiology (De Weer P, Salzberg BM, eds). Wiley, New York pp. 71–99.

Dix JA, Verkman AS (1989) Spatially resolved anisotropy images of fluorescent probes incorporated into living cells. Biophys. J. 55, 189a.

Ehrenberg B, Montana V, Wei MD, Wuskell JP, Loew LM (1988) Membrane potentials can be determined in individual cells from the Nernstian distribution of cationic dyes. Biophys. J. 53, 785–794.

Fine A, Amos WB, Durbin RM, McNaughton PA (1988) Confocal microscopy: applications in neurobiology. Trends Neurosci. 11, 346–351.

Gandin E, Lion Y, Van de Vorst A (1983) Quantum yields of singlet oxygen production by xanthene derivatives. Photochem. Photobiol. 37, 271–278.

Giloh H, Sedat JW (1982) Fluorescence microscopy: reduced photobleaching of rhodamine and fluorescein protein conjugates by n-propyl gallate. Science 217, 1252–1255.

Glazer AN (1988) Fluorescence-based assay for reactive oxygen species: a protective role for creatinine. FASEB J. 2, 2487–2491.

Glazer AN (1989) Light guides. Directional energy transfer in a photosynthetic antenna. J. Biol. Chem. 264, 1–4.

Gross D, Loew LM (1989) Fluorescent indicators of membrane potential: microspectrofluorometry and imaging. Meth. Cell Biol. 30, 193–218

Haugland RP (1989) Molecular probes: handbook of fluorescent probes and research chemicals. Molecular Probes Inc., Eugene, Oregon pp.86–94.

Hernandez-Cruz A, Sala F, Adams PR (1989) Subcellular dynamics of [Ca²⁺]$_i$ monitored with laser scanned confocal microscopy in a single voltage-clamped vertebrate neuron. Biophys. J. 55: 216a

Herman B (1989) Resonance energy transfer microscopy. Meth. Cell Biol. 30, 219–243.

Hirschfeld T (1976) Quantum efficiency independence of the time integrated emission from a fluorescent molecule. Appl. Opt. 15, 3135–3139.

Jericevic Z, Wiese B, Bryan J, Smith LC (1989) Validation of an imaging system: steps to evaluate and validate a micrscope imaging system for quantitative studies. Meth. Cell Biol. 30, 47–83.

Kang HC, Fisher PJ, Prendergast FG, Haugland RP (1988) Bodipy: a novel fluorescein and NBD substitute. J. Cell Biol. 107, 34a.

Kao JPY, Harootunian AT, Tsien RY (1989) Photochemically generated cytosolic calcium pulses and their detection by fluo-3. J. Biol. Chem. 264, 8179–8184.

Kaplan NO (1960) The pyridine coenzymes. In The Enzymes, 2nd. ed. (Boyer PD, Lardy H, Myrbäck K, eds). Academic Press, New York. pp. 105–169.

Koziol J (1971) Fluorometric analyses of riboflavin and its coenzymes. Meth. Enzymol. 18B, 253–285.

Kurtz I, Balaban RS (1985) Fluorescence emission spectroscopy of 1,4-dihydroxyphthalonitrile: A method for determining intracellular pH in cultured cells. Biophys. J. 48, 499–508.

Kuwahara M, Verkman AS (1988) Direct fluorescence measurement of diffusional water permeability in the vasopressin-sensitive kidney collecting tubule. Biophys. J. 54, 587–593.

Kuwahara M, Berry CA, Verkman AS (1988) Rapid development of vasopressin-induced hydroosmosis in kidney collecting tubules measured by a new fluorescence technique. Biophys. J. 54, 595–602.

Lakowicz JR (1983) Principles of fluorescence spectroscopy. Plenum, New York.

Lewis GN, Lipkin D, Magel TT (1941) Reversible photochemical processes in rigid media. A study of the phosphorescent state. J. Am. Chem. Soc. 63, 3005–3018.

Lindqvist L (1960) A flash photolysis study of fluorescein. Arkiv för Kemi 16, 79–138.

Liphardt B, Liphardt B, Lüttke W (1982) Laserfarbstoffe mit intramolekularer Triplettlöschung. Chemische Berichte 115, 2997–3010.

Liphardt B, Liphardt B, Lüttke W (1983) Laser dyes III: concepts to increase the photostability of laser dyes. Optics Communications 48, 129–133.

Manitto P, Speranza G, Monti D, Gramatica P (1987) Singlet oxygen reactions in aqueous solution. Physical and chemical quenching rate constants of crocin and related carotenoids. Tetrahedron Lett. 28, 4221–4224

Matheson IBC, Rodgers MAJ (1982) Crocetin, a water soluble carotenoid monitor for singlet molecular oxygen. Photochem. Photobiol. 36, 1–4.

Mathies RA, Stryer L (1986) Single-molecule fluorescence detection: a feasibility study using phycoerythrin. In Applications of Fluorescence in the Biomedical Sciences (Taylor DL, Waggoner AS, Murphy RF, Lanni F, and Birge RR, eds). AR Liss, New York. pp 129–140.

Matthews MM, Sistrom WR (1959) Function of carotenoid pigments in nonphotosynthetic bacteria. Nature (Lond.) 184, 1892–1893.

Minta A, Kao JPY, Tsien RY (1989) Fluorescent indicators for cytosolic calcium based on rhodamine and fluorescein chromophores. J. Biol. Chem. 264, 8171–8178.

Nguyen DC, Keller RA, Jett JH, Martin JC (1987) Detection of single molecules of phycoerythrin in hydrodynamically focused flows by laser-induced fluorescence. Analyt. Chem. 59, 2158–2161.

Oi V, Glazer AN, Stryer L (1982) Fluorescent phycobiliprotein conjugates for analyses of cells and molecules. J. Cell Biol. 93, 981–986.

Peck K, Stryer L, Glazer AN, Mathies RA (1989) Single molecule fluorescence detection: autocorrelation criterion and experimental realization with phycoerythrin. Proc. Natl. Acad. Sci. USA 86, in press for June.

Reyftmann JP, Kohen E, Morliere P, Santus R, Kohen C, Mangel WF, Dubertret L, Hirschberg JG (1986) A microspectrofluorometric study of porphyrin-photosensitized single living cells – I. Membrane alterations. Photochem. Photobiol. 44, 461–469.

Schäfer FP (1983) New developments in laser dyes. Laser Chem. 3, 265–278.

Schneider MB, Webb WW (1981) Measurement of submicron laser beam radii. Appl. Opt. 20, 1382–1388.

Sheetz MP, Koppel DE (1979) Membrane damage caused by irradiation of fluorescent concanavalin A. Proc. Natl. Acad. Sci. USA 76, 3314–3317.

Smith SJ, Augustine GJ (1988) Calcium ions, active zones and synaptic transmitter release. Trends Neurosci. 11, 458–464.

Strickler SJ, Berg RA (1962) Relationship between absorption intensity and fluorescence lifetime of molecules. J. Chem. Phys. 37, 814–822.

Tinoco I, Mickols W, Maestre MF, Bustamante C (1987) Absorption, scattering, and imaging of biomolecular structures with polarized light. Annu. Rev. Biophys. Biophys. Chem. 16, 319–349.

Tsien RY (1988) Fluorescence measurement and photochemical manipulation of cytosolic free calcium. Trends Neurosci. 11, 419–424.

Tsien RY (1989a) Fluorescent probes of cell signaling. Annu. Rev. Neurosci. 12, 227–253.

Tsien RY (1989b) Fluorescent indicators of ion concentrations. Meth. Cell Biol. 30, 127–156.

Tsien RY, Poenie M (1986) Fluorescence ratio imaging: a new window into intracellular ionic signaling. Trends Biochem. Sci. 11, 450–455.

Uster PS, Pagano RE (1986) Resonance energy transfer microscopy: observations of membrane-bound fluorescent probes in model membranes and in living cells. J. Cell Biol. 103, 122–1234.

Vigers GPA, Coue M, McIntosh JR (1988) Fluorescent microtubules break up under illumination. J. Cell Biol. 107, 1011–1024.

Wages J, Packard B, Edidin M, Brand L (1987) Time-resolved fluorescence of intracellular quin-2. Biophys. J. 51, 284a.

Waggoner A, DeBiasio R, Conrad P, Bright GR, Ernst L, Ryan K, Nederlof M, Taylor, D (1989) Multiple spectral parameter imaging. Meth. Cell Biol. 30, 449–478.

Watt RM, Voss EW Jr (1977) Mechanism of quenching of fluorescein by anti-fluorescein IgG antibodies. Immunochemistry 14, 533–541.

White JC, Stryer L (1987) Photostability studies of phycobiliprotein fluorescent labels. Analyt. Biochem. 161, 442–452.

White JG, Amos WB, Fordham M (1987) An evaluation of confocal versus conventional imaging of biological structures by fluorescence light microscopy. J. Cell Biol. 105, 41–48.

Wilson EO: Sociobiology. Harvard University Press, Cambridge, Massachusetts. pp. 38–43.

Wories, HJ, Koek JH, Lodder G, Lugtenburg J, Fokkens R, Driessen O, Mohn GR (1985) A novel water-soluble fluorescent probe: synthesis, luminescence and biological properties of the sodium salt of the 4-sulfonato-3,3',5,5'-tetramethyl-2,2'-pyrromethen-1,1'-BF$_2$ complex. Recl. Trav. Chim. Pays-Bas 104, 288–291.

Chapter 17

Image Contrast in Confocal Light Microscopy

P.C. Cheng and R.G. Summers

Advanced Microscopy Laboratory*, Department of Anatomical Sciences, State University of New York at Buffalo, Buffalo, NY 14214 USA

INTRODUCTION

For any form of microscopy, one needs not only an imaging system which has enough resolution to reveal the fine details of a specimen, but also, a suitable contrast mechanism to "see" the structures of interest. As defined by the New Webster's Dictionary, contrast is the difference between light and dark areas of a negative or print. In other words, contrast is the difference in signal strength between various parts of an image or between details of interest and "background". To be slightly more scientific, the detected contrast is proportional to the brightness difference, ΔI, between two image areas divided by the average image brightness, $\bar{I}$.

$$\text{Contrast} = \frac{\Delta I}{\bar{I}}$$

In the confocal microscope, contrast emerges because of differences in the way that the various subvolumes of the specimen (voxels) interact with the focused illumination. This interaction may include absorption, fluorescence, refraction, reflection, phase-shift, scattering, or changes in polarization. This chapter will concentrate on the contrast characteristics of the two modalities that have been most fully investigated thus far: fluorescence and reflection. It will also consider the deleterious effects on the confocal image produced by the absorptive, refractive and reflective properties of features that are between the plane-of-focus and the objective lens, as all of these topics are relevant to epi-illuminated operation. Confocal imaging in transmission contrast is covered in Chapters 8 and 11.

SOURCES OF CONTRAST

The interaction of an incident light beam with the sample is a complex event. Figure 1 shows a simplified version of such an interaction and the effect of voxels above and below the voxel being sampled.

Ideally, the transmitted intensity (I) of the incident light (I_o) through structures (voxels) above the voxel being sampled is:

$$I = I_o \, e^{-\mu x}$$

where μ is the absorption coefficient of the structure, and x is the thickness of the absorption path (the total thickness of the voxel). In the situation of a heterogeneous structure, the absorption coefficient, μ_T is:

$$\mu_T = \sum_{i=1}^{m} f_i \, \mu_i$$

Here the absorber (specimen) is composed of m different subunits, each containing a certain percentage of the total mass, f_i, and their individual absorption coefficients, μ_i, where μ_T is the absorption coefficient which is associated with the light attenuation by the structure (Fig. 1). In addition to the absorption phenomenon, reflection and scattering from structures with refractive indices different from those of the surrounding medium also attenuate the transmitted light.

The detectable fluorescent intensity resulting from the voxel is a function of the quantum efficiency of the fluorochrome (for a given excitation wavelength), the incident intensity and the self-absorption within the voxel, the absorption characteristic of the structures between the voxel and objective and the solid angle of the detector (objective).

If the voxel above the sampled voxel has a significant difference in refractive index from the bathing medium, refraction causes the incident ray to be deviated from the original path

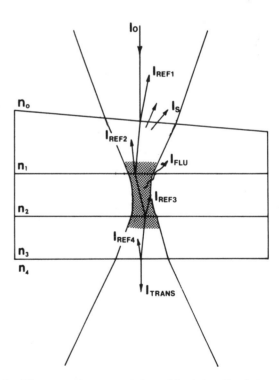

FIG. 1. Diagrammatic representation of the interaction between an incident light beam and a specimen. The shaded space in the diagram represents the volume (voxel) which is imaged by the confocal microscope to form an image pixel. Reflectal (I_{REFn}) results from media interfaces (e.g. n_1 and n_2 interface) and their intensity is a function of the difference in refractive indices between the interfacing media. I_s: intensity of scattered light. I_{TRANS}: intensity of transmitted light. I_{FLU}: intensity of fluorescence. I_o: incident intensity.

*A joint facility of the School of Medicine and Biomedical Sciences and the School of Engineering and Applied Sciences, SUNYAB.

which can cause a sampling error (i.e. imaging of a different voxel).

It is clear that for any kind of microscopy, the image contrast is the result of the proper choice of the methods for specimen preparation and the optical arrangement of the microscope. Confocal light microscopy is a special type of contrast enhancement for optical microscopy. In phase contrast and differential interference contrast (DIC) modes, image contrast is the result of the phase effects produced by differences in the refractive indices of structures at or near the plane of focus within a specimen. In confocal microscopy, a special arrangement of optics and pinholes is used to further restrict the information depth, and hence increase the contrast of the in-focus image (Wijaendts van Resandt et al., 1984). It is the intention of this paper to discuss the various factors which affect the contrast of a confocal image.

Basically, the contrast of a confocal image is caused by (1) intrinsic factors and/or (2) extrinsic factors. Intrinsic factors are physical properties of the specimen such as refractive index, color (selective absorbance), birefringence, etc. The extrinsic factors are those chemical and physical contrast mechanisms that can be used to label one or more specific properties of the specimen. For example, certain molecules within a cell, such as chlorophyll fluoresce when excited with a proper light source (an intrinsic factor). The contrast of an autofluorescent image is the result of the proper selection of excitation wavelength, microscope optics and the use of specific properties of the specimen.

On the other hand, fluorochrome-conjugated antibodies can be used to chemically "tag" specific molecules in a cell which then become fluorescent when the specimen is excited by a suitable light source. This is extrinsic contrast because it requires the binding specificity of fluorescent probes to produce the image contrast in mapping target molecules or structures. To obtain a good confocal microscopic image, one should combine both extrinsic and intrinsic factors to selectively improve the image signals and decrease the "background" signals. This can be done by improving optical performance and by using special optical contrast methods, but one must also pay particular attention to the proper preparation of the specimen (see Chapter 18).

At the present time, confocal microscopes with both reflective and epifluorescent capabilities are commercially available; this paper will discuss the various factors which affect the contrast of the final images produced by each method.

CONFOCAL MICROSCOPY IN BACKSCATTERED MODE

Signal Formation

One of the basic modes of confocal microscopy utilizes backscattered or reflected light. The image is the result of differences in reflective signals, both direct reflection and scattering, from a specimen. The signal strength is highly dependent upon the type of specimen being studied.

In geometric optics, when light travels from one medium to another of different refractive index, the light is separated into two components: the reflected ray and refracted ray. The degree of reflection is dependent on the gradient of the refractive index between the two media. The refracted ray changes its propagation angle (θ_r) with respect to the incident beam (θ_i) as described by Snell's law:

$$\frac{\sin \theta_i}{\sin \theta_r} = n_{21}$$

where constant n_{21} is the refractive index of the second medium relative to the first medium and can be expressed in terms of the refractive indices of n_1 and n_2.

$$n_1 \sin \theta_i = n_2 \sin \theta_r$$

In the event that the incident angle, θ_i, is greater than the critical angle, θ_c, where

$$\sin \theta_c = n_{21} \qquad (n_{21} < 1)$$

then total reflection results.

In reflective confocal microscopy, the reflectance (the ratio between illuminating intensity and reflective intensity) of the specimen is one of the key factors which determines the signal strength. The reflectance is determined by the ratio of the difference of the squares of the refractive indices of the two media.

$$\frac{I_{ref}}{I_o} = \left(\frac{n_1 - n_2}{n_1 + n_2}\right)^2$$

Therefore, the less the difference between the refractive indices of the two media, the less the reflectance. This is generally the case for living biological specimens where the refractive indices of various cellular structures differ very little from that of the surrounding water. Hence, a biological specimen gives much poorer reflectance than most materials-science specimens. For instance, the reflectance of a gold-coated glass surface (a mirror or an intergrated circuit (IC) chip) can be as high as >0.95 ($>95\%$) and that of the metallic silver deposited in a Golgi-stained neuron may be $\sim 10\%$, but the typical reflectance of the surface of a corn leaf (interface with air) is approximately 3×10^{-4} of the reflectance of a mirror surface. Human bone imaged under a confocal microscope with a N.A.$=0.8$ objective gives a signal strength approximately 1×10^{-4} that of a mirror surface. The reflectance of living specimens such as tissue culture cells is even lower. However, the signal can be significantly improved when light resulting from total-reflection is detected. This can be achieved in many situations by using high numerical aperture objectives (Fig. 2). Despite the low reflectance, confocal images of tooth enamel prisms and Golgi-stained (silver impregnated) Purkinje cells have been obtained (Boyde et al., 1985). Recently, Watson et al. (1989) demonstrated real-time imaging of an internal section of a tooth being abraded by a dental burr by using a tandem scanning confocal microscope (TSRLM) operated in reflective mode.

In addition to the reflectance of the sample, the local orientation of the structure and overall surface profile of the specimen have a profound effect on the image contrast in confocal microscopy. The local tilting of structural surfaces within a specimen affects the reflective signal strength (Fig. 3). If the surface tilt is high enough so that no directly reflected light enters the objective, then this part of the surface appears dark (or absent) in the image. A metallic surface perpendicular to the optical axis will give maximum signal strength.

It is clear that this type of image contrast is highly dependent on the solid angle of the detector (i.e. the N.A. of the objective) and the degree of tilting of surfaces within the sample. The use of high N.A. objectives minimizes this type of topographic contrast (Fig. 2). On the other hand, such contrast could be increased if the detector were placed not directly behind the pinhole but in the diffraction plane of a lens focussed on the

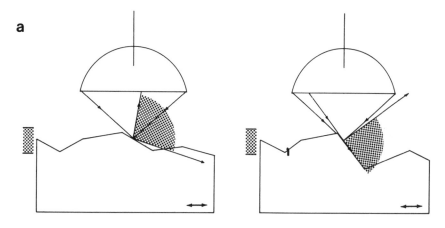

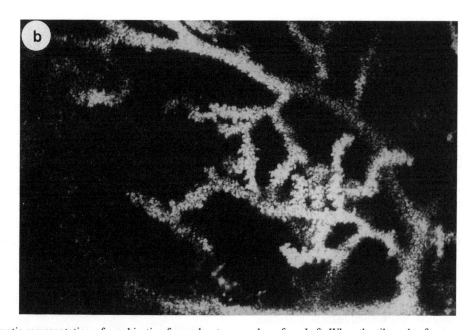

Fɪɢ. 2. (a) Diagrammatic representation of an objective focused onto a rough surface. Left: When the tilt angle of a structure within the specimen is low, a certain percentage of reflective light (shaded angle) can enter the solid angle of the objective. Right: If the local tilt is high, then all the reflected rays miss the solid angle of the detector, therefore, the only signals detected are those of scattered light.
(b):   Confocal image of the dendritic tree of a Purkinje cell of the rat. The punctate appearance is the result of varying the orientation of the surface of the dendrite. The reflective image was obtained by using a BioRad MRC 500 laser scanning system. (Specimen courtesy of Dr. R. Pentney, Dept. of Anatomical Sciences, SUNYAB)

pinhole. A four-segment detector in this position could give independent signals proportional to reflective surfaces tilted in four different directions. A 2-dimensional CCD array would be an ideal detector for this purpose.

Backscattered Light Contrast on Stained Specimens

For the reasons described above, reflective imaging of silver-impregnated nerve cells presents a "punctate" appearance even though the dendrites are continuous structures. Therefore, a small "gap" between nerve fibers seen in the reflective confocal mode may not mean that they lack physical contact or continuity (Fig. 3b) but only that the reflecting surface is tilted so steeply that the reflected light does not strike the objective. For a low-reflectance planar specimen placed perpendicular to the optical axis, signals resulting from total reflection can be detected if the solid angle of the detector is greater than the critical angle (θ_c) of reflection.

In biological specimens, Golgi-"stained" Purkinje cells demonstrate strong contrast. The contrast in these images is the result of strong surface reflection of the silver-decorated cells in comparison to the weakly scattered signals from the surrounding non-impregnated tissues. An important feature of the Golgi preparation is that the method stains only 1–5% of the neurons in the preparation (Barr and Kiernan, 1988; Scheibel and Scheibel, 1970). If the Golgi preparation "stained" all of the neurons in the tissue, the clear image of the dendritic tree of a single neuron (hundreds of micrometers in depth) would be replaced by an image with poor contrast and optical sectioning would be nearly impossible because the high reflectivity would prevent light from penetrating much below the surface of the specimen.

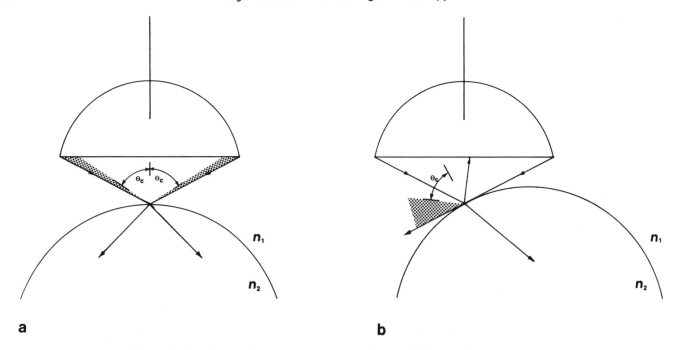

a   b

FIG. 3. Diagrammatic representation of varying signal intensity from a translucent object (n_2) embedded in a medium which has a different refractive index (n_1). The change of signal intensity depends upon the orientation of the interface with respect to the incident beam.
(a): An objective lens is focused onto the surface of a spherical structure with a refractive index, n_2, which is different from the surrounding medium, n_1. The objective lens detects signals resulting from the surface reflection and scattering. Illumination rays which have a higher incident angle than the critical angle, θ_c, result in total reflection (shaded rays). The light from total reflection contributes strongly to the image. It is clear that the greater the difference in refractive indices between the structure and bathing medium is, the smaller the critical angle. Hence, for a given objective lens, the brighter the image is.
(b): If the orientation of the structure is tilted, the objective detects only some of the reflected rays and scattered light from the structure. Therefore, the signal obtained is weaker than the situation shown in the previous example (a).

Reflection Contrast on Non-Biological Specimens

Another popular usage of reflective mode is the examination of integrated circuits. The image contrast is generally the result of differences in surface reflectivity and surface topography (Fig. 4). Note that image contrast between adjacent circuit structures is primarily due to the variation in structural heights. In certain cases, changes of refractive index within a translucent specimen are responsible for image contrast. A typical example of this is the confocal study of the optical waveguides on a Ti-doped Li-Niobate single crystal (Fig. 5). Reflective confocal imaging can also be used for composite materials such as carbon-filled polyethylene insulators although, in this case, the results are strongly modified by absorption, as discussed later, (Fig. 9b, c and d). The carbon particles embedded in a polyethylene matrix give both surface reflection and scattering.

Backscatter Contrast on Living Specimens

Imaging of living biological specimens in the reflective mode presents the same problems. Image contrast degrades as the objective lens focuses deeper into the tissue. Interfacial reflections from the various cellular components have the effect that the denser the overlying cells, the poorer the image signal. In addition, the deeper the objective lens is focussed into the specimen, the more heterogeneous the "medium" between the focal plane and the objective. Refraction produced by these inhomogeneities significantly degrades the optical performance of the objective. Figure 6a shows an epireflective image of the surface of *Stentor coeruleus*; however, the image of the macronuclei (Fig. 6b), located deep inside the cell, shows significant degradation

in image definition and contrast. The *Stentor* images were obtained in real-time (single TV frames) by using a Tracor Northern TSRLM equipped with a TV camera-coupled image intensifier (Chen and Cheng, 1989). The low reflectance of many living specimens can make real-time imaging in reflective mode difficult. However, the reflectance of biological specimens can be improved, at least in fixed tissue and cells, by the use of reflective dyes, and the use of metallic decoration or staining (Golgi preparation, etc. also Paddock 1989).

The Effect of Overlying Structures

In the optical path, especially close to the focal plane, small structures with refractive indices different from those of the surrounding medium can cause pronounced degradation in image quality and introduce sectioning artifacts. These structures can cause scattering which lowers the signal and also alters the level of the focal plane which results in a "rippled" section. The "rippling" of the sectioning plane can introduce false contrast not related to the real structures within the plane of section. Figure 7 is a model of such a situation. A glass bead was placed on the surface of a mirror and the microscope was focused on the mirror surface. Because of the difference in refractive index between the glass bead (n = 1.53) and mounting medium (water, n = 1.3), the specimen under the glass bead is no longer in focus (Fig. 7b). This type of problem can exist when imaging cells loaded with mineral crystals, lipid granules and protein bodies.

Careful selection of a mounting medium to match the refractive index of such cellular "inclusions" can significantly reduce this type of distortion, but it will also render such inclu-

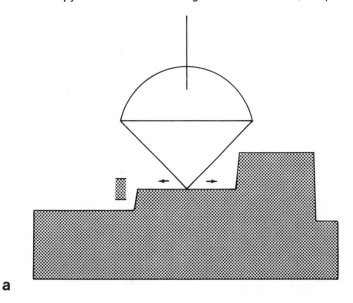

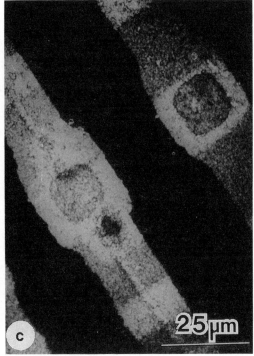

FIG. 4.   (a): Diagrammatic representation of confocal imaging of a metal-coated stepped structure (where the steps are greater than the thickness of the imaging plane [shaded bar]). The image contrast is primarily the result of variation in signal strength between in-focus and out-of-focus structures.
(b) (c): Reflective confocal images of an integrated circuit at different focal levels.

sions invisible unless they are fluorescent. Figure 7d employed the same model as in Fig. 7b, but when the mounting medium is replaced with immersion oil (n=1.53), the mirror surface below the glass bead is now in focus. (For comparison see the corresponding transmitted light images in Fig. 7c and e made by collecting light with a non-confocal detector.) In fluorescent imaging, this type of "heterogeneity" within a specimen can also cause signal loss (due to scattering, reflection, absorption and refraction) *and* alteration of the level of the focal plane.

The reflective confocal mode works particularly well in the study of various mineral deposits in cells, providing that the

tissue is processed properly. For instance, we have been using the BioRad MRC500 laser confocal microscope in the study of silicon dioxide deposits in the leaf epidermal cells of maize (*Zea mays* L.). Excellent reflective images can be obtained from the *surface* of a fresh leaf. However, due to the heterogeneity of the cell wall, the silica deposits *within* the epidermal cells are very difficult to observe in a living leaf blade. If one fixes, dehydrates and subsequently clears the leaf tissue in methyl salicylate (n= 1.535–1.538), then, the silica deposits within the epidermal cells can be imaged easily (Fig. 8). The clearing procedure produces a significant improvement in the optical properties of the tissue.

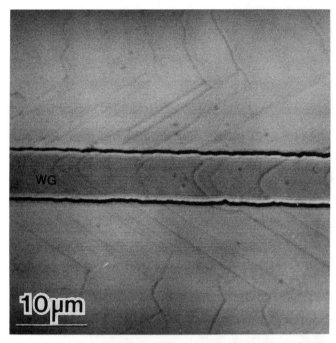

FIG. 5.   (a) Reflective confocal image of an optical waveguide (WG) on a transparent Li-Niobate crystal. The image is the result of variation of refractive index within the very top layers of the crystal. The image was obtained on a BioRad MRC500 operated in reflective mode. (Specimen courtesy of Dr. P. L. Liu, Dept. of Electrical and Computer Engineering, SUNYAB)

The reflection from the surface of the silica deposits is due to the differences in refractive index between the opaline silica (n=1.42–1.44) (Jones and Handreck, 1967) and the mounting medium (methyl salicylate, n=1.535 − 1.538) whereas the non-mineral components of the plant cells, after clearing, have a refractive index closer to that of methyl salicylate. Proper selection of a clearing and mounting medium in terms of refractive index is essential for tuning reflective signals to improve image contrast.

Absorption Contrast

Absorption properties of a specimen, in terms of color or opacity, can have a negative impact on image contrast in the reflective mode. For instance, the nearly opaque carbon particles in the polyethylene insulator shown in Fig. 9 cause a significant loss in signal intensity by attenuating both the illuminating beam and reflected signal. Deep coloration in biological specimens such as that from pigment granules and chloroplasts also significantly attenuates both the **illuminating beam** and **reflected signal** by scattering and absorption. This problem can be minimized by proper selection of the wavelength so that the absorption is kept at a minimum. For instance, when imaging plant cells heavily loaded with chloroplasts, green illumination will do much better than blue or red. Similarly, near-infrared (700–1200nm) radiation can be used to study the internal structure of insects, since the insect cuticle is relatively translucent in the IR spectrum.

Artificial Contrast

In disk-scanning confocal microscopes that utilize a single-sided scanning method (see Chapter 10), image contrast is also

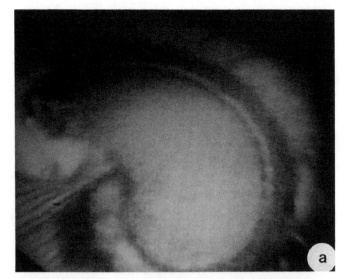

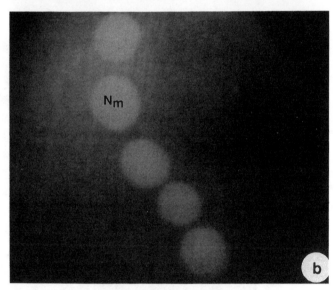

FIG. 6.   Reflective confocal image of a living *Stentor coeruleus* obtained by using a tandem scanning confocal microscope (Tracor Northern TSM) equipped with a TV camera -coupled image intensifier. The images are single-frame TV images.
(a): Surface membranelle
(b): Image of the macro nuclei (N_m) within the cell.

affected by inadequately trapped light reflected from the **surface** of the spinning disk, as this increases background signal level. This is particularly serious when the reflectance of the specimen is low (i.e., the signal strength is weak). In the single-sided confocal microscopes constructed by Kino (Xio et al., 1988) and us (Cheng et al., 1989), the light reflection from the surface of the spinning disk is removed by a polarizer (Glan-Taylor polarizer) and analyzer. In addition, slightly tilting the disk can also remove a significant amount of surface reflection. The degree of scattering from the surface of the disk depends on the surface finish of the disk. Coherent reflection is easier to remove than scattered light so a disk with a highly polished surface is desirable.

Reflection from lens elements is a serious problem in confocal microscopy operated in reflective mode. The on-axis reflection of coherent light from the lens surfaces can result in a bright spot and a series of diffraction fringes in the center of

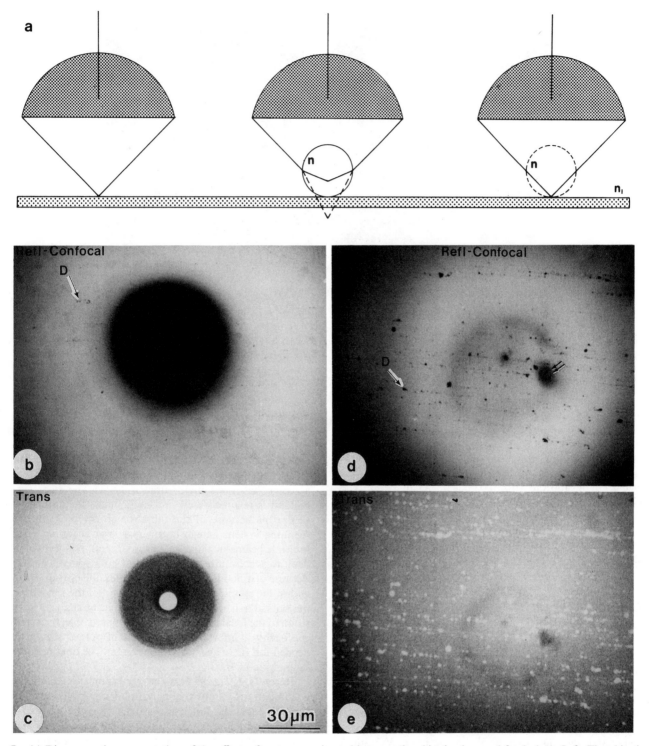

FIG. 7.   (a) Diagrammatic representation of the effects of a structure situated between the objective lens and focal plane. Left: The objective is focused onto the first surface of a mirror. Middle: The focal plane of the objective is deviated if a spherical structure, with a refractive index n, different from the surrounding medium (n_1), is introduced into the optical path. The focal plane moves upward when $n > n_1$ or downward when $n < n_1$ (dotted rays). Right: When the refractive index of the spherical structure (n) is the same as the surrounding medium (n_1), the focal plane of the objective remains on the mirror surface.
(b):   Confocal image of the first surface of a partially aluminized mirror (with defects, D) with a 67μm glass sphere (n=1.53) was suspended in water (n=1.3) on the surface of the mirror. Some of the area covered by the glass bead is "out-of-focus" and appears dark. (Compare diameter with 30μm scale bar.)
(c):   Non-confocal transmission image of the situation shown in (b).
(d):   Confocal image of a partially aluminized mirror surface (with a defect, D) with a glass sphere (n=1.53) suspended in immersion oil (n=1.53) on the mirror. Because of the matching of reflective indices of the glass bead and "mounting medium", the mirror surface which directly lay under the glass bead remains in focus. The small dark spot (double arrows) is the result of an air bubble (n=1) within the glass bead. Darkening at corners of image is caused by curvature of field in the objective lens.
(e):   Non-confocal transmission image of the situation shown in (d).
Photographs (b), (c), (d) and (e) have the same magnification.

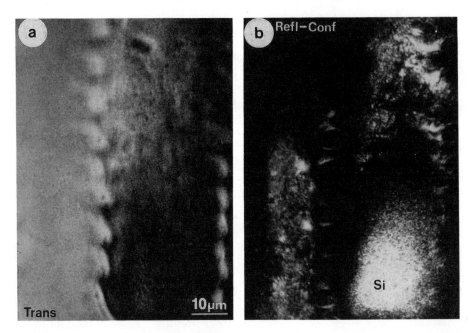

FIG. 8.   Silica deposits (n=1.42–1.44) in the leaf epidermal cell of maize. The leaf was fixed according to the procedure described by Cheng et al. (1979), dehydrated in EtOH and cleared in methyl salicylate (n=1.53).
(a):   Transmission image of the leaf blade.
(b):   Reflective confocal image showing silica deposits (Si). The image was obtained by using a BioRad MRC500 laser scanning system.

the image (Fig. 10a). Many investigators use the off-axis scanning method to eliminate the "ghost" spot in the image (the "PAN" option in the BioRad system). But this approach sacrifices the size of the field of view and produces image degradation by using off-axis portions of the optical system. (See Chapter 7.) In our BioRad MRC500 system, a Glan-Taylor type polarizer (a double calcite prism) was used in the laser beam to achieve high polarization extinction (10^{-5}) for the illuminating beam, and then, a 1/4 wavelength retardation plate was inserted into the optical path just above the objective to change the linearly polarized illuminating beam to a circularly polarized form. An analyzer is placed just in front of the detector. This arrangement (Fig. 10b) removes most of the unwanted reflection from the microscope lens elements (Fig. 10c). However, there is still a small amount of surface reflection from the lower surfaces of the objective lens. An objective with a built-in 1/4 wave retardation plate on its front surface may be the answer.

Vibrations resulting from the mechanical scanning system in the confocal microscope and/or vibrations from external sources can both have a serious negative effect on image quality. For instance, both internal and external vibration can alter the position of the specimen relative to the focal plane of the objective lens and produce artificial contrast which does not convey accurately the 3D structure of the specimen. Vibration-induced variation of the relative positions of the pinholes can cause similar artifacts. Figure 11 shows the effects of mechanical vibration on a confocal image of a dirty first-surface mirror (imaged on a BioRad MRC500, epireflective mode). The image shows vibration contrast due to poor vibration isolation from the building. An actively-isolated optical bench can significantly improve the situation.

TRANSMITTED CONFOCAL IMAGE

The straight-forward approach to the design of a trans-illuminated, confocal microscope is to mount two confocal microscopes with one serving as the light source and the other as the detector. The two microscopes are positioned on a common optical axis with both objective lenses focussed on a common point in a specimen. Raster images are obtained by scanning the specimen with an X-Y mechanical stage. It is clear that such a design has some major drawbacks: 1) The stage scanning method is relatively slow and not suitable for most biological specimens because of the vibration involved. 2) In a beam-scanning system (single beam in a laser scanning system or multiple beams in a disk-scanning system), it is technically difficult to synchronize the scanning of both systems perfectly. 3) Because of differences in refractive index and optical path length within the specimen, a small translation of the specimen along the optical axis (z) can result in significant changes in the position of the focal points of the two opposed objectives, reducing confocality. Unfortunately, the sets of optical section images needed for 3D image processing can only be obtained by translation in z.

Recently, Art (1989 personal communication) demonstrated a simple trans-illuminated confocal design utilizing folded optics (Fig. 12a). The design uses a high N.A., infinity-focus second objective which is coaxial and confocal with the primary objective so that light transmitted through the specimen is captured by this second objective. A mirror normal to the optical axis and placed behind the second objective reflects the transmitted light back to the first objective via the same path. The confocal configuration is achieved as long as the second objective remains confocal with the primary objective.

The difficulty is to maintain the confocal configuration when a heterogeneous specimen is translated in the z direction between the two objectives. Based on the notion that focal point misalignment, caused by variations in reflective index and path length within the specimen, causes a rapid drop-off in image intensity, we have developed a computer-controlled, precision piezo-electric/mechanical system which allows precise posi-

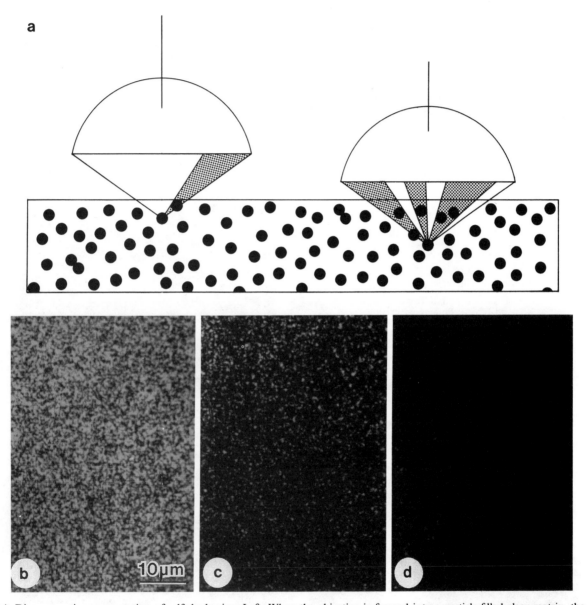

FIG. 9.   (a): Diagrammatic representation of self-shadowing. Left: When the objective is focused into a particle-filled clear matrix, the scattered and reflected rays from the structure of interest are modulated by the particles located between the objective and focal plane. Right: When the objective is focused deeper into the specimen, the detected signal strength deteriorates when more particles are encountered.
(b), (c) and (d): Reflective confocal image of a 30% carbon-filled polyethylene insulator. (b): Image obtained near the surface of the sample. (c) and (d): Image obtained approximately 20 and 30um from the surface respectively. (D. M. Shinozaki, P. C. Cheng and Haridoss).

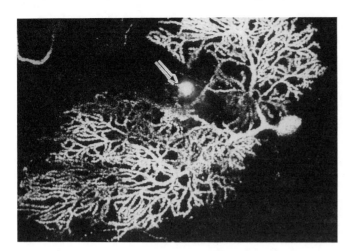

FIG. 10. Effects of lens reflection in reflective confocal mode.
a: Reflection from lens elements causes a bright spot in the center of the image (arrow).
b: Diagrammatic representation of our method for removing reflection from lens elements. A Glan-Taylor polarizing prism is placed in the illuminating laser beam and rotated to achieve maximum transmission intensity. A 1/4 wavelength retardation plate is placed just above the objective. A dichroic sheet polarizer is used as an analyzer and placed in front of the detector. The analyzer can be rotated to achieve maximum extinction of reflected light from the lens elements. PMT: photomultiplier tube.
c: By using a Glan-Taylor polarizer, a 1/4 wavelength retardation plate and an analyzer, the strong surface reflection from the lens elements was removed. (The Purkinje cell specimen is courtesy of Dr. R. Pentney, Dept. of Anatomical Sciences, SUNYAB).

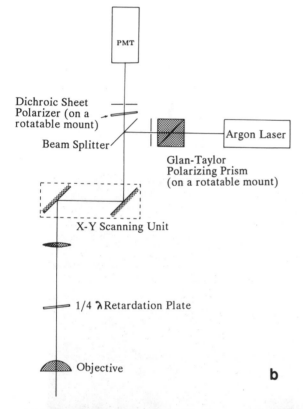

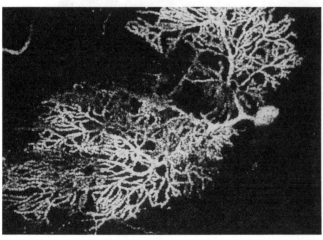

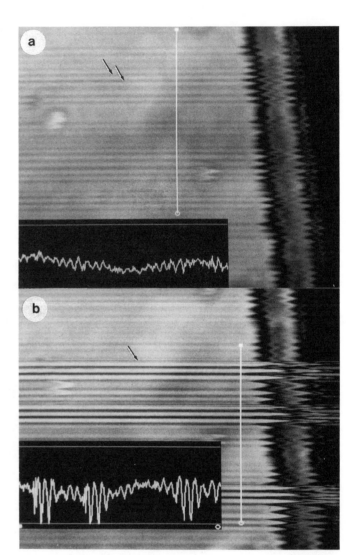

FIG. 11. The effect of mechanical vibration on a confocal image of a dirty mirror surface. a) Resonant vibration of the microscope system produces periodic line structures on the image as the mirror surface moves above and below the focus plane. Arrows mark one period of the most prominent frequency of the vibration (total picture height is 1 second). Insert shows the intensity plot along the vertical, white line. b) Effect of transient vibration on the image. Arrow shows the onset of the vibration as a result of the author walking near the microscope. Insert shows the intensity plot of the image along the white line: several resonant frequencies are indicated.

tioning of the second objective lens by monitoring the intensity changes of the captured image. (Fig. 12a)

Figure 12b shows two of a series of optical sections of a sea urchin embryo (*S. purpuratus*) obtained in the trans-illuminated, confocal mode using a laser scanning system. The set of images were obtained by re-aligning the folding optics after each focus change (4 μm). The image contrast present in these images is primarily the result of specimen absorption of the light summed over both passes but there is a small contribution of back-scattered light and interference effects between the two beams are also possible. The effect of the back-scattered light in the image can be easily removed by subtracting a pure back-scatter (reflected) image from the absorption image.

A wide variety of interference contrast mechanisms can be used with this basic optical system by adding the appropriate optical components into the back focal plane of one or both objectives or simply by using mirrors that only cover parts of the focal plane. As such images can in principle be collected in addition to, and independently of, any fluorescent signals (see Chapters 2 and 9) developments in this field should be watched with interest.

To optimize the optical conditions of both objectives, the specimen has to be sandwiched between two cover-slips instead of a microscope slide and cover glass. In addition, it is easier to operate using a microscope in which the stage focusses without affecting the position of either objective.

One of the bonus features of this trans-illuminated configuration is an improvement in the signal strength when the microscope operates in epi-fluorescent mode. The folded optical path provides double excitation and, in addition, fluorescent light captured by the lower objective lens is returned to the detector. The system provides an increase in fluorescent signal strength of 3 to 4×, (depending on the transmittance of the second objective). The configuration is particularly useful with the disk-scanning microscopes where fluorescent image intensity is relatively low compared to laser scanning systems.

CONFOCAL MICROSCOPY IN EPI-FLUORESCENT MODE

The use of confocal microscopy in the fluorescent mode has generated great excitement in the biological community. In fluo-

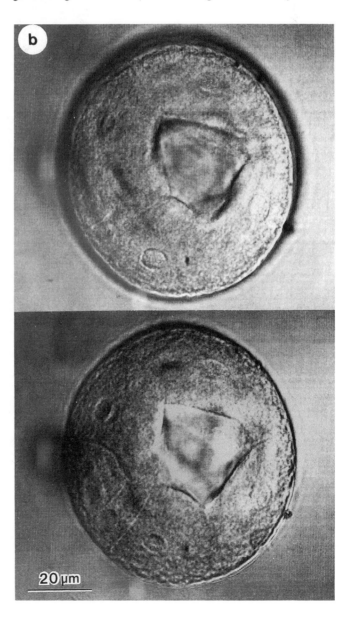

FIG. 12.   a: Diagrammatic representation of a laser scanning, folded-optics, trans-illuminated confocal light microscope. In the case of disk-scanning trans-illuminated confocal microscopes, the upper portion of the microscope (above the first objective lens) is replaced by a disk scanning system. b: A set of trans-illuminated confocal images of a sea urchin embryo (*S. purpuratus*). The optical sections were obtained at 4 μm apart. The specimen was fixed in 3:1 (ethanol/acetic acid), stained by the Feulgen method, dehydrated and cleared in methyl-salicylate.

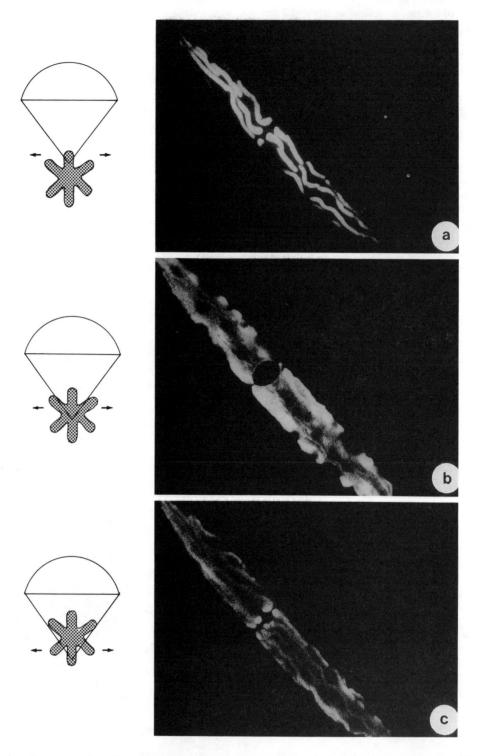

FIG. 13. Self-shadowing phenomenon in epifluorescent mode. The specimen attenuates both the excitation and the resulting fluorescent intensity. Therefore, detected fluorescent intensity is lower for structures located in the deeper part of the specimen. This phenomenon is particularly pronounced when the specimen is very densely stained or pigmented.

(a), (b) and (c): Epi-fluorescent confocal images of a living alga, *Closterium*. Three images were obtained under the same conditions. (a): Optical section showing chlorophyll autofluorescence near the top of the specimen. (b): From the middle of the specimen (~35μm from the top of the surface) and (c): From the bottom of the specimen (~70μm from the top of the surface). Note the reduction of the fluorescent signal (particularly in the center of the specimen where there is maximum shading).

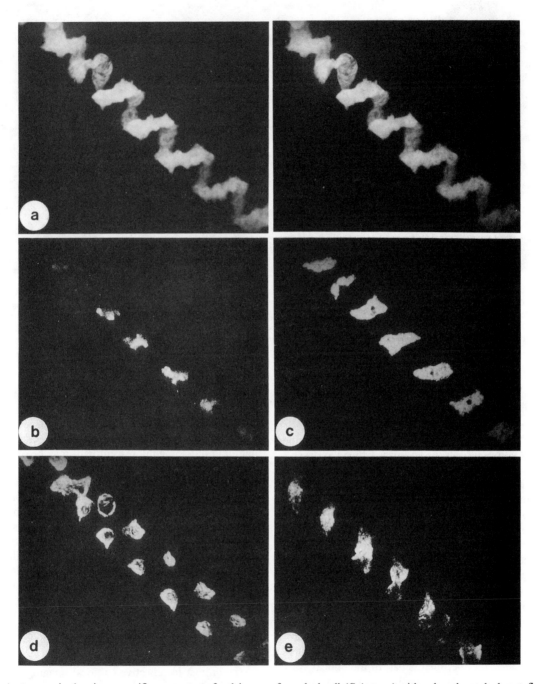

FIG. 14. (a): A stereo-pair showing an epifluorescent confocal image of an algal cell (*Spirogyra*) with a loosely packed, autofluorescent spiral chloroplast. (b): Epi-fluorescent confocal image obtained from the top surface of the autofluorescent algal chloroplast. (c) and (d): Optical sections at various depths (20μm and 40μm respectively). e: Fluorescent image obtained from the bottom of the algal cell (60μm). Due to loose packing of the chloroplast, the effects of self-shadowing are minimal.

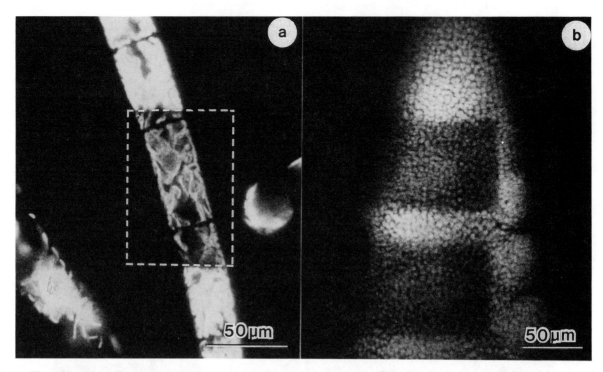

FIG. 15.   a: Photo-bleaching of chlorophyll autofluorescence in living *Zygnema* cells. The rectangular region of the specimen was scanned by the illuminating laser beam for 90 sec (by a BioRad MRC500), and then an image was taken at low zoom setting to show the resulting photo-bleaching. b: Young terminal inflorescence of maize (*Zea mays L.*). The two rectangular regions of the specimen were scanned by the illuminating laser beam for 120 sec each (by a BioRad MRC500, 20 optical sections were obtained) and then an image was taken to illustrate the effect of photo-bleaching on the fluorochrome. The specimen was fixed in 1:3 acetic acid-EtOH, stained with the Feulgen reaction, dehydrated in EtOH and cleared in methyl-salicylate.

rescent microscopy, the microscope images a light-emitting volume which has been excited by the excitation illumination. In conventional epi-fluorescent microscopy, the light-emitting volume imaged by the objective lens includes both in-focus and out-of-focus subvolumes, producing an image which has excessive glare and lack of contrast. Glare occurs in proportion to specimen thickness and staining density, thus limiting the effective use of conventional epifluorescence to thin specimens (e.g., tissue culture cells). In confocal contrast mode, the out-of-focus signals are removed nearly completely resulting in an image with exceptionally high contrast (Wijaendts van Resandt, 1984; White et al., 1987). Furthermore, advances in computer image processing have added an additional dimension to the confocal fluorescence studies in terms of signal to noise ratio (S/N) and contrast parameters.

A biological specimen can seldom be considered to be an ideal (optical) specimen. Generally, such specimens are heterogeneous in structure, absorption properties, refractive index and thickness. Because the specimen is part of the optical system, its heterogeneity creates serious problems in the performance of the microscope. Here, we consider the impact of such a heterogeneous specimen in quantitative fluorescent confocal imaging. In a situation similar to that in reflective confocal mode, reflection, refraction and scattering of the **illuminating beam** by structures situated between the focal plane and objective lens can reduce the intensity of **excitation radiation** reaching the structures of interest (the voxel being sampled). The loss of excitation intensity causes a decrease in the effective **fluorescent**

yield of the specimen. Furthermore, the **emitted** fluorescent signals can also be attenuated (by means of reflection, refraction, scattering and absorption) by the same structures on their return. The structure(s) which attenuated the incoming excitation light and out-going fluorescent light may be of little interest to the observer, or they might be the upper portion of the structure under study. This self-shadowing is another factor which can significantly reduce the image contrast by lowering the signal strength. It is particularly pronounced when observing densely packed specimens. For instance, Fig. 13 shows a confocal autofluorescent images of the chloroplast of *Closterium*. This algal cell contains two chloroplasts with fin-like laminar projections which shield the lower portion of the chloroplast from excitation light (Figs. 13b and 13c). Therefore, the images of the lower optical sections show a significant reduction in signal strength. In contrast, Fig. 14 shows a similar autofluorescent image of *Spirogyra*. The spiral arrangement of the chloroplast minimizes self-shadowing, hence, there is no significant drop in signal strength from the lower sections.

In contrast to reflective confocal imaging, the illumination (excitation) and imaging (emitting) wavelengths differ in fluorescent microscopy. Therefore, the structures within a specimen can selectively attenuate (in terms of wavelength) either the excitation radiation or fluorescent signal. For instance, in the autofluorescent imaging of the chloroplast of an algal cell, the chlorophyll within the chloroplast attenuates weakly in green (excitation) but strongly in red (fluorescent). Therefore, we believe that the loss of signal strength in the lower sections is mainly due to the self-shadowing.

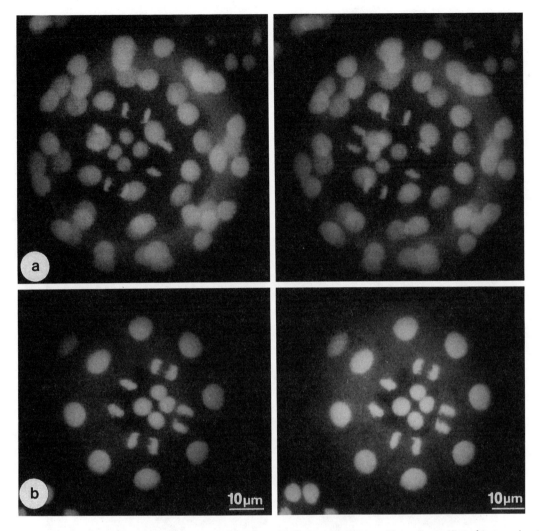

FIG. 16.   (a) and (b):   Three dimensional reconstruction of two Feulgen-stained sea urchin embryos (*Lytechinus variegatus*).

Countermeasures

An improvement in image contrast can be achieved by either increasing the signal strength from the structure of interest or by reducing the background signal. In other words, increasing the signal from a fluorescent specimen can be achieved by the delivery of higher intensity excitation radiation, the use of proper wavelength, the selection of dyes with higher fluorescent quantum efficiency, higher staining specificity and concentration as well as higher resistance to photo-bleaching. However, increased illumination intensity does have serious drawbacks. Not only might the higher intensity illumination cause photo damage to the structure of the specimen, but it will also cause unacceptable photo-bleaching of the fluorochrome. Photo bleaching is always a major problem in conventional fluorescent microscopy, and is particularly serious in confocal microscopy when high numbers of optical sections are required. The photo-bleaching phenomenon results in a gradual degradation in image contrast as the fluorescent signal diminishes during the process of image acquisition. Figure 15 shows a photo-bleached region of the chloroplast of the alga *Zygnema*, as the result of prolonged exposure to the scanning laser beam (approximately equivalent to the dosage of acquiring 100 optical sections from

this type of specimen in a BioRad MRC500 system). In this example, the image was the autofluorescent signal from the chlorophyll, hence there is no possibility of selecting a different fluorochrome. However, in fluorescent microscopy involving structures artificially tagged with fluorochromes, the selection of stable fluorescent dyes must be addressed. For instance, we have found that pararosaniline sulfate (product of the Feulgen reaction) shows better stability against photo bleaching than chromomycin A3 as the chromosomal stain in our experiment (Summers and Cheng, 1989). Figure 16 shows images of a sea urchin embryo (*Lytechinus variegatus*), fixed in Carnoy's, Feulgen-stained (Nislow and Morrill, 1988), dehydrated in ethanol and cleared in methyl salicylate.

There is a general misconception that the confocal microscope is capable of obtaining optical sections as deep into a tissue as the working distance of the objective permits. In fact, with the best objective, the image degrades even as it is focused into a transparent object particularly if a water immersion objective is not used. Objective lenses are designed to be operated under a very limited set of conditions (i.e., certain cover glass thickness and refractive indices of the immersion oil, etc.); deviation from the optimal design parameters, such as altering

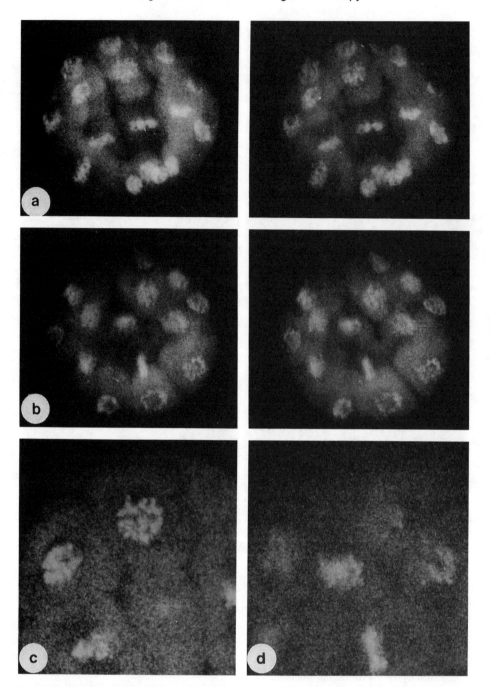

FIG. 17.   Two stereo-pairs showing the top half (a) and bottom half (b) of a sea urchin embryo (*Strongylocentrotus purpuratus*). Note the deterioration of image definition in the lower half. The specimen was Feulgen-stained, cleared in glycerol and scanned for 16 s on each of 15 sections using an MRC-500 operating at 514nm, full power with a Nikon 40× Fluor, 1.3NA lens. The *S. purpuratus* embryo (80 μm diam.) is less transparent than the species *Lytechinus variegatus* shown in Figure 14.
(c): An optical section obtained from the top of the embryo (10μm deep). (d): An optical section obtained from 70μm deep.

the required refractive index of the medium by focusing deep into a tissue, can dramatically degrade the performance of the objective, resulting in poor image definition and contrast. Figure 17 shows the degree of image degradation between optical sections obtained from the top and bottom of a sea urchin embryo. The top section is just beneath the cover glass and the bottom section is approximately 70 μm below the cover glass. Although the embryo had been cleared in glycerol and is very transparent, the loss of image definition is obvious in the lower section. (See also Chapter 7.)

Image contrast in confocal microscopy depends upon a number of variables presented in this article. The most important consideration is preparation of the specimen, which is dependent on an understanding of its physical properties in order to observe the detailed structures with appropriate contrast.

ACKNOWLEDGMENT

This work was supported by grants from the Biomedical Research Support Grant, National Institute of Health (BRSG

SO RR07066) and US Department of Energy (DE-AS08–88DP10782). We also gratefully acknowledge Dr. C. Musial for her suggestions.

REFERENCES

Barr, M. L. and J. A. Kiernan (1988): The human nervous system—An anatomical viewpoint. 5th ed. J. B. Lippincott Co., London. p. 17.

Boyde, A. (1985): The tandem scanning reflected light microscope. Part II. Pre-Micro'84 application at UCL. Proceeding of RMS, 20(3): 131–139.

Cheng, P. C., V. H-K. Chen, H. G. Kim and R. E. Pearson (1989): An epi-fluorescent spinning-disk confocal microscope. Proc. of 47th Annual meeting of EMSA.

Chen, V. K-H, and P. C. Cheng (1989): Real-time confocal imaging of *Stentor coeruleus* in epi-reflective mode by using a Tracor Northern Tandem scanning microscope. Proc. of 47th Annual meeting of EMSA.

Jones and Handreck (1967): Silica in soils, plants, and animals. Adv. Agron. 19, 107-149.

Nislow, C. and J. B. Morrill (1988): Regionalized cell division during sea urchin gastrulation contributes to archenteron formation and is correlated with the establishment of larval symmetry. Dev. Growth and Differ. 38:483–499.

Paddock, S. W. (1989): Tandem scanning reflected-light microscopy of cell-stratum adhesions and stress fibers in Swiss 3T3 cells. J. Cell. Sci. 93:143–46.

Scheibel, M. E. and A. B. Scheibel (1970): The rapid Golgi method. Indian summer or renaissance? Contemporary Research Methods in Neuroanatomy. eds. W. J. H. Nauta and S. O. E. Ebbeson, Springer-Verlag, New York, p. 1–11.

Summers, R. G. and P. C. Cheng (1989): Analysis of embryonic cell division patterns using laser scanning confocal microscopy. Proc. of 47th Annual meeting of EMSA.

Watson (1989):—Real-time confocal microscopy of high speed dental burr/tooth cutting interactions. Abstracts of the 1st International Conference on Confocal Microscopy and the 2nd International Conference on 3-D Image Processing in Microscopy. March 15-17, 1989. Amsterdam.

White, J. G., W. B. Amos and F. Fordham (1987): An evaluation of confocal vs. conventional imaging of biological structures by fluorescent light microscopy. J. Cell Biol., 105:41–48.

Wijaendts van Resandt, W., H. J. B. Marsman, R. Kaplan, J. Davoust, E. H. K. Stelzer and R. Stricker (1984): Optical fluorescence microscopy in three dimensions: microtomoscopy. J. Microscopy, 138: Pt. 1 April, 29–34.

Xiao, G. O., T. R. Corle and G. S. Kino (1988): Real-time confocal scanning microscope. Appl. Phys. Lett. 53(B): 716–718.

Chapter 18

Guiding Principles of Specimen Preservation for Confocal Fluorescence Microscopy

ROBERT BACALLAO#, MORGANE BOMSEL+, ERNST H.K. STELZER* AND JAN DE MEY+

#Division of Nephrology, UCLA Medical School, Los Angeles, Cal., *Light Microscopy Group, +and the Cell Biology Program, European Molecular Biology Laboratory (EMBL), Meyerhofstrasse 1, Heidelberg, FRG

INTRODUCTION

Traditionally, biologists have been confined to electron microscopy and light microscopy in order to correlate biochemical and molecular data with morphology. Electron microscopy provides fine ultrastructural detail, but tends to limit one to the study of cellular structures that react with electron-dense stains deposited in fixed specimens. Immunogold labeling allows one to study non electron-dense material, but the EM sections must be relatively thin, and even then there are problems with penetration of the labelled antibodies. Another problem is the necessity of making thin sections to prevent scattering of the electron beam. The electron microscopist is forced to live like a citizen of Flatland. Flatland is a story about beings that existed entirely within a plane, and were trying to figure out what the various two dimensional shapes appearing on their "world" were (Abbott, 1884). The shapes were sections of three dimensional objects passing through their plane of being. Similarly, biologists using an electron micrsoscope attempt to reconstruct the three dimensional structure of a cell based on the two dimensional cuts through the specimen. In practice, the better one's microtome, the more accurate the three dimensional reconstruction. In any event, reconstruction is a laborious process.

Traditional light microscopic methods, such as Nomarski optics and phase-contrast microscopy, tend to confine the data collected to events observable by transmitted light, such as *in vitro* studies involving cytoskeletal elements (Dabora and Sheetz, 1988; Ito, 1962; Inoué, 1986; Lee and Chen, 1988; Sheetz and Spudich, 1983). The use of vital dyes and fluorescent dyes has allowed the microscopist to make inquiries about the activities of the cell's interior both *in vitro* and *in vivo*. In addition, the development of immunofluorescence labeling has allowed researchers to correlate functional biochemical data with structural data. However, the light microscope has a lower limit of resolution than the electron microscope, and heretofore the reconstruction of three dimensional images has required sophisticated numerical deconvolutions requiring a large investment in computers.

In order to obtain high contrast images, the immunofluorescence staining protocols, (by intention or otherwise), have tended to flatten the specimens under study to reduce the effect of out-of-focus light on the final image. This tendency has pushed the biologist to study either thin cells, or cells grown in conditions that are not optimal for the expression of the cell's full phenotype.

Confocal fluorescence microscopy is an exciting advance which extends the utility of fluorescence labeling techniques. Its ability to exclude out-of-focus information from the image permits the acquisition of 3D intensity data sets which can be viewed as 3D images. The purpose of this chapter is to discuss methods for insuring that the specimens from which the data are acquired maintain the 3D structure they had *in vivo*.

We have studied MDCK cells grown on Costar™ polycarbonate membrane filter supports. The filter supports have the disadvantage that they are opaque, but they do allow the cells to be supplied with nutrients in a more physiological way. Under these growth conditions, the basal membrane has access to nutrients at all times, somewhat reproducing the growth conditions *in vivo*. MDCK cells form a more completely polarized monolayer when grown on the membrane filters. These studies have asked specific questions about cellular organization both *in vitro* and *in vivo* during the formation of an epithelial monolayer. This chapter reflects the lessons learned while attempting to study cells under growth conditions that are not generally amenable to study by immunofluorescence methods. Additionally, we will examine some of the issues involved in specimen preservation, and some of the criteria we have used to evaluate our preservation methodologies. While the methods were developed to answer a specific question in cell biology, we believe the practical lessons learned, and our approach to the problems, are more widely applicable.

CRITICAL EVALUATION OF FIXATION AND MOUNTING METHODS

Theoretical considerations

Immunofluorescence labeling methods have been widely employed in cell biology (Osborn, 1981). The major concerns when using these methods to study cell morphology have been to preserve the antigenic and structural integrity of the specimen. In general, the goal is to quickly immobilize the antigen, while preserving the cell's organization. All too frequently, the best preservation methods destroyed the epitopes required for antibody binding. This is a particular problem with glutaraldehyde fixation (Cande et al., 1977; Nakane, 1975, Weber et al., 1978). In an effort to solve this problem, formaldehyde has been used as a fixative, since this preserves antigenicity better. However, this fixative has been reported to cause morphological distortion, particularly in the preservation of microtubules in mitotic spindles (Sato et al., 1976).

The initial attempts to use the fixation and mounting methods previously described for use in epi-fluorescence microscopy, yielded images that were markedly deformed. It became apparent that these methods had been specifically designed to shrink the cells in order to reduce the out-of-focus contributions in images obtained by standard epi-fluorescence microscopy. As a result, it became necessary to meld some of the fixation methods developed for electron microscopy with the techniques employed for immunofluorescence microscopy. This meant that in addition to the requirements for structural and antigenic preservation, the spatial preservation had to be considered also. This additional concern has been a problem for workers using scanning electron microscopy or stereographic analysis of images taken by EM. Since no drying agents are used in preparing the samples for immunofluorescence microscopy, the major concern we had was shrinkage induced by fixation. This problem has been examined by several workers (Lee et al., 1979; Lee et al., 1980; Lee et al., 1982; Lee, 1984; Tooze, 1962; Wangensteen et al., 1981). It has been found that glutaraldehyde fixation induces cell shrinkage when hypertonic buffers are used. Additionally, Lee has shown that the total osmolarity of the fixative and the type of buffer used determine the extent of specimen shrinkage (Lee et al., 1982; Lee, 1984). Other fixation procedures can also affect the degree of cell shrinkage. For example, osmium tetroxide fixation causes a variable degree of volume shrinkage in erythrocytes. It has been suggested that the amount of shrinkage induced by this fixative depends upon the interplay between the electrostatic interactions between charged protein particles and osmotic forces (Tooze, 1964). A recent review and study on the effect of formaldehyde fixation on cell volume found that rat liver strips shrank in length only by 3% when fixed at room temperature. Raising the temperature to 37°C diminished the amount of shrinkage observed (Fox et al., 1985). It was also observed that increasing the concentration of formaldehyde caused increased shrinkage of rat kidney sections. Paradoxically, a 40% solution seemed to cause swelling of the sample. This paradoxical effect has not been satisfactorily explained. The shrinkage is due to the extremely high total osmolality of fixative solutions containing formaldehyde. It should be noted that a 3% solution of paraformaldehyde has a far higher osmolality than a 3% solution of glutaraldehyde (Fox et al., 1985). Taken together, the data suggests that the buffer conditions should be adjusted to bring the fixation conditions more toward isotonic conditions.

The overall approach to solve these problems was to start with fixation methods that still preserved the epitope binding sites for the antibody label. This obviously reflected a bias towards immunofluorescence studies. Once an acceptable fixation method was found in this regard, the fixation was optimized to preserve the three dimensional aspects of the specimen. The modifications were checked against the prior optimum staining protocol for preservation of antigenicity. Unfortunately, our experience has shown that there are no shortcuts through this feedback loop. In addition, some of the hard-won solutions for sample preparation problems tend to reflect the question one is studying. This means that a methodology cannot be freely transferred to another system under study. An example of this occurred when the paraformaldehyde/pH shift fixation protocol, (see below), was adopted to study microtubule/kinetochore interactions during mitosis in newt lung epithelial cells. While the microtubules were well preserved, it was found by DIC-video microscopy that the chromosomes continued to move during the low pH incubation step (A. Merdes, unpublished observation). This indicated that the cells were not immediately fixed and immobilized by the first step of the fixation and as a result, this method was not useful in these cells, for this particular study.

The Use of the Cell Height to Evaluate the Fixation Method

In order to generate three-dimensional images that accurately reflect the cellular architecture, it was necessary to employ fixation methods that minimize cell shrinkage or distortion of the cyto-architecture. To study this issue, we took advantage of the ability of the fluorescent lipid analog C6-NBD-ceramide to label the plasma membrane in vivo (Lipsky and Pagano, 1985). The plasma membrane of MDCK cells, grown to confluence on filter supports, was labeled as described by van Meer (van Meer et al., 1987). The height of the living cells was determined from randomly-selected vertical sections (Fig. 1). The samples were fixed and stained using probes which recognize either actin filaments, or microtubules. Actin staining and microtubule staining were used as markers for the cell height in the fixed cells since these networks lie close to the plasma membrane. Furthermore, the preservation of the cytoskeletal network is particularly sensitive to preservation methodology. The height of the fixed cells was examined from randomly selected sites. The mean height of the cells was determined and the two groups, (fixed vs in vivo cells), were analyzed by the Student's T test. Figure 1A and B show the plasma membrane labeling observed in cells labeled in vivo with C6-NBD-ceramide and by immunofluorescence labeling of another part of the same sample after glutaraldehyde fixation. Both samples were mounted with PBS. Notably the height and shape of both sam-

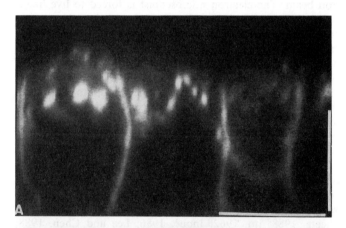

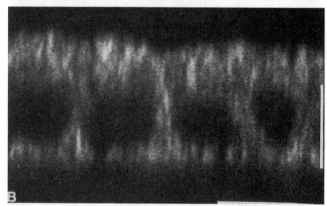

FIG. 1. Vertical optical sections of MDCK cells. MDCK cells were plated on polycarbonate filters and grown for 5 days in culture. The cells have formed a columnar epithelium of fairly uniform height. A) C6-NBD-ceramide labeling of the plasma membrane. Note the curved appearance of the apical plasma membrane. B) Microtubule staining in glutaraldehyde-fixed cells. Note that the cell height and apical membrane curvature are roughly comparable. Bar = 10 μm.

ples is quite similar. We observed that the apical dome was very sensitive to fixation artifacts. We found that glutaraldehyde fixation, with or without Triton X-100 in our buffer, preserved the cell height most accurately with very little shrinkage detected. Formaldehyde fixation, using a method adapted from Berod, caused less than 5% increase of the cell height (Berod et al, 1981). We consider this degree of distortion acceptable in some well-defined situations. Figure 2A and B shows stereo images of isolated cells fixed with methanol and the formaldehyde/pH shift method. The methanol caused a flattening of the area overlying the nucleus. In this case the methanol probably caused a 10 to 20 percent decrease in cell height. When methanol was used as a fixative or as a permeabilization agent on confluent cells, it caused a 20–50% decrease in cell height. We think it is inappropriate to use this agent in samples prepared for examination in a confocal fluorescence microscope.

The Use of Cell Height to Evaluate Mounting Media

The same strategy was employed to evaluate different mounting methods and mounting media. Gross distortion can be produced if the coverslip touches the specimen surface (Figure 4).

To avoid this we found that filter-grown cells were best mounted under a coverslip suspended by four posts made from clear nail polish. The average height of the posts was 40 μm and with a little practice the post height can be very reproducible. The best mounting media was found to be 50% glycerol and PBS. No cell shrinkage was detectable in fixed specimens compared to *in vivo* labeled cells with this mounting media. Mowoil and Gelvatol caused a 10% decrease in cell height in glutaraldehyde-fixed cells. This amount of shrinkage was considered to be significant because the apical domes, seen in polarized MDCK cells *in vivo*, were completely flattened by these mounting agents. The mounting media appeared to be a more critical parameter in formaldehyde fixed cells. This may be due to the low degree of cross-linking in formaldehyde fixed specimens.

Well-Defined Structures Can Be Used to Evaluate Fixation Methods

A second method used to evaluate fixation was to examine structures that have a well-defined morphology. Since we had an interest in the microtubule organization of epithelial cells, we examined the preservation of mitotic spindles in our sample preparations. Changes in the natural symmetry of the mitotic

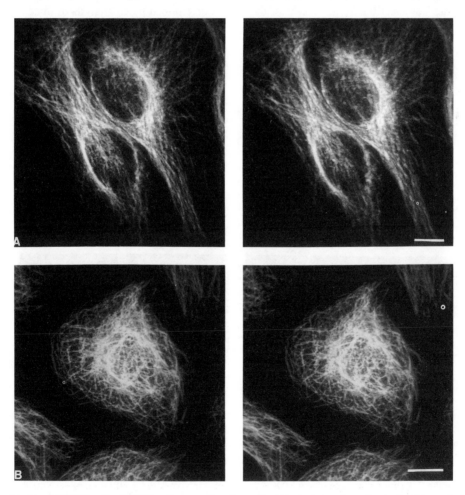

FIG. 2.   Stereo image of isolated MDCK cells. MDCK cells were plated at a low density, one day prior to fixation and staining. This image was reconstructed from a series of optical sections taken in the x-y plane from consecutive "z" positions, 0.4 μm apart. No other image processing was performed. The field is made up of 512 × 512 pixels. The image is the average of 4 scans per line. A) Microtubule staining in methanol-fixed cells. Note the flattening over the nuclear region. The distance from the top of the cell to the bottom is 4.1 μm. B) Microtubule staining in cells fixed with the formaldehyde/pH shift method. No flattening is noted and the microtubules are well preserved. The distance from the top of the cell to the bottom is 4.5 μm. Bar= 10 μm.

spindle, due to fixation or mounting artifacts, were easily detected. Breaks in the microtubules or shortening of the microtubules within the spindle could be seen readily and these changes were used to disqualify some fixation methods. In general, formaldehyde fixation yielded poorly preserved microtubules, however, the formaldehyde/pH shift fixation method described below gave acceptable microtubule preservation in the mitotic spindles.

This fixation method was compared directly with glutaraldehyde fixed cells. While the formaldehyde/pH shift method was not as good as glutaraldehyde fixation for the preservation of microtubules, it was an acceptable compromise. When the two fixation methods were compared sided by side, the staining in the formaldehyde/pH shift method was slightly lower in intensity than formaldehyde alone. However, we found it to be a useful method for double immunofluorescence labeling with antigenic epitopes that were destroyed by glutaraldehyde fixation. The periodate-lysine-formaldehyde fixation described by McLean did not preserve mitotic spindles well (McLean et al., 1974).

Comparison of *in vivo* Labeled Cell Organelles with Immunolabeled Cell Organelles

Some membrane structures can be distorted even though the fixation method used does not affect the overall height of the cell. Light microscopic observation of cell nuclei during fixation with formaldehyde, as described below, revealed marked changes in nuclear size and shape during the pH 6.5 step of the fixation. For this reason we do not use the formaldehyde/pH shift method to examine nuclear membrane antigens. We have not yet exhaustively tested this fixation method on this system. It is possible that adjustments in the tonicity of the buffers may solve the problem. The use of vital fluorescent dyes such as Rhodamine 123,3,3'-dihexyloxacarbo-cyanine (DiOC$_6$) and C6-NBD-ceramide can allow one to compare the effects of the fixation on the morphology of the mitochondria, RER and Golgi apparatus respectively (Lipsky and Pagano, 1985; Terasaki et al., 1984; Walsh et al., 1979). MDCK cells have striking changes in their Golgi apparatus morphology during the formation of a polarized epithelium (Bacallao et al., 1989). The morphology in the final polarized state was examined *in vivo* using the fluorescent lipid analog, C6-NBD-ceramide. The morphology seen *in vivo* was compared to samples that were fixed and stained using a Golgi specific monoclonal antibody generously supplied by Dr. M Bornens (Figure 3). Note that the Golgi morphology observed *in vivo* compares well with the morphology observed with a monoclonal antibody which recognizes a Golgi specific protein. The Golgi morphology observed was similar to the description of the Golgi apparatus in non-ciliated epithelial cells as determined by an analysis of thick sections at low magnifi-

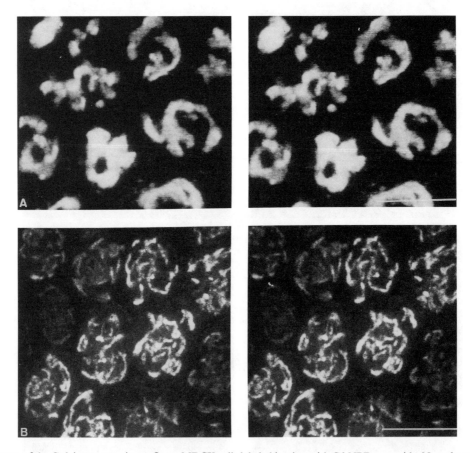

FIG. 3. A) Stereo images of the Golgi apparatus in confluent MDCK cells labeled in vivo with C6-NBD-ceramide. Note the convoluted morphology. This image was reconstructed from a series of optical sections taken in the x-y plane from consecutive "z" positions, 0.4 μm apart . No other image processing was performed. The distance from the top of the Golgi to the bottom is 6.4 μm. The field is made up of 512 × 512 pixels. The image is the average of 4 scans per line. B) Stereo images of the Golgi apparatus in confluent MDCK cells labeled by a monoclonal antibody. Cells were fixed by the formaldehyde/pH shift method described in this chapter. Note that the overall morphology is similar to the ceramide label morphology. The image was generated as described above. Bar= 10 μm.

cation (Rambourg et al., 1987). Both the glutaraldehyde fixation, and the ph shift/formaldehyde fixation protocol described below, preserved the morphology of the Golgi apparatus well.

FIXATION METHODS

The fixation methods described herein have been optimized for the confocal fluorescence microscope in studies in which MDCK cells have been grown on opaque filter supports (Bacallao and Steltzer, 1989). The cells grow to a height of 18 μm and form a dense monolayer under the growth conditions we used. These fixation and staining protocols have been tested using the criteria cited above to ensure the veracity of the data obtained.

A) Glutaraldehyde fixation

Stock solutions

- 8% glutaraldehyde E.M. grade (Polysciences)
- 80 mM K pipes, pH 6.8, 5 mM EGTA, 2 mM MgCl2, 0.1% Triton X-100
- Phosphate buffered saline without Ca_2+/Mg_2+ (PBS-)
- Phosphate buffered saline without Ca_2+/Mg_2+, pH 8.0

Preparation of stock solutions

E.M. grade glutaraldehyde was obtained from Polysciences. It is supplied as an 8% aqueous solution. When a new vial is opened, the glutaraldehyde is diluted to 0.3% in a solution of 80 mM Kpipes, pH 6.8, 5 mM EGTA, 2 mM $MgCl_2$, 0.1% Triton X-100. The aliquots are stored at $-20°$ C. Prior to each experiment, a fresh aliquot is used soon after thawing. These aliquots are never frozen again or reused, since this caused a loss of preservation efficacy. PBS, pH 8.0 is made by adding a few drops of 6N NaOH to normal PBS.

Fixation Protocol

1. Warm 100 ml of 80 mM Kpipes, pH 6.8, 5 mM EGTA, 2 mM $MgCl_2$ to 37° C in a beaker.
2. Pour off the media in the apical well of the Costar filter. Dip the entire filter plus filter holder in this modified 80 mM Kpipes buffer for 5 seconds.
3. Transfer the filter to the 6-well plate supplied with the polycarbonate filters to permit convenient fixation and washing steps.
4. Fix the cells for 10 min with 0.3% glutaraldehyde + 0.1% Triton X-100 at room temperature. The glutaraldehyde fixative is added to both the apical (2 ml) and basal (3 ml) portion of the filter. During all the incubation steps and washes, the 6-well plate is agitated on a rotary shaker.
5. During the fixation period, weigh out 3–10 mg aliquots of fresh $NaBH_4$ per filter. The $NaBH_4$ should be kept in an anhydrous state, preferably under dry nitrogen gas, since it is a very strong reducing agent. When combined with water, hydrogen gas is released. Explosions in the laboratory setting have been reported so this agent should be used with care. The $NaBH_4$ should be weighed out immediately prior to use.

The $NaBH_4$ is poured into 50 ml, sterilized, conical tubes with screw caps.

6. Aspirate the fixative, and dip the entire filter successively in 3,100 ml beakers containing phosphate buffered saline, without Calcium or Magnesium (PBS-).
7. Add PBS- pH 8.0 to the $NaBH_4$. (Final concentration 1 mg/ml). Add 3 ml to the apical portion of the cell, and 4 ml to the basal chamber. Incubate 15 minutes at room temperature. Repeat this step two more times using freshly dissolved $NaBH_4$. The adjustment of the pH to 8.0 increases the half life of $NaBH_4$ in the solution. This step is essential to decrease the autofluorescence of the glutaraldehyde fixed cells. You should see gas bubbles in the solution during this step.
8. Wash the cells with PBS- by dipping in 3 beakers containing PBS-. Return the filters to the 6 well plate with PBS- bathing the apical and basal side. The filter is now ready for immunofluorescence staining.

B) The pH shift/Formaldehyde fixation

Stock solutions

- 40% formaldehyde (Merck) in H_2O
- 80 mM Kpipes, pH 6.5, 5 mM EGTA, 2 mM $MgCl_2$
- 100 mM NaB_4O_7, pH 11.0
- Phosphate Buffered Saline w/o Ca_2+/Mg_2+ (PBS-) pH 8.0
- Phosphate Buffered Saline w/o Ca_2+/Mg_2+ (PBS-) with or without 0.1% Triton X-100

Preparation of the stock solutions

The preparation of the formaldehyde stock solution is based on the description by Robertson (Robertson et. al.; 1963). 40 g of formaldehyde is added to 100 ml of H_2O. While continuously stirring, the mixture is heated to greater than 70° C. A few drops of 6 N NaOH is added to dissolve the formaldehyde. The stock solution is divided into aliquots and stored at $-20°$ C. Prior to use, aliquots are thawed by warming in a water bath. Above 75° C, the formaldehyde will go into solution. The formaldehyde solution should not be allowed to boil, however. The formaldehyde is diluted to 2–4% in both the Kpipes and NaBorate buffers. For our purposes, a 3% solution of formaldehyde was adequate for preserving both the structure and antigenic determinants of a wide variety of cell organelles. The pH of the Kpipes buffer is brought to 6.5 with 1N HCl after the formaldehyde has been added.

PBS-, pH 8.0 is made by adding a few drops of 6 N NaOH to normal PBS, made without calcium or magnesium. 100 mM NaBorate is titrated to pH11.0 by adding 6N NaOH to the buffer.

Fixation Protocol

1. Pour off the media in the apical well of the filter.
2. Dip the filters in 80 mM Kpipes pH 6.8, 5 mM EGTA, 2 mM $MgCl_2$ pre-warmed to 37° C.
3. Add 3 ml of 3.0% formaldehyde in 80 mM Kpipes pH 6.5, 5 mMEGTA, 2 mM $MgCl_2$ to the basal chamber of the filter

in a 6 well dish, and add 2 ml of the fixative on the apical surface of the cells. Incubate the cells with agitation on a rotary table for 5 min at room temperature.

4. Aspirate the formaldehyde/Kpipes solution. Add 3 ml of 3% formaldehyde in 100 mM NaB_4O_7, pH 11.0 to the basal side and 2ml to the apical side of each filter. Incubate with agitation on a rotary table for 10 min. at room temperature.

5. Weigh out two 10 mg aliquots of $NaBH_4$ for each filter and store in a conical tube with a screw cap.

6. Aspirate the fixation solution. Wash the filters by successively dipping the filters in 3 beakers containing 100 ml of PBS-.

7. Dissolve each aliquot of $NaBH_4$ in 10 ml PBS-, pH 8.0 (Final concentration of $NaBH_4$ should be 1 mg/ml). Vortex the solution briefly, and add the solution to the apical (2ml) and basal (3 ml) portions of the filters. Incubate 15 min while shaking the filters on a rotary table. Repeat this step one more time using a fresh solution of $NaBH_4$/PBS-, pH8.0.

8. Wash the filters by successively dipping the filters in 3 beakers containing 100 ml of PBS-. The filters can be stored overnight at 4° C with PBS-/0.1% NaN_3.

9. The sample is permeabilized with PBS(-) + 0.1% Triton X-100. Wash the sample for 5 minutes.

C) Immunofluorescence staining

1. Cut the filter from it's plastic holder. Be sure to note which side of the filter has the cells layered on it! Cut the filter into four squares using a sharp scalpel, keeping the filter wetted with PBS while cutting. To ensure that the cell side of the filter can be readily identified, we routinely cut a slit in the right upper corner of the filter. The filter is cut into squares because this tends to give a flat field of cells after the filter has been mounted. Dividing a filter into wedges with one rounded edge causes the filter to ripple during mounting of the specimen and results in cells oriented vertically and horizontally in the same focal plane.

2. Wash the filter squares in PBS- containing 0.2% Fish skin gelatin (FSG), (Sigma Inc), and the appropriate percentage of detergent. Wash the filter squares in a 6 well plate. All washes are done in 4 ml of solution, at room temperature, with agitation. Unless otherwise stated, the filters are washed for 15 minutes after every change of washing buffer.

3. Place a 50 μl drop of the first antibody diluted in PBS- containing 0.2% FSG on a piece of parafilm on the bottom of a Petri dish.

4. Place a filter square, cell-side down, on the antibody solution. Place a piece of wet Whatman filter paper in the Petri dish, well away from the antibody solution. Cover the Petri dish, to form a small, humidified chamber.

5. Incubate at 37° C for 1 hour (for specimens that are less than 10 μm thick, 35 minutes is an adequate incubation time).

6. Wash the filter twice with PBS- containing 0.2% FSG. Follow this with 3 successive washes with PBS-.

7. Wash the filter once more with PBS- containing 0.2% FSG.

8. Add the second antibody as described for the first antibody.

9. Incubate at 37° C for 1 hour.

10. Wash the filters in PBS- containing 0.2% FSG twice.

11. Wash 3 times in PBS-.

12. Incubate once in PBS containing 0.1% Triton X-100 for 5 min.

13. Wash twice in PBS- for 5 min each time.

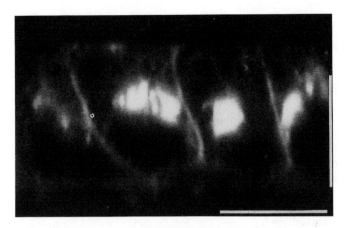

Fig. 4. Deformation of a sample due to improper mounting. A confluent monolayer of MDCK cells was labeled *in vivo* with C6-NBD-ceramide. The coverslip was placed on the acrylic spacing mounts incorrectly. The apical surface has been completely flattened. The basolateral membranes are no longer vertical probably due to shearing. Bar= 10 μm.

The filter squares are ready for mounting. In this protocol FSG is used as a carrier protein instead of albumin.

D) Mounting the specimen

Place 4 drops of clear acrylic nail polish on a microscope slide to make support mounts for a coverslip. Each drop should be at a point corresponding to the corner of a coverslip. We use 22 X 22 mm coverslips. The size of the coverslip used should be as small as possible, since the lens objective can mechanically deform the coverslip while focussing. This can distort an otherwise good sample. The acrylic, when dry, should be no thicker than 40 μm. Place the filter square in the center of the area demarcated by the nail polish. Take care to ensure that the cells are facing up. Put a drop of 50% glycerol/2× PBS/0.1% NaN_3/100 mg/ml DABCO (1,4-diazabicyclo [2.2.2] octane, Sigma Co.) on the filter. Carefully place the coverslip over the filter. Avoid trapping air bubbles in the specimen mount. Make sure that the corners lie on the drops of acrylic polish. Aspirate the excess glycerol/PBS/NaAzide/DABCO. Put 4 drops of nail polish on the 4 corners of the coverslip to stabilize the mount. Once the nail polish has dried, the entire mount can be sealed with nail polish. The specimen should be viewed within 24 hours since these are not permanent mounts. Semi-permanent samples can be made by post-fixing the filter in 4% formaldehyde dissolved in 100 mM NaCacodylate pH7.5 for 30 minutes at room temperature followed by quenching with 50 mMNH$_4$Cl in PBS for 15 minutes. Post-fixed samples have maintained excellent labeling characteristics for over 6 months when stored at 4° C or at −20° C. Figure 4 shows the unfortunate result of an improper mounting method. In this case the coverslip was not adequately supported by the acrylic nail polish because they were set too far apart. This shows how small attention to the details of the mounting procedure can determine the success or failure of specimen preservation.

GENERAL NOTES

The repeated use of borohydride in these fixation protocols was found to significantly decrease endogenous cellular fluorescence. Other quenching agents such as ammonium chloride and lysine were tried in an effort to diminish the endogenous fluorescence, but borohydride worked best. This was a crucial obstacle to overcome in our work because our specimens had high cell densities when the MDCK cells grew to confluence on membrane filter supports. High endogenous background fluorescence caused our initial images to be have poor contrast and we lost important details. These fixation methods work very well with cells grown on coverslips, but some shortening of the fixation time is necessary. Typically, a four minute incubation in the pH 6.5 buffer and an eight minute fixation in the pH 11.0 buffer worked well with glass-grown cells using the formaldehyde pH shift fixation described above. One caveat that should be noted is the tendency of formaldehyde to induce vesiculation of cell membranes. Fortunately, this artifact is not observed in all tissues fixed with formaldehyde.

Both saponin and Triton X-100 have been used as permeabilization agents in the formaldehyde fixation method. Triton X-100 has been most effective when used after the fixation is completed, while saponin worked best when included with the borate buffer. NP40 worked very well for specimens in which the microtubules were stained with monoclonal antibodies to alpha and beta tubulin.

We have used DABCO, (1,4-diazabicyclo [2.2.2] octane, Sigma Co.) at a concentration of 100 mg/ml as an anti-bleaching agent (Langanger et al., 1983) Yellowing of the specimen occurs one month after mounting when DABCO is included with the mounting media. We have not noted a significant change in the images produced from sample mounts that have yellowed. A recent paper suggested that NaN_3 is a better anti-bleaching agent than DABCO (Bock et al., 1985), however, in our experience, we found that DABCO prevented bleaching of our samples better then NaN_3 (A. Merdes, manuscript in preparation). N-propyl-gallate has been tried as an anti-bleaching agent but in our hands it caused a dimming of the fluorescent signal. p-Phenylenediamine has not been used as an anti-bleaching agent because this agent destroys the sample over time (Langanger et al., 1983). These comments are the result of our preliminary observations; an exhaustive study of anti-bleaching agents has not been performed.

Labeling Samples With Two Or More Probes

One of the unique aspects of three dimensional imaging is that it gives one the power to determine spatial relationships. However, this is an inherent weakness also. For example, in our early work using C6-NBD-ceramide to study the Golgi morphology, we found ourselves dissatisfied with the images. One frequently wanted to know where the Golgi apparatus was located in reference to other cellular structures (see Figure 3). Our early attempts to label other structures simultaneously led to unforeseen difficulties. The first major pitfall was the finding that FITC and rhodamine could not be used in combination with the filter sets available at EMBL. Although the cut-off filters were supposed to eliminate signals above 530 nm, we were unable to cleanly separate the FITC image from the rhodamine image. This was due in part to the wavelengths available for excitation with our argon-ion laser. The confocal microscope at EMBL has an argon-ion laser with lines at 528.7 and 476.5 mm. When the 528.7 line is used, FITC is excited and the cut off filters could not completely eliminate the FITC signal. At

the lower wavelength, we experienced problems with fluorescence energy transfer because the light emitted from the FITC was exciting the rhodamine. This problem was partially overcome by combining FITC with Texas Red fluorescent dyes for double-labeling experiments. The two wavelengths were used to excite the different fluorophores, but at 528.7 nm, a higher cut off filter (580 nm) was used to block out the FITC signal. There were no detectable problems with fluorescence energy transfer with this combination. However this combination presented another difficulty. Although the laser we use has lines available at 528.7 and 476.5 nm, the power at these wavelengths varies markedly. Switching between the two excitation wavelengths yields images with are not matched in intensity. To overcome this problem, the gain is adjusted to "normalize" the images. This is done so the image intensities match when the data sets are mapped together using our image processing software. Future designs of the EMBL confocal microscope will automatically compensate for differences in power output at different lines. Another useful combination was Lucifer Yellow and Texas Red, which has been used to study the endocytic compartments in filter-grown MDCK cells *in vivo*.

Some consideration must be given as to what structures will be labeled prior to the experiment. In our experience, and perhaps because of the higher quantum efficiency of the detector or the lower diffraction limit, FITC appears to give images with better contrast than does Texas Red, so structures with fine detail, (such as microtubules), tend to yield a better image when stained with FITC. In samples which have been labeled with both FITC and Texas Red, the FITC image must be obtained first, followed by the Texas Red image, because FITC bleaches rapidly even with anti-bleaching agents present. Some microscopes now permit the simultaneous acquisition of images produced by these fluorophores.

One promising method for triple labeling involves the use of the new immunogold, silver-enhancement labeling techniques (Bastholm et al., 1986; Birrell and Hedberg, 1987; Danscher et al., 1987; Holgate et al., 1983; Lackie et al., 1985; Scopie and Larsson, 1985). This labeling method has been used successfully to stain cell adhesion plaques. Potentially, one could add a third label to double-labeled fluorescent samples using immunogold conjugated antibodies and imaging in the reflection mode. Image processing techniques should allow one to overlay the successive images. Once again, the cellular structures one wants to study should be matched with the particular labeling method employed to reveal the structural details. In our initial attempts to study mitotic spindles using immunogold labels, the gold acted as a mirror preventing us from obtaining an image below the upper half of the spindle. Another difficulty was the tendency of unlabeled thick samples, (greater than 12 μm in thickness), to give poorly resolved images in the optical sections far from the surface. Overall, the method will probably work best with sparsely-located antigens in specimens with a thickness of less than 12 μm.

Ramifications Of Techniques To Preserve The Specimens

In our experience, glutaraldehyde fixation best preserved the structural and spatial integrity of the cell. The main difficulty with glutaraldehyde fixation is the frequent loss of epitope antigenicity. Given this constraint, formaldehyde fixation may be an acceptable compromise but we would recommend a different approach. We recommend that monoclonal antibodies be screened with glutaraldehyde-fixed samples. Frequently, the clones are screened with samples fixed with methanol or formaldehyde. Monoclonal antibodies used for detailed structural studies on a confocal microscope should be tested in glutaraldehyde-fixed samples.

CONCLUSION

The spatial organization of organisms is rapidly becoming a major subject for analysis in molecular cell biology. For example, the temporal sequence of morphogenetic changes readily observable in embryos, would make an excellent system to test the effect of gene deletions, protein over-production and changes in transcriptional control in the development of an organism. The ability of the confocal microscope to render accurate, three dimensional images using classical immunofluorescence techniques means that it will be a major tool in the analysis of morphogenesis. Structural morphology obtained by various preservation methods should, (where possible), be compared to the morphology observed in vivo. In some cases, a compromise will have to be made with respect to fixation methods in order to preserve the antigenicity of a particular protein. These compromises should only be made if the *in vivo* data suggests that the compromise does not affect the accuracy of one's data. Only vigorous attention to these details, and in particular, constant comparison between living and prepared specimens, can ensure that an accurate analysis of the three dimensional structure of the cell is achieved.

ACKNOWLEDGEMENTS

The authors would like to thank Clemens Storz, Reinhard Pick, and Reinner Stricker for their superb technical assistance. R. Bacallao is a recipient of a Physician Scientist Award, NIH grant DK01777–02.

REFERENCES

Abbott, E. (1884) Flatland: A Romance of Many Dimensions, 2nd ed,. Dover, London.

Bacallao, R., Dotti, C., Antony, C., Stelzer, E.H.K., Karsenti, E and K. Simons, (1989) Subcellular organization of MDCK cells during the formation of a polarized epithelium, J. Cell Biol. (109, 2817–32).

Bacallao, R., Jesaitis, L., Karsenti, E and J. De Mey, (1990) The Effects of Fixation On Shrinkage-Induced Artifacts. Submitted, J. Histochem & Cytochem.

Bacallao, R., Steltzer, E. H. K., (1989) Preservation of BIOLOGICAL Specimens for Observation in a Confocal Fluorescence Microscope, Operational Principles of Confocal Fluorescence Microscopy Methods in Cell Biology, Vol. 31, 437–452

Bastholm, L., Scopsi, L., and Nielsen, M.H. (1986) Silver-enhanced immunogold staining of semithin and ultrathin cryosections, J. Electron Microsc. Technique, 4, 175–6.

Berod, A., Hartman, B.K. and Pujol, J.F. (1981) Importance of fixation in immunohistochemistry, J. of Histochem and Cytochem. 29: 844–50.

Birrell, G.B. and K.K., Hedbert (1987) Immunogold labeling with small gold particles: Siver enhancement provides increased detectability at low magnifications, J. Electron Microsc. Technique, 5, 219–20.

Bock, G., Hilchenbach, M., Schauenstein, K., and G. Wick (1985) Photometric analysis of anti-fading reagents for immunofluorescence with laser and conventional illumination sources, J. Histochem. Cytochem., 33, 699–705.

Bomsel, M., Prydz, K., Parton, R.G., Gruenberg, J., and K. Simons, Functional and topological organization of apical and basolateral endocytic pathways in MDCK cells, manuscript submitted.

Cande, W.Z., Lazarides, E., and J.R. McIntosh (1977) Composition and distribution of actin and tubulin in mammalian mitotic spindle as seen by indirect immunofluorescence, J. Cell. Biol., 72, 552–567.

Dabora, S.L. and M.P. Sheetz (1988) The microtubule-dependent formation of tubulovesicular network with characteristics of the endoplasmic-reticulum from cultured cell extracts, Cell, 54, 27–35.

Danscher, G., Rytter Nørgaard, J.O., and E. Baatrup (1987) Autometallography-tissue metals demonstrated by a silver enhancement kit, Histochemistry, 71, 1–16.

Fox, C.H., Johnson, F.B., Whiting, J., and P.P. Roller (1985) Formaldehyde fixation, J. Histochem. Cytochem., 33, 845–53.

Holgate, C.S., Jackson, P., Cowen, P.N., and C.C. Bird (1983) Immunogold-silver staining: New method of immunostaining with enhanced sensitivity, J. Histochem. Cytochem., 31, 938–44.

Inoué, S., (1986) Video Microscopy, New York and London: Plenum Press

Ito, S., (1962) Light and electron microscopic study of membranous cytoplasmic organelles, In *The Interpretation of Ultrastructure*, R.J.C. Harris, ed. New York: Academic Press, pp. 129–148.

Lackie, P.M., Hennessy, R.J., Hacker, G.W., and J.M. Polak (1985) Investigation of immunogold-silver staining by electron microscopy, Histochemistry, 83, 545–50.

Langanger, G., De Mey, J., and H. Adam (1983) 1,4-Diazobizyklo-[2.2.2]oktan (DABCO) verzogest das Ausbleichen von immunofluoreszenzpraparaten, Mikroskopie, 40, 237–41.

Lee, C., and L.B. Chen (1988) Dynamic behavor of endoplasmic-reticulum in living cells, Cell, 54, 37–46.

Lee, R.M.K. (1984) A critical appraisal of the effects of fixation, dehydration and embedding on cell volume, in *The Science of Biological Specimen Presevation for Microscopy and Microanalysis.*, ed Revel, J-P., Barnard, T., Haggis, G.H., and S.A. Bhatt, SEM Inc., AMF O'Hare, Chicago, Ill.,61–70.

Lee, R.M.K., Garfield, R.E., Forrest, J.B., and E.E. Daniel (1979) The effects of fixation, dehydration and critical point drying on the size of cultured smooth-muscle cells, Scanning Electron Microsc. 179, III, 439–448.

Lee, R.M.K., Garfield, R.E., Forrest, J.B., and E.E. Daniel (1980) Dimensional changes of cultured smooth muscle cells due to preparatory processes for transmission electron-microscopy, J. Microsc., 120, 85–91.

Lee, R.M.K., McKenzie, R., Kobayashi, K., Garfield, R.E, Forrest, J.B., and E.E. Daniel (1982) Effects of glutaraldehyde fixative osmolalities on smooth-muscle cell-volume and osmotic reactivity of the cells after fixation, J. Microsc., 125, 77–88.

Lipsky, N. and Pagano, R.E. (1985) A vital stain for the Golgi apparatus, J. Cell Biol. 100: 27–34.

McLean, I.W. and P.K. Nakane (1974) Periodate-lysine-formaldehyde fixative-a new fixative for immunoelectron microscopy, J. Histochem.Cytochem. 22, 1077–1083.

Merdes, A., and J. De Mey, manuscript in preparation.

Nakane, P. (1975) Recent progress in peroxidase-labeled antibody method, Ann. N.Y. Acad. Sci., 254, 203–210.

Osborn, M. (1981) in Techniques in Cellular Physiology part 1, ed. P.F.Baker, Elsevier North Holland Inc., New York, N.Y., 107/1–28.

Paddock, S.W., Tandem scanning reflected light microscopy of cell substratum adhesions and stress fibers in Swiss 3T3 cells, J. Cell Science, 93: 143–146.

Rambourg, A., Clermont, Y., Hermo, L., and D. Segretain (1987) Tridimensional structure of the Golgi apparatus of non-ciliated epithelial cells of the ductuli efferentes in rat—an electron microscope stereoscopic study, Biology of the Cell, 60, 103–116.

Robertson, J.D., Bodenheimer, T.S., and D.E. Stage (1963) Ultrastructure of Mauthner cell synapses and nodes in goldfish brains, J. Cell Biol., 19, 159–199.

Sato, H., Ohnuki, Y., and K. Fujiwara (1976) Immunoflourescent antitubulin staining of spindle microtubules and critique for the technique, in *Cell Motility*. R. Goldman, T. Pollard, and J. Rosenbaum, editors. Cold Spring Harbor Laboratory, Cold Spring Harbor, N.Y., 419–33.

Scopsi, L., and L.-I. Larsson (1985) Increased sensitivity in immunocytochemistry-effects of double amplification of antibodies and of silver intensification on immunogold and peroxidase-antiperoxidase staining techniques, Histochemistry, 82, 321–29.

Sheetz, M.P. and Spudich, J.A. (1983) Movement of myosin-coated fluorescent beads on actin cables in vitro, Nature, 303, 31–35.

Terasaki, M., Song, J., Wong, J.R., Weiss, M.J., and L.B. Chen (1984) Localization of endoplasmic-reticulum in living and glutaraldehyde-fixed cells with fluorescent dyes, Cell, 38, 101–108.

Tooze, J. (1964) Measurements of some cellular changes during fixation of amphibian erythrocytes with osmium tetroxide solutions, J. Cell Biol., 22, 551–63.

van Meer, G., Stelzer, E.H.K., Wijnaendts van Resandt, R.W., Simons, K. (1987) Sorting of glycolipids in epithelial (Madin-Darby canine kidney) cells, J. Cell Biol., 105: 1623–35.

Walsh, M.L., Jen, J., and L.B. Chen (1979) Transport of serum components into structures similar to mitochondria, Cold Spring Harbor Conf. Cell Prolif., 6, 513–20.

Wangesteen, D., Bachofen, H., and E.R. Weibel, (1981) Effects of glutaraldehyde or osmium tetroxide fixation on the osmotic properties of lung cells, J. Microsc., 124, 189–96.

Weber, K., Rathke, P.C., and M. Osborn (1978) Cytoplasmic microtubular images in glutaraldehyde-fixed tissue culture cells by electron microscopy and by immunofluorescence microscopy, Proc. Natl. Acad. Sci. USA., 75, 1820–24.

Chapter 19

A Comparison of Various Optical Sectioning Methods: The Scanning Slit Confocal Microscope

CHARLES J. KOESTER, PH.D.

Columbia University, College of Physicians & Surgeons, Department of Ophthalmology, 635 West 165th Street, New York, New York 10032

INTRODUCTION

The term "Confocal Microscopy" has been applied primarily to instruments using circular field stops, e.g. single pinholes or arrays of pinholes in the illumination and imaging systems. Other aperture shapes can of course be utilized, and the slit is an attractive alternative. In a number of circumstances the slit aperture confocal system can have advantages over circular aperture systems.

When Marvin Minsky (1961) described the confocal microscope for the first time one of his principal goals was to produce a system for "rejecting all scattered light except that emanating from the central focal point, i.e., the illuminated point of the specimen." This important principle defines one major method for achieving optical sectioning. However, in general usage, the term "optical sectioning" enjoys a somewhat broader definition. In this broader sense optical sectioning refers to the formation of an image that has minimal disturbance from light scattered, refracted, reflected, or generated by fluorescence at planes other than the focal plane. In this definition there may be scattered or reflected light from out-of-focus planes as long as it does not adversely affect the in-focus image.

The second part of this paper is a comparison of confocal systems employing pinholes with those employing slits. Before undertaking this detailed comparison it is useful to review some of the alternative methods for achieving optical sections.

NON-CONFOCAL OPTICAL SECTIONING

It has been found that differential interference contrast (DIC) microscopy developed by Nomarski (1955) yields images that are sharp over a remarkably shallow depth. [Inoué 1986 and Chapter 1, Fig. 6]. The reason is that in DIC the image contrast is generated by interference of light waves forming the image. A small departure from the focused plane leads to rapid departures from the precise phase relationships that produce the interference contrast. Therefore, the out-of-focus image has little or no information content, i.e. is nearly uniform in intensity. Video techniques (and certain photographic techniques) allow a uniform background to be subtracted from the image, thereby restoring the contrast in the in-focus image.

Tomography has been used by Agard and Sedat (1983 and Chapter 13) and by Fay, et al. (1985 and Chapter 14) to reconstruct optical sections with shallow depth of field as well as good lateral resolution. This allows the reconstruction of three-dimensional images of fluorescent components, by utilizing information present in light contributions from nearby planes.

Fourier analysis of images can also be used to produce a form of optical sectioning. When multiple images are obtained at several focal planes Agard and Sedat (1983 and Chapters 13 and 14) and Gruenbaum et al. (1984) showed that the Fourier components from out-of-focus details of adjacent images are nearly the same. On the other hand, the Fourier components from the in-focus plane change rapidly from one image to the next. Hence, the former can be subtracted out of the image, while the Fourier components that define the in-focus image are retained. These methods are discussed and examples are shown by Inoué (1986, pp. 375, 376, 418).

In ophthalmology a form of optical sectioning has been in use for many years: the slit lamp biomicroscope (Fig. 1). The name derives from the use of an illuminated slit that is re-imaged at the surface of the cornea or at a position within the eye. The bundle of rays forming the image can be reduced in width in the direction perpendicular to the slit length, thereby producing essentially a sheet of light extending into the eye. Light scattered from this thin illuminated section is examined from the side by means of a low power microscope. The angle between the illuminating beam and the microscope can be varied to suit the task, from examining the cornea and the lens, to the vitreous or the retina. This versatile device has recently been adapted to project the narrow slit beam to the retina at the maximum angle permitted by the pupil of the eye. The beam is photographed as it traverses the half-millimeter thickness of the retina [Zeimer, 1989]. The photograph is then analyzed to

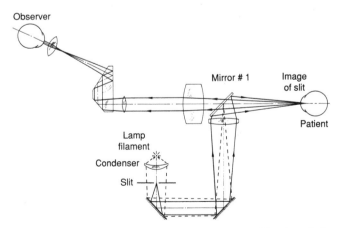

FIG. 1. Optics of the slit lamp (biomicroscope). The illuminated slit is imaged at the patient's eye, forming a thin sheet of illumination at the cornea. The viewing microscope can be rotated about an axis that passes through the focus of the slit beam. The microscope remains in focus at the patient's eye (from Campbell et al 1974).

provide a measurement of retinal thickness, an important parameter in the early detection of diseases such as glaucoma and macular edema.

When the slit lamp is used for the cornea and lens and the thin illuminated layer is examined at an angle, as described above, only one section can be in focus at any one time. Therefore, it is necessary to move the microscope to examine the various regions in detail. This is not a major difficulty for clinical exams, because of the smooth motions provided for positioning the microscope and the relatively low magnification. But for quantitative analysis of scattering within the lens (the early sign of cataract formation), an optical system devised by Scheimpflug [see Kingslake, (1983) p. 58] is used. By tilting both the imaging lens and the image plane (photographic film or video camera face) at the proper angles relative to the illuminated object plane, it is possible to have the entire image plane in focus simultaneously. This becomes a form of optical sectioning in which the focal plane is inclined rather than perpendicular to the axis of the microscope.

CONFOCAL OPTICAL SECTIONING

A confocal system for examination of the retina has been developed by Webb, et al. (1987). (See Fig. 2) A laser beam (visible or infrared) is passed through the first pinhole, then scanned raster fashion across the retinal surface by means of rotating and oscillating mirrors and appropriate lenses. The light returning from the retina passes through the system in reverse and is incident on a pinhole at the image plane, to be received by a detector. By using a sensitive detector it is possible to reduce the average power incident on the retina to a fraction of that required in a conventional ophthalmoscope and to use an undilated pupil. The optical sectioning provided by the confocal pinholes eliminates scattered light from the ocular media, an important advantage in cases of incipient cataract or corneal cloudiness.

For studies of the cornea *in vitro,* David Maurice (1974) developed a slit-scanning transmission microscope in which the image of a stationary illuminated slit was projected onto the specimen by the condenser (Fig. 3). A confocal slit in the image plane passed the light from the illuminated strip. The specimen was moved slowly in a direction perpendicular to the slit, and photographic film was moved synchronously behind the second slit.

Excellent optical sectioning was achieved by this technique, and well resolved cells could be seen in the stroma as well as in the endothelial and epithelial cell layers of the cornea (Gallagher and Maurice, 1977). However, the full image was not available in real-time, and therefore could not be utilized for focusing the microscope.

A slit system with a rapid scan was designed and patented by Baer (1970). He described several schemes for synchronously moving two slits in the plane of the illumination field stop and the image plane respectively. One scheme utilized a spinning disc with pairs of diametrically opposite slits for the illumination and imaging systems. Another employed a mechanically resonant structure that caused the two slits to oscillate in directions perpendicular to their long axes, in synchrony.

Baer even proposed the use of stationary slits, with chromatic dispersing prisms between the slits and the specimen. The il-

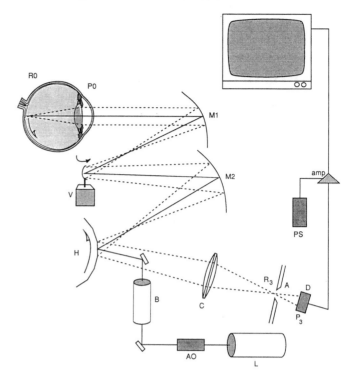

FIG. 2. Schematic drawing of the scanning laser ophthalmoscope. R_0 and P_0 are the Retina and Pupil of the eye—the object plane and entrance pupil. R_3 and P_3 are optically conjugate planes where the confocal aperture (A) and the detector (D) are situated. The aperture is actually an indexed wheel containing several sizes of "pinhole" and their opaque inverses. The SLO uses a confocal stop as much as 10 times the size of the illuminating spot at the retina, for control of scattered light rather than for optical sectioning. The inverse stop allows imaging in *only* scattered light—a dark field effect. The vertical scanner, V, is a galvanometer-mounted mirror scanning at 60 Hz in a sawtooth pattern. The horizontal scanner is a 25 facet polygon rotating at 37800 rpm, for standard TV rate imaging. AO is an acousto-optic modulator for impressing text or pictures on the illumination raster—which the patient sees, since it is focused on her retina. B is a beam expander, L the laser—*any* laser will work. Between H and collector lens C is a small turning mirror (actually a 1.5 mm ellipse) which separates the incident and return beams and blocks reflected light from the cornea. This beam separator is unique to the scanning laser ophthalmoscope, separating the pupil into coaxial 1.5 mm input and 7 mm output pupils (after Webb et al, 1987).

lumination system would form an image of the slit at different wavelengths across the specimen. Each chromatic slit image would be passed by the confocal slit in the imaging system, but light scattered in other planes would be lost at the second slit. The light passing through the second slit is viewed through a third dispersing prism to give an image consisting of a spectrum with image details superimposed. I am not aware of any publication in which Baer's systems were employed, but the patent stands as a useful contribution of ideas in this field.

Systems involving slit illumination combined with a split objective aperture were developed in response to the need to examine the endothelial cell layer of the cornea. Because of the very low reflectance of these cells, approximately 0.02%, and the presence of reflective and scattering material both anterior and posterior to this cell layer, it was necessary to separate the illumination and imaging light paths.

Maurice (1968) accomplished this by bringing the illumination through one half of the objective aperture, leaving the

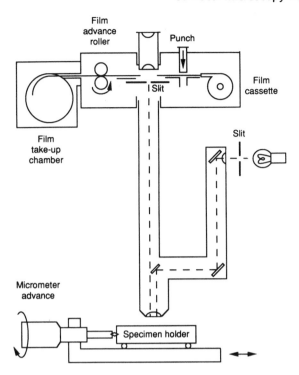

FIG. 3. The Maurice scanning slit microscope. The scanning action was provided by synchronous motors driving the specimen holder and the film advance rollers. The microscope could be focused on the specimen by viewing through a hole punched in the photographic film. This feature was also useful for adjusting the width of the slit in the camera to correspond to that in the illumination system (Maurice, 1974).

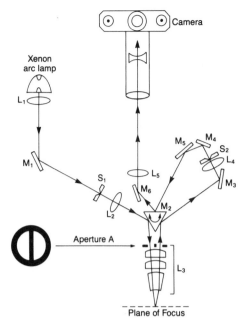

FIG. 4. Schematic diagram of the scanning mirror/slit microscope. The light source is a xenon arc lamp with a built-in parabolic reflector. The arc image is focused at slit S1 by lens L1. Lens L2 adjusts the optical tube length, and together with the objective L3 images slit S1 on the focal plane. As mirror M2 rotates in an oscillatory fashion the image of S1 is scanned across the focal plane. See text for explanation of remainder of the optical system. The aperture A is placed at or near the second focal plane of the objective. It serves as the aperture stop for the objective, but the central divider also blocks rays from passing through the central portion of the aperture plane.

other half available for the imaging rays. It was also necessary to image an illuminated slit at the object plane, which limited the field to a width of 100 to 150μm.

Scanning Mirror/Slit Microscope

The scanning mirror/slit microscope (5) utilizes a divided aperture and slit illumination, as illustrated in Figure 4. But in this case the illuminated slit image is scanned across the focal plane by the oscillating mirror M2. The light reflected or scattered by the object is focused by the other half of objective L3 to an image at the plane of the second slit S2. Reflected light from the image of the illuminated slit is passed by slit S2. Light scattered or reflected from other planes is blocked by the jaws of the slit. Because the imaging rays are reflected from the second facet of the oscillating mirror M2, the image of the illuminated slit is stationary at S2.

The function of the remaining optics is to form an enlarged image of slit S2 and to scan that image across the film plane, thereby laying down the final image strip by strip. The mirror M2 is mounted on a torsion rod that is resonant at 1000 Hz and is driven magnetically by a feedback circuit. Because of the rapid scan rate the image appears to be continuous.

It should be emphasized that the slits S1 and S2 may be wider than the resolution limit, since image detail is preserved within the width of the slit. That is, when a finite width of the object plane is illuminated and re-imaged at S2, two-dimen-

sional image detail is preserved, and is transferred to the image plane. As the mirror scans, adjacent strips of image are laid down in succession on the image plane, in a continuous manner. Therefore, the widths of slits S1 and S2 are parameters that can be optimized for optical sectioning or for image illuminance; they do not limit image quality. In ophthalmological applications a typical width of slit S2 is 1.5mm.

Optical sectioning is accomplished by a combination of two effects. The first is the spread of the illumination beam as the slit image goes out of focus below or above the focal plane. As in the pinhole confocal system this effect operates in both the illumination and the imaging systems.

Second, the aperture A contains a central opaque divider, the function of which is to block all illumination and imaging rays that have less than a predetermined angle with respect to the axis of the objective lens. To accomplish this, the aperture stop and the opaque divider must be at or close to the second focal plane of the objective. Selection of the optimum width for this divider is discussed below. The opaque divider has an additional benefit in that it eliminates those incident rays that could otherwise reflect from the centers of the glass elements in the objective and produce unwanted stray light in the image.

Figure 2 shows details of the light paths in the region of the focal plane. Illumination rays are contained within the lines marked by single arrowheads, pointing down. Imaging rays lie within the lines with double arrowheads, pointing upwards. The outermost ray in each case is at an angle Θx corresponding to the NA of the objective. The innermost ray is at an angle Θ_n that is determined by the width of the opaque divider. The intersection of the illumination and imaging bundles is indicated by the crosshatched area. Only in this region can light from the illumination beam be scattered or reflected directly into the imaging bundle.

As the image of slit S1 scans across the focal plane, the diamond-shaped region generates a layer of thickness 2h, the optical section. Its thickness can be calculated from the geometry of Figure 5:

$$2h = w/\tan \Theta_n$$

where w is the width of the slit image at the focal plane.

Since the widths of slits S1 and S2 can be adjusted, the thickness of the optical section is under the control of the investigator. The slit width also controls the image luminance. It is useful to employ wide slits for an initial search to locate the area of interest. A thin optical section is inconvenient for this searching. When the desired area is located the slit widths can be optimized for best optical section thickness vs. image luminance. Image luminance is also determined by the width of the scanned image. If desired, the scan width can be reduced, to give a smaller but brighter image.

The width of the central divider affects the optical sectioning characteristics, the image luminance, and the resolution of the objective, particularly in the direction perpendicular to the divider. The trade-offs are discussed by Koester (1980). For an objective aperture stop 5mm in diameter, a central divider width of 1 to 1.5mm is optimum.

If there is reflecting or scattering material outside of the optical section, the only way for it to contribute stray light to the image is by multiple scattering. That is, after initial scattering outside the optical section, the light must then be scattered again at some point within the bundle of imaging rays, and in a direction that lies within that bundle.

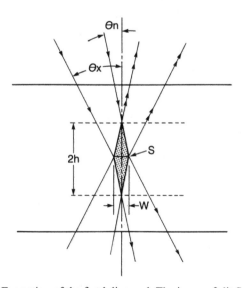

FIG. 5. Formation of the focal diamond. The image of slit S1 is at S, in the plane of focus. The width of the slit image is w. Angle θn is the minimum angle of rays in the illumination and imaging bundles, measured relative to the optical axis. Angle θx is the maximum angle of rays, determined by the NA of the objective. The overlap of illumination and imaging bundles is indicated by crosshatching. 2h is the total thickness of the optical section.

OPTICAL SECTIONING: EXPERIMENTAL AND THEORETICAL

In this section experimentally determined optical sectioning characteristics are compared with theoretical calculations based on geometrical optics, first for the slit and then for the pinhole confocal systems. The purpose is to determine the extent to which the theoretical calculations predict the experimental results. For experimental purposes the slit widths and pinhole sizes used are large enough to give reliable light level measurements. We then utilize the computer programs to compare the slit and pinhole systems using smaller aperture sizes, comparable to those that are useful in biological research.

Scanning Mirror/Slit System

Figure 6 illustrates the experimental arrangement for measuring optical sectioning characteristics of the scanning mirror/slit system. The aluminzed mirror is mounted perpendicular to the axis of the objective and moved axially by the adjustable slide. The detector is located in the center of the field and mea-

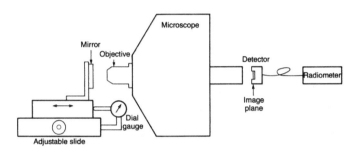

FIG. 6. Schematic diagram of the experimental setup for measuring optical sectioning characteristics of the slit system. The detector was a 1cm square silicon detector.

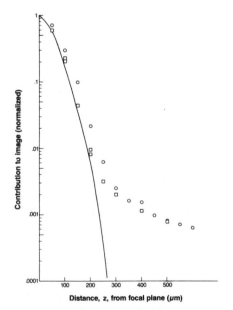

FIG. 7. The contribution of stray light to the image from an out-of-focus plane, in the slit confocal system with divided aperture. Objective: 20×, NA 0.4. Central divider width: 1.5mm, which gave a minimum angle of Θn = 4.8 degrees. Slit width 1mm, optical section half-thickness, h = 300µm. Curve: calculated stray light contribution. Circles represent measured values when the mirror was between the focal plane and the objective. Squares represent data obtained with the mirror beyond the focal plane.

sures the image illuminance. Measurements were taken at intervals of 50μm, in both directions from best focus.

Experimental results obtained with an Olympus 20×, NA0.4 objective are shown as open circles and squares in Figure 7. Circles represent measurements taken with the mirror between the focal point and the objective, squares represent data obtained with the mirror beyond the focal point. Care was taken to avoid backlash by moving in the same direction to make each setting.

At a given distance from the focal plane the readings that were obtained closer to the objective (circles) are consistently higher than those obtained farther from the objective (squares). There are at least two possible explanations. First, the central divider is not located precisely at the second focal plane of the objective. When the central divider is outside the second focal point, the optical section has a greater thickness in the direction toward the objective. Second, the paths of the outermost rays through the objective are quite different for the two cases. Some stray light is generated when the outermost rays strike the edges of lenses and/or the walls of the lens mounts and then scatter back into the image forming bundle. This contribution to stray light could conceivably be larger when the mirror is to the right of the focal point (Figure 6).

The solid line in Figure 7 represents the calculated contribution to the image due to a reflector at various distances from the focal plane. Calculations were carried out as follows. First the distribution of incident light at the plane of the mirror was calculated. A typical illuminance distribution is illustrated as the solid curve in Figure 8. At each point across this distribution the fraction accepted by the objective and the second slit was calculated. The dotted line indicates the product of the illuminance and the fraction accepted by the imaging optics. The contribution to the image is proportional to the area under the dotted curve.

Returning to Figure 7, the calculated contribution to the image is seen to fall rapidly toward zero at a distance h from the focal plane, in this case 300μm. The experimental points always lie above the theoretical curve, indicating that there is stray light reaching the image from sources other than the out-of-focus mirror. The relative amount increases as the distance z is increased. In the region beyond about 250μm the experimental data follow a very different curve than the theoretical line, indicating that the dominant source of stray light is not the out-of-focus reflector. This is easily verified by visual inspection of the back aperture of the objective, which exhibits scattered light coming from several sources: the edge of the objective aperture, dust particles, and a dim blue glow that is presumed to be due to interreflections between coated lens surfaces. Some of these sources of stray light could be reduced, but the value is already low in this objective compared to others that are not designed for incident light applications.

Confocal Pinhole System

Figure 9 illustrates the experimental arrangement for measuring optical sectioning characteristics of the confocal pinhole system. The same 20×, NA0.4 Olympus objective was used. The beamsplitter was slightly tilted so that reflected light from the outside prism surface did not reach the detector. Pinhole 2 was made conjugate to pinhole 1 by first setting its distance from the beamsplitter equal to that of pinhole 1, then adjusting

its lateral position to coincide with the image of pinhole 1 as reflected by the mirror and imaged by the objective.

Figure 10 shows experimental data and theoretical curves for the confocal 200μm diameter pinhole system. As in Figure 7, the circles are for the mirror located between the focal point and the objective; the squares are for the mirror located beyond the focal point. For a given distance, z, there is a greater contribution when the mirror is located closer to the objective (circles). Possible explanations are the same as those given above for the case of the slit system.

Two theoretical curves are given in Figure 10 for the pinhole confocal system. The upper theoretical curve is for a diffusely reflective out-of-focus plane. In this case, where the full aperture is used for illumination and imaging, there is a difference in the calculations for diffuse and specular reflecting surfaces. Details of the calculation are to be published elsewhere (Koester and Khanna, 1989).

The experimental data obtained with the mirror surface fall above the theoretical curve for the mirror, as in the case of the slit confocal system in Figure 7. This indicates the presence of stray light from sources other than the out-of-focus mirror.

The theoretical curves exhibit the general shape calculated by Wilson and Sheppard (1984). At large distances they approach the inverse square law as predicted by these authors.

Theoretical Comparison of Slit and Pinhole Systems

In Figure 11 theoretical curves are shown for pinhole and slit systems in which the dimensions are appropriate for the study of biological systems: 50μm diameter pinholes and 50μm

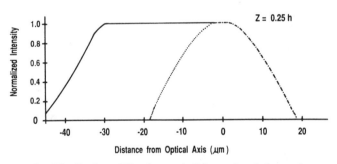

FIG. 8. Distribution of illuminance (solid curve) and the portion accepted by the imaging system (dotted curve) for an out-of-focus surface in the slit system. The illuminance is not symmetrical in this case because of the half circle shape of the illumination aperture.

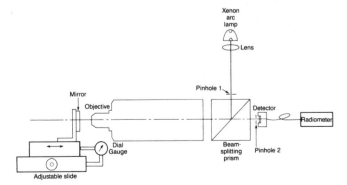

FIG. 9. Schematic of the setup for optical sectioning measurements with the pinhole system. In this case the detector accepted all the light passed by the second pinhole.

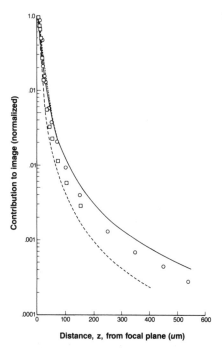

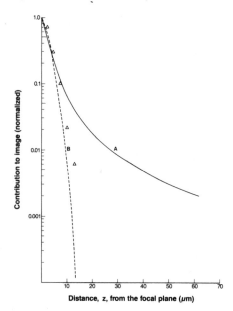

FIG. 10. Optical sectioning characteristic of the pinhole confocal system. Same objective as in Figure 3. Pinhole diameter: 200μm. The solid curve represents calculations for a diffusely reflecting surface, while the dashed curve represents calculations for a specular reflector. Circles and squares are experimental points obtained with a mirror surface, as in Figure 6. Note that at large distances from the focal plane the curve closely follows the inverse square law, represented by the dotted line.

FIG. 11. Comparison of the slit and pinhole systems for (slit width) = (pinhole diameter) = 50μm. The diffuse reflection calculation was used for the pinhole system. For the slit system with divided aperture the theoretical contribution falls to zero at 15μm, whereas the contribution of the pinhole system is 0.03 at the same distance. Points represented by triangles were obtained by scaling the experimental points represented by circles in Figure 7.

wide slits. With the 20× objective, these correspond to a 2.5 μm diameter pinhole image and a 2.5 μm wide slit image at the focal plane. At small distances from the focal plane the pinhole curve is slightly lower, indicating slightly better optical sectioning. Beyond about 4μm the curves separate and the theoretical optical sectioning of the divided aperture slit system is clearly superior.

Experimental data have not been obtained with these field stop dimensions, but if we *assume* that experimental data would fall above the theoretical curve in the same ratio as in Figure 7, then we obtain the points shown as triangles. These pseudo experimental points indicate that the divided aperture slit system has substantial advantages over the pinhole system at distances beyond about 7μm. Obviously it will be desirable to obtain actual experimental data for comparable slit width and pinhole diameters. To the extent that it is possible, this should be done with commercially available systems rather than with laboratory mockups.

Another advantage of the slit system is that the light throughput will be many times that of the pinhole system. For a slit 50μm wide, 18mm long, the ratio is approximately 18/.05 = 360. (This comment is pertinent for incandescent and arc sources, but has less relevance when a laser source is used with the pinhole system.)

Is this a fair comparison of the two systems? One could argue that tandem scanning systems (Petráň et al. 1968) have many pinholes in the field at any one time, thereby increasing the light throughput. For the slit system we could increase light throughout by increasing the number of slits in the field, or by increasing the width of the original slit.

Other considerations are also important. The resolution limit in the slit system is reduced by a factor of about 2.5 in

the direction perpendicular to the central divider, because the objective aperture is reduced by this factor, as seen in Figure 4. On the other hand, the image in the slit system, like that from the disk-scanning confocal microscopes, can be received directly by high resolution imaging devices such as photographic film or the eye, so that there is little or no further loss in resolution. The image in the slit system is not modulated by the presence of scan lines such as are common in the original images obtained from pinhole systems.

A POSSIBLE IMPROVEMENT IN PINHOLE CONFOCAL SYSTEMS

The optical sectioning capability of the slit system is due in large part to the separation of the illumination and imaging beams, as illustrated in Figures 4 and 5. The central divider, located at aperture A in Figure 4, serves to block illumination rays that are close to the axis. These rays can contribute strongly to stray light in the image because of reflections from lens or coverglass surfaces. Also, the greatest luminance in an out-of-focus image of a slit (or pinhole) is normally on the axis, therefore this region contributes most strongly to stray light in the image.

Pinhole confocal systems can also benefit from such a central aperture stop. In this case it should be an opaque circular stop located on axis, at the second focal plane of the objective. As in the slit system, this central stop serves to block rays that are close to the axis and thereby eliminate their contribution to stray light in the image.

While this benefit can be significant, it does not provide the theoretical absolute cutoff to the optical section that is achieved with the divided aperture system (Figures 4, 5 and 7). The explanation is facilitated by referring to Figure 2. With a slight modification in the interpretation of this diagram, the ray paths

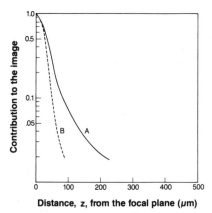

FIG. 12. Comparison of pinhole confocal system with an unmodified objective (A) and with the addition of a central obstruction (B). These are experimental data, obtained with a modified Nikon objective, 13×, NA 0.22. A mirror was used as the object. At a value of 0.03 on the vertical scale, the abscissa of curve A is 166μm, whereas curve B is at 74μm, indicating an improvement in optical sectioning by a factor greater than two.

can be seen to correspond to those for the pinhole confocal system with an opaque central stop. The modification is that rays are now travelling *both* directions within the bounds indicated by single arrows or double arrows. The diagram now represents a cross-section through a three-dimensional structure that has radial symmetry about the axis. The rays that have been blocked by the opaque central stop are those with an angle less than Θ_n.

The major difference between this system and the divided aperture system can now be seen. In the region bounded by the single arrowheads, for example, both illumination and imaging rays are present. Therefore scattered or fluorescent light that is generated *anywhere* in this region can contribute light to the image. This comment applies to the entire hollow cone of illumination rays. Thus the region of overlap is not confined to the focal diamond (the cross-hatched area in Figure 2), and therefore the contribution does not fall off to zero at a particular distance from the focal plane. That advantage can only be achieved when the illumination and imaging beams are separated everywhere except in the immediate region of the focal plane as would happen in a confocal system only if the illuminating and imaging rays passed through separate halves of the unmasked annulus at the entrance pupil of the objective lens. Such a system would have certain advantages. For example, if the object has horizontal specular reflecting planes at several different levels such as an integrated circuit chip, then specular reflections from planes that are sufficiently out of focus will be eliminated. Only if a reflecting plane crosses the focal diamond will it contribute light to the image.

This principle was tested briefly with a simple 13× NA.22 objective, using a central stop about 1.5 X 1.5mm square. Results are shown in Figure 12. The central stop reduced the optical section thickness substantially: greater than a factor of 2 at a stray light level of 0.02.

Such a central stop would not be without its effect on the image. Central obstructions in telescope and reflection objectives are known to produce an altered Airy disc pattern from a point source: a slightly narrower central disc but a greater fraction of light in the rings (Kingslake 1983, pp. 259-261). The effect on imaging is to aid slightly the resolution of simple structures that are near the resolution limit, but to adversely affect images with intermediate spatial frequencies.

A POSSIBLE IMPROVEMENT IN THE SLIT SCANNING SYSTEM

To overcome the reduction in resolution imposed by the divided aperture in the slit system, it is possible to utilize both sides of the objective aperture for both illumination and imaging. The central divider would have an effect on resolution similar to that described above for the case of the pinhole system, except that the effect would not be circularly symmetric. But the resolution limit would be set by the *full* aperture of the objective in both meridians, rather than by a 40% aperture in one meridian.

The disadvantage of this approach is that it does not separate the illumination and imaging bundles as they pass through the objective. Reflection and back scattering from lens surfaces can be much more damaging than when the paths are separated. This comment applies equally to the pinhole systems that typically employ full aperture for both illumination and imaging.

EXAMPLES OF IMAGES OBTAINED WITH THE DIVIDED APERTURE SCANNING SLIT SYSTEM

Figure 13 illustrates the image obtained with the slit scanning system in an ophthalmological application: examination of the single cell layer on the interior surface of the cornea. Normal cells are hexagonal in shape and uniform in size. In this case the cells are larger than normal, variable in size, and many are abnormal in shape, indicating that the intra-ocular lens and/or the surgery caused some damage to this cell layer.

Another application of the scanning slit system is a study of the response of cells in the inner ear to various acoustic frequencies. The optical sectioning property permits the hair cells and pillar cells within the cochlea to be visualized through the intact round window membrane. (See Figure 14). As described by Khanna et al. (1989), a laser beam is then projected through the same objective lens, focused on the structure of interest, and the returning beam is analyzed utilizing a heterodyne interferometer, in order to deduce the amplitude and phase of the vibration.

SUMMARY COMPARISON OF SLIT AND PINHOLE CONFOCAL SYSTEMS

From the above discussion it is apparent that an absolute comparison of slit scanning and pinhole confocal systems is difficult, in part because evolutionary improvements may be made in each. Nevertheless it may be useful to list those advantages that are inherent in each system, together with the advantages of each when the systems are compared as they exist today. Perhaps these can serve as a guide to selecting the best system for a given application.

Slit system

Inherent advantages

- Freedom from scan lines in the image.
- Ability to change optical section thickness during an experiment.
- Predictable resolution based on optical considerations, i.e. no electronic signal and/or image processing required.

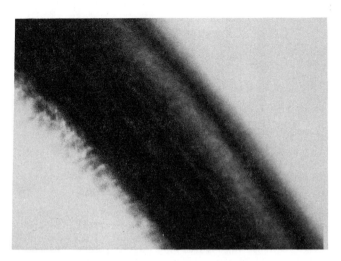

FIG. 13.   Corneal endothelial cells in a patient with an early model intraocular lens. The slit scanning system was used to obtain this photomicrograph *in vivo*, with an exposure time of 1/60 sec to minimize the effect of eye movements. The bar indicates 100μm.

FIG. 14.   The organ of Corti and adjacent structures in the inner ear of a cat, photographed through the intact round window membrane, *in vivo*. Rows of hair cells are seen on either side of a central band, which represents pillar cells, slightly out of focus.

Practical advantages of divided aperture system as described

- Better optical sectioning, in that, when using the divided aperture system, the stray light contribution due to an out-of-focus plane goes to zero, in principle, at a predictable distance.
- Separation of illumination and imaging light beams within the objective and in the anterior region of the specimen.
- Relatively simple optical system requiring only one scanner and no beamsplitters. (A beamsplitter would be required if the full aperture modification were implemented.)

Single pinhole confocal systems

Inherent advantages

- Easy application of lasers as point sources.
- Possibility of enhanced resolution when pinhole diameters can be reduced below the size of the Airy disc.
- For systems in which image processing is to be performed, the electronic signal is immediately available (no necessity for scanning a photograph, for example).
- Theoretical resolution limited only by the objective numerical aperture, in all meridians.

REFERENCES

Agard D and JW Sedat (1983) Three dimensional architecture of a polytene nucleus. Nature 302:676–681

Agard DA (1984) Optical sectioning microscopy: Cellular architecture in three dimensions. Annu. Rev. Biophys. Bioeng. 13:191–219

Baer S (1970) Focal plane specific microscopy. U.S. Patent No. 3,547,512

Campbell, CJ, Koester, CJ, Rittler, MC and Tackaberry, RB, 1974. *Physiological Optics,* Harper & Row, Hagerstown, Md., page 179

Fay FS, KE Fogarty, and JM Coggins (1985) Analysis of molecular distribution in single cells using a digital imaging microscope. In:

Optical Methods in Cell Physiology (P. DeWeer and B.M. Salzberg, eds.) Wiley, New York

Gallagher B and D Maurice (1977) Striations of light scattering in the corneal stroma. J. Ultrastructure Res. 61:100–114

Gruenbaum Y, M Hochstrasser, D Mathog, H Saumweber, DA Agard, JW Sedat (1984) Spatial organization of the Drosophila nucleus: A three-dimensional cytogenic study. J. Cell Sci. Suppl. 1:223–234

Inoué S (1986) Video Microscopy, Plenum Press, New York. p. 410

Khanna SM, CJ Koester, SM van Netten (1989) Integration of the Optical Sectioning Microscope and Heterodyne Interferometer for Vibration Measurement. Acta Otolaryngologica Supplement 1989, in press.

Kingslake R (1983) Optical System Design. Academic Press, London pp. 260–261

Koester CJ (1980) A scanning mirror microscope with optical sectioning characteristics: Applications in ophthalmology. Appl. Optics 19:1749–1757

Koester CJ and Khanna SM (1989) Optical sectioning characteristics of confocal microscopes. Optical Society of America, Technical Digest, October, 1989

Maurice DM (1968) Cellular membrane activity in the corneal endothelium of the intact eye. Experientia 15:1094–1095

Maurice DM (1974) A scanning slit microscope. Invest. Ophthalmol. 13:1033–1037

Minsky M (1961) Microscopy apparatus. U.S. Patent No. 3,013,467

Nomarski G (1955) Microinterféromètre différentiel à ondes polarisées. J. Phys. Radium 16:S9-S13

Petráň M, M Hadravský, MD Egger, and R Galambos (1968) Tandem scanning reflected light microscope. J. Opt. Soc. Am. 58:661–664

Webb RH, GW Hughes, FC Delori (1987) Confocal laser scanning ophthalmoscope. Appl. Optics 26:1492–1499

Wilson T and C Sheppard (1984) Theory and Practice of Scanning Optical Microscopy. Academic Press, London. p. 72

Zeimer RC, MT Mori, and M Shahidi (1989) New noninvasive method to measure changes in the nerve fiber layer thickness: Methodology and reproducibility in normal subjects. Invest. Ophthalmol. Vis. Sci. Suppl. 30:175

The author has a proprietary interest in the scanning mirror/slit system. A model for ophthalmic applications is manufactured by Alcon Surgical, Inc., Irvine, California.

Work supported in part by NIH program project grant 2P01-NS22334–04.

Bibliography on Confocal Microscopy

Robert Webb

Eye Research Institute of Retina Foundation, 20 Staniford Street, Boston, MA 02114

This is a bibliography, as of Fall 1989, of accessible papers on confocal microscopy. Not included are conference reports and other documents not likely to be available in most technical libraries. Summaries are given where possible, often a shortening of the author's own abstract. Some are more complete for historical or instructive value, others are absent when titles are adequately descriptive, or when an earlier paper covers the same material. Patents are listed at the end.

1. Amos W.B., White J.G. and Fordham M., *Use of confocal imaging in the study of biological structures.* Appl.Opt. **26,** 3239–3243 (1987).

A good general review, and a description of the MRC (Biorad) microscope.

2. Ash E.A., Ed., *Scanned Image Microscopy,* Academic Press, 1980.

The Proceedings of a conference on scanning optical, scanning acoustic, thermal, photoacoustic and X-ray microscopes which contains a number of useful early papers on scanning optical microscopes and the principles of related scanning microscopes:

2a. Brakenhoff G.J., Binnerts J.S. and Woldringh C.L., *Developments in High Resolution Confocal Scanning Light Microscopy* (CSLM).

Early experiments on the scanning optical microscope with standard and annular lenses, showing good images of live and fixed E. coli bacteria.

2b. Kino G.S., *Fundamentals of Scanning Systems.*

Develops simple criteria for two point resolution of scanning microscopes and compares the results to those for standard microscopes and synthetic aperture imaging systems.

2c. Sheppard C.J.R., *Imaging Modes of Scanning Optical Microscope.*

A review of the theory developed elsewhere by Wilson and Sheppard.

2d. Welford W.T., *Theory and Principles of Optical Scanning Microscopes.*

A review of the basics of scanning optical microscopy, and comparison of CRT, laser and thermal sources.

3. Åslund N., Liljeborg A., Forsgren P.O., and Wahlsten S., *Three-dimensional digital microscopy using the PHOIBOS scanner.* Scanning **9,** 227–235 (1987).

Consecutive optical sections obtained by confocal scanning are used to generate a basis for digital three-dimensional microscopy. Some representative results are presented. The method can also be used to study surface topologies either in fluorescent or reflected light.

4. Baak, J.P.A., F.B.J.M. Thunnissen, C.B.M. Oudejans, and N.W. Schipper. *Potential clinical uses of laser scan microscopy.* Appl.Opt. **26** 3413–3416, (1987).

Detection of low amounts of proto-oncogene mRNA which are minimally detectable by conventional microscopy. Evaluation of Grimelius-stained sections of lung cancer by CLSM with antiflex permits detection of previously undetected granula.

5. Baddely A.J., Howard C.V., Boyde A., Reid S.A.
Three-dimensional analysis of the spatial distribution of particles using the tandem scanning relected light microscope. Acta Stereologica **6** Suppl. 2: 87–100 (1987).

6. Balasubramanian N., *Optical Design Considerations in Laser Scanning Systems.* J.Opt.Soc.Am. **69,** 1479 (1979).

7. Barnett M.E., *Image formation in optical and electron transmission microscopy.* J.Microscopy **102,** 1–27 (1974).

8. Bertero M., C. De Mol, E.R. Pike and J.G. Walker, *Resolution indiffraction-limited imaging.* IV. The case of uncertain localization or non-uniform illumination of the object. Opt.Acta. **31,** 923–946(1984).

The resolution of the type-II confocal scanning microscope may be improved by recording the full image and by inverting the data.

9. Bertero M., Brianzi P., and Pike E. R., *Super-resolution in confocal scanning microscopy.* Inverse Probl. **3,** 195–212 (1987).

Proposes a numerical method which can be easily implemented and, in principle, applied to the practical problem addressed in the previous paper. Shows that by using a rather small number of data points on the image plane, it is possible to obtain the improvement in resolution (by a factor of two) predicted in the previous analysis.

10. Bertero B., De Mol C., and Pike E. R., *Analytic inversion formula for confocal scanning microscopy.* J.Opt.Soc.Am. A **4,** 1748–1750 (1987).

A simple analytic expression for the inverse of an operator is related to the problem of data reduction in confocal scanning microscopy. Potential applications of this result to the practical scanning microscope problem are outlined.

11. Box H.C., and Freund H.G., *Flying-Spot Microscope Adapted for Quantitative Measurements.* Rev.Sci.Instrum. **30,** 28–30 (1959).

215

12. Boyde A., Petran M., and Hadravsky M., *Tandem scanning reflected light microscopy of internal features in whole bone and tooth samples.* J.Micros. **132**, 1–7 (1983).

The TSM has a small depth of focus and gives high contrast for features such as osteocyte lacunae and canaliculi in bone, and prism boundaries in dental enamel.

13. Boyde A., Ali N.N., and Jones S.J., *Optical and scanning electron microscopy in the single osteoclast resorption assay.* Scanning. Electron Microsc. **3**, 1259–1271 (1985).

Optical microscopy was found to be complementary to SEM, enabling vital microscopy of unstained and stained cells. In particular, oblique illumination light microscopy and tandem scanning reflected light microscopy (TSRLM) proved to be of paramount value for this purpose. Fixed coated specimens could be most rapidly scanned for resorption lacunae using darkfield reflected LM or TSRLM.

14. Boyde A., *Stereoscopic images in confocal (tandem scanning) microscopy.* Science **230**, 1270–1272 (1985).

Stereoscopic pair images with parallel projection geometry are obtained by through-focusing along two inclined axes while recording two (summed and stacked) images with a microscope with a very shallow depth of field. The two stack images sample the same depth slice of translucent or reflective specimens. This is a direct method for recording stereo images than can be used to the limit of resolution in optical microscopy.

15. Boyde A., *The Tandem Scanning Reflected Light Microscope.* Part 2—Pre-MICRO 84 applications at UCL. Proc.Roy.Microsc.Soc. **20** 130–139 (1985).

16. Boyde A., Reid S. A. *3-D analysis of tetracycline fluorescence in bone by tandem scanning of reflected microscopy.* Bone **7** 148–149 (1986).

17. Boyde A., *Applications of Tandem Scanning Reflected Light microscopy and 3-dimensional imaging.* Ann. New York Acad. Sci. **484** 428–439 (1987).

18. Boyde A. and Martin L., *Tandem scanning reflected light microscopy of primate enamel.* Scanning.Micros. **1**, 1935–1948 (1987).

Examination of enamel prism packing patterns in modern and fossil primate teeth, and the preliminary results of a survey of enamel structural diversity in the Order Primates. The phylogenetic implications of these findings are also discussed. The TSM has allowed these data to be obtained nondestructively, which has permitted the inclusion of rare fossil primates in this survey. The specimens are not etched or otherwise prepared.

19. Boyde A., *Colour-coded stereo images from the tandem scanning reflected light microscope (TSRLM).* J.Micros. **146 pt2**, p137-p142 (1987).

Stereo-pair images are coded in colour for depth within the field imaged. Images are recorded photographically whilst focusing vertically through the layer to be imaged. A horizontal component of motion is applied at the same time, but in opposing senses for the two images. Coding for depth is obtained by changing colour filters so that reflective features lying at different depths are imaged in corresponding colours.

20. Boyde A., *Combining confocal and conventional modes in tandem scanning reflected light microscopy.* Scanning **11** 147–152 (1989).

21. Brakenhoff, G.J., van der Voort, H.T.M., van Spronsen, E.A., Nanninga, N. *3-dimensional imaging of biological structures by high resolution confocal scanning laser microscopy.* Scanning Microsc. **2**, 33–40 (1988).

22. Brakenhoff G.J., Blom P., and Barends P., *Confocal scanning light microscopy with high aperture immersion lenses.* J.Miscros. **117pt 2**, 219–232 (1979).

The imaging characteristics of a confocal scanning light microscope (CSLM) with high aperture, immersion type, lenses (N.A.=1.3) are investigated. In the confocal arrangement, the images of the illumination and detector pinholes are made to coincide in a common point, through which the object is scanned mechanically. Results show that for point objects the theoretically expected improved response by a factor of 1.4 in comparison with standard microscopy can indeed be realized. Low side lobe intensity and absence of glare permits the imaging at high resolution of weak details close to strong features. A further improvement by a factor of 1.25 in point resolution in CSLM is found after apodization with an annular aperture. Due to the scanning approach, all possibilities of electronic image processing become available in light microscopy.

23. Brakenhoff G.J., *Imaging modes in confocal scanning light microscopy (CSLM).* J.Micros. **117**, 233–242 (1979).

A number of imaging modes is considered in which the confocal scanning approach can be incorporated. In a scanning instrument, the measured data become available sequentially in time.

The optical arrangement for confocal scanning light microscopy can be incorporated in various imaging modes. Light microscopical specimens can be imaged with contrast enhanced, under gamma-control, inverted, etc in interference, conditions can be set such that either pure phase or pure amplitude images result. Stereoscopic images at arbitrary aspect ratios can be realized in CSLM by electronic processing of the data obtained when the specimen is sampled with more than one confocal point concurrently. Also forms of differential imaging either amplitude or phase are possible. The coupling of these imaging modes with the improved resolving powers of CSLM results in some unique imaging opportunities, especially of value for high-resolution microscopy of living specimens.

24. Brakenhoff G.J., van der Voort H.T.M., van Spronsen, E.A., Linnemans W.A.M., and Nanninga N., *Three-dimensional chromatin distribution in neuroblastoma nuclei shown by confocal scanning laser microscopy.* Nature **317**, 748–749 (1985).

The exceptionally short depth of field of this imaging technique provides direct optical sectioning which, together with its higher resolution, makes CSLM extremely useful for studying the three-dimensional morphology of biological structures.

25. Brakenhoff G.J., Van Der Voort H.T.M., Van Spronsen, W.A.M., and Nanninga N., *Three-dimensional imaging in fluorescence by confocal scanning microscopy.* J.Micros. **153** 151–159 (1989).

26. Carlsson K., Danielsson P.E., Lenz R., Liljeborg A., Majlof L., and Åslund N., *Three-dimensional microscopy using a confocal laser scanning microscope.* Opt.Lett. **10**, 53–55 (1985).

In Fluorescent light the depth-discriminating property of-confocal scanning has been used to carry out optical slicing of a thick specimen. The recorded digital images constitute a three-dimensional raster covering a volume. The specimen has been visualised in stereo and rotation by making look-through projections of the digital data in different directions. The contrast of the pictures has been enhanced by generating the gradient volume. This permits display of the border surfaces between regions instead of the regions themselves.

27. Carlsson K. and Liljeborg A., *A Confocal Laser Microscope Scanner for Digital Recording of Optical Serial Section,* J.Micros. **149**, 957 (1988)

Description of a mirror scanned confocal laser scanning microscope, used for direct imaging and fluorescence imaging.

28. Carlsson, K. and N. Åslund. *Confocal imaging for 3-D digital microscopy.* Appl.Opt. **26** 3232–328, 1987.

Optical serial sectioning based on the depth-discriminating ability of confocal laser scanning can be combined with digital image processing to realize fast and easy-to-use 3D microscopy. A great advantage as compared with traditional methods, e.g., using a microtome, is that the specimen is left undamaged. An account is given of an instrument designed for this purpose and of feasibility studies that have been carried out to assess the usefulness of the method in fluorescence microscopy.

29. Chen J., Baba N., and Murata K., *Quantitative measurement of a phase object by fringe scanning interference microscopy.* Appl.Optics **28**, 1615–1617 (1989).

30. Chou C.H. and Kino G.S., *The evaluation of V(z) in a type II reflection microscope.1 IEEE. Trans.Ultrason.Ferroelectr.& Freq.Control.* **34**, 341–345 (1987).

A more complete theory is developed for the V(z) characteristic of an acoustic microscope. This theory is non-paraxial and treats the effect of finite ka, where a is the radius of the aperture. It explains well the asymmetry of the V(z) curve for a perfect reflector, which has been observed experimentally and has been difficult to explain theoretically. The results obtained are also of importance to the scanning optical microscope.

31. Cohen-Sabban J., Rodier J.C., Roussel A., and Simon J., *Scanning Ophthalmoscope.* Innov.Tech.Biol.Med. **5**, 24 (1984).

A Scanning Laser Ophthalmoscope with two galvo mirrors.

32. Corle T.R., Chou C.-H., and Kino G.S., *Depth response of confocal optical microscopes.* Opt.Lett. **11**, 770–772 (1986).

The on-axis intensity response for an objective of numerical aperture 0.9. The data compare favorably with theoretical calculations obtained by numerical integration of the standard theory, provided that lens aberrations are taken into account. The invariance of the shape of the central lobe to surface roughness and tilt is also demonstrated.

33. Cox I.J., Sheppard C.J.R., and Wilson T., *Improvement in resolution by nearly confocal microscopy. The theory of the direct-view confocal microscope.* J.Micros. **124**, 107–117 (1981).

In a conventional confocal microscope the resolution is improved over that attainable in a conventional instrument. A further improvement in resolution is produced when the detector pinhole is offset, resulting in nearly confocal operation. For the case where the pinhole is placed over the first dark ring in the Airy disk in the detector plane, dark-field conditions are produced by a very simple method. A theory is presented which describes imaging in both conventional and scanning microscopes, embracing conventional microscopes with partially coherent source and scanning microscopes with partially coherent effective source and detector, including confocal microscopes. The theory is applicable to the direct-view confocal microscope of Petran, the design of which is discussed. This microscope combines the resolution and depth discrimination improvements of confocal microscopy with the ease of operation of the conventional microscope.

34. Cox I.J., Sheppard C.J.R., and Wilson T., *Super-resolution by confocal fluorescent microscopy.* Optik **60**, 391–6 (1982).

In the confocal coherent microscope a spatial frequency bandwidth twice as wide as in the conventional coherent microscope is achieved. A confocal incoherent microscope may be constructed by destroying the coherence in the object plane, and this system has a bandwidth four times that of the conventional coherent instrument. The coherence may be destroyed by imaging fluorescence either from the specimen itself or from a subsidary fluorescent material. Transfer functions for these systems are presented. The two-point resolution is also examined and it is shown that an improvement of more than a factor of two may be obtained.

35. Cox I.J., Sheppard C.J.R., and Wilson T., *Reappraisal of arrays of concentric annuli as super resolving filters.* J.Opt.Soc.Am. **72**, 1287–1291 (1982).

The superresolving filter design of Toraldo di Francia (Atti.Fond.Giorgio ronchi 7, 366 (1952)), which consists of an array of concentric annuli of finite width, is studied. Such a filter compares favorably with other superresolving filter designs while being considerably more simple to fabricate. In particular, for given input energy, the intensity at the focal point is usually greater than for optimized filter designs. The manufacturing tolerances of such a filter are discussed.

36. Cox I.J., and Sheppard C.J.R., *Scanning optical microscope incorporating a digital framestore and microcomputer.* Appl.Opt. **22**, 1474–1478 (1983).

A scanning optical microscope is particularly well suited for image digitization since the image is already in the form of an electronic signal. A mechanically scanned optical microscope is described, which is controlled by a microcomputer and the image displayed on a framestore. The results of several simple digital image-processing algorithms applied to the micrographs are presented.

37. Cox, I.J., *Scanning optical fluorescence microscopy.* J.Miscrosc. **133**, 149–154 (1984).

Advantages include improved resolution, reduction in background and auto-fluorescence, an increase in the available fluorescence spectrum and simple modification for automated fluorescence studies.

38. Cox, I.J., and Sheppard, C.J.R., *Information capacity and resolution in an optical system.* J.Opt.Soc.Am. A **3**, 1152–8 (1986).

The concept of invariance of information capacity is discussed and applied to the resolution of an optical system. Methods of obtaining superresolution in microscopy are discussed, and scanning microscopy has many distinct advantages for such applications.

39. Cunha A., Friedman M., Leith E.N., Lopez J., Reid E., and Silverman K., *Tandem coherent-incoherent filtering in scanning optical microscopy.* Appl.Opt. **28**, 2993–2995 (1989).

A method of imaging through inhomogeneities using the principles of scanning optical microscopy is described. The authors describe and analyze a system comprising a confocal scanning system, a coherent spatial filtering system, followed by detection and then a second spatial filtering system.

40. Davidovits P., and Egger M.D., *Scanning laser microscope.* Nature 223, **831** (1969).

41. Davidovits P. and Egger M.D., *Scanning laser microscope for biological investigations.* Appl.Opt. **10**, 1615–1619 (1971).

42. Dilly P.N., *Tandem scanning reflected light microscopy of the cornea.* Scanning. **10**, 153–156 (1988).

Ex vivo rabbit and human eyes, and one live human cornea.

43. Draaijer A., and Houpt P.M., *A standard video-rate confocal laser- scanning reflection and fluorescence microscope.* Scanning. **10**, 139–145 (1988).

A confocal laser-scanning microscope (CLSM) differs from a conventional microscope by affording an extreme depth discrimination, as well as a slightly improved resolution. The CLSM developed at TNO has standard video-rate imaging, and is capable of working in reflection and in fluorescence mode simultaneously.

44. Dyer D.L., and Fuller C.H., *Vidicon Microscope for Counting Fluorescent Particles.* Rev.Sci.Instrum. **42**, 508–509 (1970).

45. Egger M.D., and Petran M., *New reflected-light microscope for viewing unstained brain and ganglion cells.* Science **157**, 305–307 (1967).

46. Egger M.D., Gezari W., Davidovits P., Hadravsky M. and Petran M., *Observation of Nerve Fibers in Incident Light.* Experientia 25, 1225 (1969).

47. Goldstein S., *A no-moving-parts video rate laser beam scanning type 2 confocal reflected/transmission microscope.* J. Micros. **153**, 1–2 (1989).

48. Hadni A., Bassia J.M., Gerbaux X., and Thomas R., *Laser scanning microscope for pyroelectric display in real time.* Appl.Opt. **15**, 2150–2158 (1976).

49. Hamilton D.K., Wilson T., and Sheppard C.J.R., *Experimental observations of the depth-discrimination properties of scanning microscopes.* Opt.Lett. **6**, 625–626 (1981).

Experimental confirmation of the predicted improved depth-discrimination properties of confocal microscopy in which detail outside the focal plane is rejected from the image. This optical sectioning is of direct importance to the microscopy of thick biological tissue.

50. Hamilton D.K., and Wilson T., *Three-dimensional surface measurement using the confocal scanning microscope.* Appl.Phys.B. (Germany) **27**, 211–213 (1982).

The use of the depth discrimination property of the confocal scanning microscope for surface profiling has been adapted to provide a method of high-resolution three-dimensional surface profilometry. Measurements on a semiconductor specimen demonstrate the technique, depth variations of the order of 0.1 μm are clearly resolved.

51. Hamilton D.K., and Wilson T., *Surface profile measurementusing the confocal microscope.* J.Appl.Phys. **53**, 5320–5322(1982). The method utilizes the depth discrimination properties ofthe confocal scanning optical microscope.

52. Hamilton D.K., Sheppard C.J.R., and Wilson T., *Improved imaging of phase gradients in scanning optical microscopy.* J.Micros. **135**, 275–286 (1984).

Previous work has used a circular large area split detector for phase gradient imaging; it is shown that substituting an annular split detector offers improvements in frequency response, particularly for weak pulse gradients. Transfer functions are calculated and transmission and reflection micrographs demonstrate the different imaging properties. Other forms of detector are also considered, some of these possessing certain advantages.

53. Hamilton D.K., and Wilson T., *Two-dimensional phase imaging in the scanning optical microscope.* Appl.Opt. **23**, 348–352 (1984).

It is shown that an image of absolute object phase may be produced by integrating a differential phase contrast image produced by a large area split detector. Even though integration is being carried out only along the scan lines,a full 2d phase image is produced by surrounding the object with a medium of uniform path length and resetting the integrator at the beginning of each scan line. Images of a buccal epithelial cell demonstrate the technique.

54. Hamilton D.K., and Wilson T., *Edge enhancement in scanning optical microscopy by differential detection.* J.Opt.Soc.Am. A **1**, 322–323 (1984).

A simple method of optically producing edge-enhanced images in a scanning optical microscope is described. The method uses a coded photodiode detector from which the conventional unenhanced image may be obtained simultaneously.

55. Hamilton D.K., and Wilson T., *Optical sectioning in infra-red scanning microscopy. Scanning optical microscopy by objective lens scanning.* J.Phys.E. **19**, 52–54 (1986).

Presents confocal reflection infra-red images of semiconductor devices and shows that the confocal microscope's unique optical sectioning property results in images of greater clarity and contrast when features are being examined through large thicknesses of semiconductor. Polarization effects may be exploited to give similar results. Mechanically scanning the objective for heavy or awkwardly shaped objects.

56. Hamilton D.K. and Wilson T., *Optical sectioning in infra-red scanning microscopy.* IEEE Proc. I **134**, 85–86 (1987).

Confocal reflection infra-red images of semiconductor devices show that the unique optical sectioning property results in images of greater clarity and contrast when features are being examined through large thicknesses of semiconductor. Polarization effects may be exploited to give similar results.

57. Hamilton D.K. and Wilson T., *Infrared sub-band-gap photocurrent imaging in the scanning optical microscope of defects in semiconductor devices.* Micron.Microsc.Acta. **18**, 77–80 (1987).

An optical beam induced contrast (obic) image of a gallium phosphide light emitting diode, produced using radiation of quantum energy less than the material's energy gap, shows sub-surface crystallographic defects which are not imaged with conventional obic. These defects show strong correspondence with a region of low intensity emission from the diode.

58. Hansen, E.W., Allen, R.D., Strohbehn, J.W., Chaffee, M.A., Farrington, D.L., Murray, W.J., Pillsbury, T.A., and Riley, M.F., *Laser scanning phase modulation microscope,* J.Micros. **140(3)**, 371–381 (1985).

Describes the concept and first implementation of a laser scanning microscope for quantitative polarized light imaging. Combines a phase modulation feedback loop for precise measurement of birefringence, etc., with laser scanning and digital image acquisition.

59. Hegedus Z.S., and Sarafis V., *Superresolving filters in confocally scanned imaging systems.* J.Opt.Soc.Am. A **3**, 1892–6(1986).

The constraints on superresolving filters in the nonscanning imaging mode are discussed. It is shown theoretically and verified experimentally that simply designed complex-amplitude filters can be used effectively to double the exit pupil of a confocal imaging system and thus improve resolution. Super-resolution can be achieved with acceptable energy losses, and within manufacturing tolerances.

60. Horikawa Y., Yamamoto M., and Dosaka S., *Laser scanning microscope: differential phase images.* J. Microsc. **148**, 1–10(1987).

A TV rate acousto-optic deflector laser scanning microscope for differential phase contrast images using the split-detector technique. The design and associated correction system allows transfer of the necessary pupil information during beam deflection. Differential phase images of surface details of crystals are simply obtained without silver coating or etching, necessary in a normal DIC. Biological specimens are also observed.

61. Hook, G.R., and C.O. Odeyale. *Confocal scanning fluorescence microscopy: A new method for phagocytosis research.* J.Leuk.Biol. **45** 277–282, 1989.

Demonstrated using fluorescent microspheres ingested by murine macrophages. CSFM, in combination with Nomarski differential interference contrast microscopy (DIC), can resolve microspheres inside cells from microspheres attached to the surface of cells. Further, combined CSFM and DIC images can quantitate phagocytosis by individual cells aggregated together. No other method offers these capabilities. A comparison of CSFM and conventional epifluoresc-

ence light microscopy (EFM) images shows that CSFM produces significantly higher-resolution images of microspheres than EFM, primarily because CSFM excludes the out-of-focus light artifacts of EFM.

62. Howard V., Reid S., Baddeley A., and Boyde A., *Unbiased estimation of particle density in the tandem scanning reflected light microscope.* J.Micros. **138, pt 2**, 203–212 (1985).

An unbiased 3D counting rule for the TSRLM, which is applied to the estimation of osteocyte lacunar density in whole bone is an extremely efficient way of making such an estimate.

63. Jones, S.J., and A. Boyde. *Scanning microscopic observations on dental caries.* Scanning Microsc. **1** 1991–2002, 1987.

64. Jungerman R.L., Hobbs P.C., and Kino G.S., *Phase sensitive scanning optical microscope.* Appl.Phys.Lett. **45**, 846–848 (1984).

An electronically scanned optical microscope which quantitatively measures amplitude and phase is described. The system is insensitive to mechanical vibrations. The phase information makes it possible to measure surface height variations with an accuracy of better than 10 nm and can be used to improve the lateral resolution.

65. Kermisch D., *Principle of equivalence between scanning and conventional optical imaging systems.* J.Opt.Soc.Am. **67**, 1357–1360 (1977).

Very theoretical. An equivalence based on fundamental physical laws, makes it possible to analyze or design a scanning system in terms of a corresponding conventional imaging system.

66. Koester C.J., *Scanning mirror microscope with optical sectioning characteristics: applications in ophthalmology.* Appl.Opt. **19**, 1749-1757 (1980).

Optical sectioning is the simultaneous illumination and viewing of only a thin region of a specimen. An illuminated slit is imaged at the plane of interest and is swept laterally by the action of an oscillating mirror. The light returning from the specimen reflects from a second facet of the oscillating mirror and forms a stationary image of the illuminated slit. At this stationary image a second slit is placed, which passes light from the desired plane and rejects scattered light from other depths within the specimen. Light passing through the second slit is reflected from the third facet of the oscillating mirror and is focused to the final image plane. The image is reconstructed as the image of the second slit sweeps across the image plane. An important ophthalmological application is the examination of the endothelial cell layer of the cornea, either by contact or noncontact techniques. Optimization for image illuminance and resolution is discussed.

67. Laeri F., and Strand T.C., *Angstrom resolution optical profilometry for microscopic objects.* Appl.Opt. **26**, 2245–2249 (1987).

An instrument capable of recording the amplitude and phase of reflected light with a phase resolution of better than lambda/3000 and the lateral resolution of a confocal scanning microscope was built. The instrument is based on a commercial microscope body and uses regular interference contrast optics. The modifications consisted of adding a co-herent (heterodyne) detector and a confocal laser scanning system. Two-dimensional surface images of amplitude, slope, and profile were taken with a step height resolution of typically 0.5–2 Angstrom. The instrument is described, and its characteristics for surface profilometry are discussed.

68. Lemp M.A., Dilly P.N., and Boyde A., *Tandem-scanning (confocal) microscopy of the full-thickness cornea.* Cornea. **4**, 205–209 (1985).

Studies the full-thickness morphology of the intact cornea in an excised human eye bank eye and in freshly sacrificed rabbit eyes in situ, layer by layer in extremely thin sections, only disturbing the tissue with an applanating tip. Demonstrates the cells of the corneal surface, subsurface cells, the topography of Bowman's membrane, corneal lamellae, stromal keratocytes, and the cornea lendothelium.

69. Magiera A., and Magiera L., *Remarks on point spread function in confocal scanning microscope with apodized pupil.* Opt.Appl. (Poland.) **15**, 107–110 (1985).

The effective intensity point spread function can be improved by using an annular pupil. A further improvement of the resolution can be achieved if one of the two pupils applied gives a point spread function with a prescribed localization of zeros.

70. Marsman H.J.B., Stricker R., Wijnaendts van Resandt R.W., Brakenhoff G.J., and Blom P., *Mechanical scan system for microscopic applications.* Rev.Sci.Instrum. **54**, 1047–1052 (1983).

A high-speed mechanical scanning stage for microscopic applications has been designed and constructed. It is especially suitable for high-resolution confocal UV microscopy. It is a feedback design using electromagnetic actuators and piezoelectric sensors with motor-driven screws for coarse adjustment. Scanning of areas up to 1 mm square at up to 300 lines per second is possible with positional resolution of better than 0.01 mm. An exceptionally stable optical system is also described.

71. Masters, B.R., and Paddock, S. *In vitro confocal imaging of the rabbit cornea* J.Micros. **157**, 1–8 (1989).

Scanning laser microscope (BioRad) on ex vivo rabbit corneas. No contact lens, with strong anterior corneal reflex needing to be blocked, is center of image.

72. Matthews, H.J., Hamilton, D.K., Sheppard, C.J.R. *Aberration measurement by confocal interferometry* J.Mod.Opt. **36**, 233–80 (1989)

The aberrations and apodization of microscope objectives have been measured by observation of the defocus signal in a confocal interference microscope system. Phase distortions can be measured to approximately $\lambda/100$, and quantitative information is given about the imaging performance of the lenses in situ in the optical system.

73. Maurice D.M., *A Scanning Slit Optical Microscope,* Investigative Ophthalmology, **13**, 1033–1037 (1973)

A pioneer paper describing an early form of confocal microscopy for imaging layers in the cornea of the eye. This system used a scanning slit 3 μm wide to give depth definition, and scanning was carried out by moving a photo-graphic film and the specimen in opposite directions. High quality images of the cornea were obtained, which took about 20 minutes to form.

74. McLaren J.W., and Brubaker R.F., *A Scanning ocular spectrofluorophotometer.* Invest.Ophthalmol.Vis.Sci. **29**, 1285–93 (1988).

We describe an instrument called a scanning ocular spectrofluorophotometer (SOSF) that measures fluorescence in a two-dimensional cross-section through the anterior chamber and cornea and provides the ability to change excitation and emission wavelengths rapidly. The output of a xenon arc lamp is filtered by a diffraction grating monochromator which has a bandpass of 4 nm and a range of 400 to 800 nm. Light emitted from the fluorophore is filtered by a variable wavelength interference filter which has a bandpass of approximately 11 nm and a range of 400 to 700 nm. To demonstrate the versatility of the instrument, we measured the spectra of fluorescein, fluorescein glucuronide andrhodamine B in the anterior chambers and corneas of pigmented rabbits after topical administration. We also measured simultaneously and independently the redistribution and disappearance of a mixture of fluorescein-labeled dextran and rhodamine B after intra cameral injection. Rhodamine B was very rapidly absorbed by the cornea and lens while fluorescein-dextran was not measurable in the cornea before 4 hr. The SOSF provides a means of carrying out spectrofluorophotometry in the living eye and carrying out kinetic experiments which would otherwise be awkward or impossible.

75. Mendez E.R., *Speckle contrast variation in the confocal scanning microscope. Hard-edged apertures.* Opt.Acta **33**, 269–278 (1986).

The speckle contrast variation as a function of defocus, and the statistical properties of random diffusing objects is studied. It is assumed that the number of scattered contributions is very large, so that the central limit theorem can be applied. The diffuser is modelled as a thin phase screen which introduces Gaussian distributed and Gaussian correlated phase fluctuations. The main results are plotted, discussed and compared with some experimental data.

76. Mickols W., and Maestre M.F., *Scanning differential polarization microscope: its use to image linear and circular differential scattering.* Rev.Sci.Instrum. **59**, 867–872 (1988).

A differential polarization microscope that couples the sensitivity of single-beam measurement of circular dichroism and circular differential scattering with the simultaneous measurement of linear dichroism and linear differential scattering. Uses a scanning microscope stage and single-point illumination, and can operate in the confocal mode as well as in the near confocal condition that can allow one to program the coherence and spatial resolution of the microscope. Has been used to study the change in the structure of chromatin during the development of sperm in Drosophila.

77. Minsky M., *Memoir on inventing the confocal scanning microscope.* Scanning **10**, 128–138 (1988).

A valuable historical document, and enjoyable reading. Minsky's patent ran out before the world was ready for the idea, but his early ideas have all proved out well.

78. Oud J.L., A. Mans, G.J. Brakenhoff, H.T.M. van der Voort, E.A. van Spronsen and N. Nanninga. *Three-dimensional chromosome arrangement of crepis-capillaris in mitotic prophase and anaphase as studied by confocal scanning laser microscopy.* J.CellSci. **92(3):** 329–340, 1989.

79. Petran M., Hadravsky M., Benes J., Kucera R., Boyde A., *The tandem scanning reflected light microscope.* Part 1 — The principle, and its design. Proc.Roy.Micros.Soc. **20:** 125–129 (1985b).

80. Petran M., and Hadravsky M., *Tandem-scanning reflected-light microscope.* J.Opt.Soc.Am. **58,** 661–664 (1968).

81. Petran M., Sallam-Sattar M. *Microscopical observations of the living (unprepared and unstained) retina.* Physiologia bohemoslov **23:** 369 (1974).

82. Petran M., Hadravsky M., and Boyde A., *The tandem scanning reflected light microscope.* Scanning **7,** 97–108 (1985). Summarizes the TSM.

83. Petran M., and Boyde A., *New horizons for light microscopy.* Science **230,** 1258–1262 (1985). Summarizes the TSM.

84. Petran M., Hadravsky M., Benes J., and Boyde A., *In vivo microscopy using the tandem scanning microscope.* Ann.NY.Acad.Sci **483,** 440–447 (1986).

85. Petran M., Hadravsky M., Boyde A., and Müller M., *Tandem scanning reflected light microscopy.* Science of Biolgical Specimen Preparation 85–94 (1987).

86. Ploem, J.S., *Laser scanning fluorescence microscopy.* Appl.Opt. **26** 3226–3231, (1987).

Another general description of CSM. Very strong excitation light can be concentrated on small spots (0.5 mm). The low levels of autofluorescence generated in the microscope objective and in the immersion oil in LSM provide images of great contrast, even with weakly fluorescent specimens. Combination of images stored in computer memory allow the comparison of phase contrast and fluorescence images of the same area of the specimen enabling multiparameter analysis of cells.

87. Reid S.A., Smith R., Boyde A., *Some scanning microscopies off ibrogenesis imperfecta ossium.* Bone **6** 275–276 (1985).

88. Reimer L., Egelkamp S.T., and Verst M., *Lock-in technique for depth-profiling and magneto optical Kerr effect imaging in scanning optical microscopy.* Scanning **9,** 17–25 (1987).

Describes the scanning optical microscope with lock-in techniques for depth-profiling and the magneto optical Kerr effect imaging of magnetic domains which allow the separation of depth information and magneto optical effects independent of surface topography and local light reflectance.

89. Salam-Satter M., Petran M., *Dynamic alterations accompanying spreading depression in chick retina.* Physiologia behemoslov **23,** 373 (1974).

90. See Chung Wah and Iravani Mehdi Vaez, *Differential amplitude scanning optical microscope: theory and applications.* Appl.Opt. **27,** 2786–2792 (1988).

Differential means two adjacent spots, to catch small changes of height or index. This is a dynamic range stretcher for those quantities.

91. Shack R.V., Bartels P.H., Buchroeder R.A., Shoemaker R.L., Hillman D.W., and Vukobratovich D., *Design for a fast fluorescence laser scanning microscope.* Anal.Quant.Cytol.Histol. **9,** 509–520 (1987).

The design of a fast fluorescence laser scanning microscope is described and illustrated, with discussion of the design consideration of the principal components, including the optical elements. The system is expected to provide very-high-speed scanning, at a high spatial sampling density, of large object areas while retaining a flexibility of applications. The projected scanning rate approximates the rate achieved by flow cytometry; the projected rates of information generation should be orders of magnitude higher.

92. Sheppard C.J.R., and Choudhury A., *Image formation in the scanning microscope.* Opt.Acta. **24,** 1051–1073 (1977).

Fourier imaging in the scanning microscope is considered. It is shown that there are two geometries of the microscope, which have been designated type 1 and type 2. Those of type 1 exhibit identical imaging to the conventional microscope, whereas those of type 2 (confocal microscopes) display various differences. Imaging of a single point object, two-point resolution and response to a straight edge are also considered. The effect of various arrangements using lenses with annular pupil functions is also discussed. It is found that type 2 microscopes have improved imaging properties over conventional microscopes and that these may be further improved by use of one or two lenses with annular pupils.

93. Sheppard C.J.R., and Wilson T., *Image formation in scanning microscopes with partially coherent source and detector.* Opt.Acta. **25,** 315–325 (1978).

The effect of partial coherence of both the source and the detector in a scanning microscope is investigated. The transfer function for the system is derived and various special cases discussed. If the effective source and effective detector are coherent and incoherent respectively, the microscope (type 1) is of the form of the scanning transmission electron microscope (stem). If the effective source and the effective detector are both coherent, the microscope (type 2) is of the form of the scanning acoustic microscope. Scanning optical microscopes of both these types may be constructed.

94. Sheppard C.J.R., and Wilson T., *Depth of field in the scanning microscope.* Opt.Lett. **3,** 115–117 (1978).

Various definitions of depth of field in the microscope are discussed. The variation in the integrated intensity in the image of a point object outside the focal plane shows how the microscope discriminates against such objects. The power diffusely scattered by a translucent object is also considered. A Type-2 scanning microscope is found to have a much reduced depth of field according to these criteria, which makes it useful for studying thick biological slices. These results do not contradict the claim that depth of field may be much increased in such a microscope by using lenses with annular pupil functions.

95. Sheppard C.J.R., and Wilson T., *The theory of scanning microscopes with gaussian pupil functions.* J.Micros. **114,** 179–197 (1978).

The theory of imaging in scanning microscopes with lenses, source and detector all having gaussian pupil function is developed. This assumption is useful as the expressions may be evaluated analytically. It is shown that type 2 microscopes exhibit superior performance to those of type 1. Effects of defocus are considered. It is found that defocus can be used in a type 2 microscope to observe phase information without the limitation in resolution associated with stopping down the collector of a conventional microscope. It is also found that a type 2 microscope discriminates against light scattered by parts of the object outside of the focal plane, allowing observation of detail within a thick object.

96. Sheppard C.J.R., and Wilson T., *Imaging properties of annular lenses.* Appl.Opt. **18**, 3764–3769 (1979).

An improvement in resolution in a conventional microscope has been shown to result if an annular condenser is employed. Here fourier imaging in the presence of defocus and spherical aberration is considered, and the image of a straight-edge calculated. Imaging in confocal microscopes is superior to that in conventional microscopes and may be further improved by the use of one lens with annular aperture. Again fourier imaging with defocus and spherical aberration is considered, resulting in an imaginary part being introduced into the transfer function. The straight edge response is very sharp.

97. Sheppard C.J.R., and Wilson T., *Effect of spherical aberration on the imaging properties of scanning optical microscopes.* Appl.Opt. **18**, 1058–1063 (1979b).

The effect of primary spherical aberration and defocus on the imaging properties of scanning optical microscopes with weak objects is considered. Optically there are two types of scanning microscope. Type 1 scanning microscopes behave identically to conventional microscopes, but in type 2 scanning microscopes an imaginary part is introduced into the transfer function. In general, therefore, it is important that the lenses be adequately corrected, but for objects with very weak amplitude contrast the effect may be a useful way of obtaining phase imaging. Experimental demonstration of the effect of spherical aberration is reported.

98. Sheppard C.J.R., and Wilson T., *Image formation in confocal scanning microscopes.* Optik **55**, 331–342 (1980).

Image formation in conventional and scanning microscopy is compared and contrasted, with emphasis on the fourier imaging approach. The effects of aberrations on the transfer function are discussed

99. Sheppard C.J.R. and Wilson T., *Multiple traversing of the object in the scanning microscope.* Opt.Acta. **27**, 611–624 (1980).

An arrangement is proposed in which the beam in a microscope traverses the object more than once. This results in the image of a single point for two passes through the object being 2.4 times as sharp as that in a conventional microscope, the side lobes also being extremely small. In the microscope in which the beam passes through the object twice the image amplitude behaves similarly to the image intensity in a conventional partially coherent microscope. Theoretical images of various objects are calculated, and the effects of using annular lenses discussed.

100. Sheppard C.J.R., *Fourier imaging of phase information in scanning and conventional optical microscopes.* Philos.Trans.R.Soc.London. A **295**, 513–536 (1980).

The imaging performance of scanning microscopes may be improved by introducing a pinhole in the detector plane, thus forming a confocal (or type 2) scanning microscope. A general imaging theory is developed from which the performance of scanning and conventional microscopes may be investigated. Various methods of obtaining phase imaging are considered, including the effects of defocus, zernike phase contrast, and interference and resonant microscopy.

101. Sheppard C. J. R., and Wilson T., *The theory of the direct-view confocal microscope.* J Micros. **124 pt2**, 107–117 (1981).

A theory is presented which describes imaging in both conventional and scanning microscopes. This theory embraces conventional microscopes with partially coherent source and scanning microscopes with partially coherent effective source and detector, including confocal microscopes. The theory is applicable to the direct-view confocal microscope of Petran, the design of which is discussed. This microscope combines the resolution and depth discrimination improvements of confocal microscopy with the ease of operation of the conventional microscope.

102. Sheppard C.J.R., and Wilson T., *The image of a single point in microscopes of large numerical aperture.* Proc.R.Soc. London ser. A **379**, 145–158 (1982).

The image of a single small hole in an opaque screen in a microscope of large numerical aperture is calculated. Both conventional microscopes and scanning optical microscopes are considered, the general trend being that the central peak is broadened, the outer rings strengthened and the minima made shallower as the numerical aperture is increased. In the conventional microscope the image is no longer independent of the illumination, as it is for paraxial theory.

103. Sheppard C.J.R., Hamilton D.K., and Cox I.J., *Optical microscopy with extended depth of field Observation of optical signatures of materials.* Appl.Phys.Lett. **41**, 604–606 (1982).

Depth of field may be extended, in principle without limit, while high-resolution, diffraction-limited imaging is retained. Experimentally, an extension of more than two orders of magnitude has been achieved. A new technique for the study of surfaces is described, whereby materials with different optical properties may be identified from characteristics responses, and which may be developed to give measurements of the optical properties. The technique is similar to one already used in acoustic microscopy.

104. Sheppard C.J.R., Cox I.J., and Hamilton D.K., *Edge detection in micrometrology with nearly confocal microscopy.* Appl.Opt. **23**, 657–658 (1984).

The technique appears particularly well suited for metrology of line structures and also in establishing dark-field conditions for a confocal microscope. An advantage of this method is that the imaging properties may be altered at will by a simple adjustment to produce greater resolution or dark-field conditions.

105. Sheppard C.J.R., and Cox I.J., *Resolution of scanned optical systems.* Acta Polytech.Scand.Appl.Phys.Ser. (Finland) **149**, 279–81 (1985).

By consideration of the invariance of the information capacity of an imaging system, the extreme noise-sensitivity of the analytical continuation method is illustrated. The flare contribution to noise is 105 times smaller for a confocal scanning microscope compared with a conventional microscope. The applicability of scanning microscopy to superresolution methods is discussed.

106. Sheppard C.J.R., and Wilson T., *Reciprocity and equivalence in scanning microscopes.* J.Opt.Soc.Am. A **3**, 755–756 (1986).

The application of the principle of reciprocity and methods of Fourier optics to imaging in conventional and scanning microscopes is discussed. It is concluded that their behavior is identical even for objects thick enough for multiple scattering to occur, provided that there is no inelastic scattering or birefringence present.

107. Sheppard C.J.R., and Wilson T., *On the equivalence of scanning and conventional microscopes.* Optik **73**, 39–43 (1986).

The principle of reciprocity and methods of Fourier optics are applied to imaging in conventional and scanning microscopes. It is concluded that their behaviour is identical even for objects thick enough for multiple scattering to occur, provided that there is no inelastic scattering or birefringence. Degradation of images by flare is also onsidered, it is found that scanning microscopes can be made superior to conventional instruments in this respect.

108. Sheppard C.J.R., *Super-resolution in confocal imaging.* Optik **80**, 53–54 (1988).

A new explanation for the imaging improvement of confocal microscopy is presented. A method of further increasing the imaging performance is also discussed.

109. Sheppard C.J.R., Mao X.Q., *Confocal microscopes with slit apertures.* J.Modern Optics **35** 1169–1185 (1988).

Using slit apertures, rather than pinholes, to construct a confocal imaging system has some advantages. The signal level is increased and, if a detector array is used, a line image can be generated in real time. Slit apertures can also be used in a direct-view confocal (tandem scanning) microscope.

110. Sheppard, C.J.R., *Aberrations in high aperture conventional and confocal imaging systems* Appl.Opt. **27** 4782–6 (1988).

An appropriate form for the expansion of an aberration function for an optical system of high numerical aperture is considered. The effects on the defocus signal of a confocal imaging system of aberrations, high aperture, finite Fresnel number, system configuration, and surface tilt are discussed.

111. Shoemaker R.L., Bartels P.H., Hillman D.W., Jonas J., Kessler D., Shack R.V., and Vukobratovich D., *An ultrafast laser scanner microscope for digital image analysis (cytology application).* IEEE. Trans.Biomed.Eng. **BME-29,** 82–91 (1982).

The design of an ultrafast laser scanner microscope has been completed and an experimental model has been constructed. The instrument is described and the considerations that led to the authors' choice of scanning method and optical and electronic system design are discussed. The scanner incorporates numerous new technologic features, and promises to make high resolution cell analysis practical at data rates comparable to those obtained now only in flow cytometry.

112. Shotten D.M., *Confocal scanning optical microscopy and its applications for biological specimens.* J. Cell. Sci. **94** 175–206 (1989).

A major, recent review article (180 references) concentrating on the uses of laser-scanning confocal microscopy (LSCM) in biology. There are interesting comparisons with other modern microscopical techniques. Most important aspects of LSCM are discussed, though seldom compared critically.

113. Shuman H., *Contrast in confocal scanning microscopy with a finite detector.* J Micros. **149,** 67–71 (1988).

The optical properties of a general scanning microscope are determined within the framework of Fourier imaging theory. For a simple model optical system, with Gaussian lens and detector apertures, the contrast transfer function can be expressed in terms of elementary functions. The theory predicts that spatial resolution and depth discrimination vary continuously with detector aperture and that defocus phase contrast is present in transmission images obtained with a symmetric objective, collector lens confocal microscope.

114. Takamatsu, T., and S. Fujita. *Microscopic tomography by laser scanning microscopy and its three-dimensional reconstruction.* J.Micros. **149** 167–174, 1988.

A confocal laser scanning microscope equipped with two galvanometer mirrors which swing the laser beam. The scanning apparatus of the system can eliminate mechanical vibration and sweep widely, to obtain images at a low magnification.

115. Toraldo di Francia G., *Resolving power and information.* J.Opt.Soc.Am. **45,** 497–501 (1955).

An often-referenced early paper: The degrees of freedom of an image formed by any real instrument are only a finite number, while those of the object are an infinite number. Several different objects may correspond to the same image. It is shown that in the case of coherent illumination a large class of objects corresponding to a given image can be found very easily. Two-point resolution is impossible unless the observer has a *priori* an infinite amount of information about the object.

116. Valkenburg, J.A., C.L. Woldringh, G.J. Brakenhoff, H.T. van der Voort, and N. Nanninga. *Confocal scanning light microscopy of the Eschericia coli nucleoid: comparison with phase-contrast and electron microscope images.* J.Bacteriol. **161** 478–483, 1985.

The nucleoid of living and OsO_4- or glutaraldehyde-fixed cells of Escherichia coli strains was studied with a phase-contrast microscope, a confocal scanning light microscope, and an electron microscope. The trustworthiness of the images obtained with the confocal scanning light microscope was investigated by comparison with phase-contrast micrographs and reconstructions based on serially sectioned material of DNA-containing and DNA-less cells. This comparison showed higher resolution of the confocal scanning light microscope as compared with the phase-contrast microscope, and agreement with results obtained with the electron microscope. The effects of fixation on the structure of the nucleoid were studied in E. coli B/r H266.

117. van der Voort H.T.M., Brakenhoff G.J., Valkenburg J.A.C. and Nanninga N., *Design and use of a computer controlled confocal microscope for biological applications.* Scanning **7**, 66–78 (1985).

An instrument under computer control and with extensive image processing capabilities is described. Various biological applications are given including computer generated stereo images of biological structures with submicron resolution.

118. van der Voort H.T.M., Brakenhoff G.J., and Janssen G.C.A.M., *Determination of the 3-dimensional optical properties of a Confocal Scanning Laser Microscope.* Optik **78**, 48–53 (1988).

Measurements of the 3-dimensional imaging properties of a Confocal Scanning Laser Microscope (CSLM) operating in reflection and fluorescence mode are described. The CSLM was equipped with high numerical aperture objectives and a finite sized detector pinhole. To determine the properties in the fluorescence mode, a special test object consisting of fluorescent bars with submicron dimensions was developed. The results, obtained with the test object and small reflecting gold spheres, indicate that the reflection point spread function can be used to test the performance of the microscope in fluorescence mode. Also, they may provide a basis for quantitative evaluation of 3D fluorescence images.

119. van Meer, G., E.H.K. Stelzer, R.W. Wijnaendts van Resandt, and K. Simons. *Sorting of sphingolipids in epithelial (Madin-Darby canine kidney) cells.* J.Cell Biol. **105** 1623–1635,1987.

An analysis of the fluorescence pattern by means of a confocal scanning laser fluorescence microscope revealed that the fluorescent marker most likely concentrated in the Golgi complex itself.

120. van Spronsen, E.A., V. Sarafis, G.J. Brakenhoff, H.T.M. van der Voort, and N. Nanninga. *Three-dimensional structure of living chloroplasts as visualized by confocal scanning laser microscopy.* Protoplasma. **148** 8–14, 1989.

121. Wallen, P., K. Carlsson, A. Liljeborg, and S. Grillner. *Three-dimensional reconstruction of neurons in the lamprey spinal cord in whole-mount, using a confocal laser scanning microscope.* J.Neurosci.Methods. **24** 91–100, 1988.

122. Watson T.F., and Boyde A., *Tandem scanning reflected light microscopy: applications in clinical dental research.* Scanning Microsc. **1**, 1971–1981 (1987).

Summarizes the TSM.

123. Watson T.F., and Boyde A., *The tandem scanning reflected light microscope (TSRLM) in conservative dentistry.* J.Dent.Res. **62** 512 (1984).

124. Watson T.F., and Boyde A., *Tandem scanning reflected light microscopy: A new method for in vitro assessment of dental operative procedures and restorations.* Clinical Materials **2** 33–34 (1987).

125. Watson T.F., *A confocal optical microscope study of the morphology of the tooth/restoration interface using Scotchbond 2 dentin adhesive.* J.Dent.Res. **68** 1124–1131 (1989).

126. Webb R. H., Hughes G. W., and Pomerantzeff O., *FLYING SPOT TV OPHTHALMOSCOPE.* Appl.Opt. **19**, 2991–2997 (1980).

A Scanning Laser Ophthalmoscope run at TV rates with much less incident light than conventional techniques.

127. Webb R.H., and Hughes G.W., *Scanning Laser Ophthalmoscope.* IEEE. Trans.Biomed.Eng. **BME-28**, 488–492 (1981).

128. Webb R.H., *Optics for laser rasters.* Appl.Opt. **23**, 3680–3683 (1984).

A number of instruments use rasters generated by deflecting one or more laser beams with some scanning device. Optics for shaping and manipulating these beams are described, with particular attention to the dual role of each element in terms of the (instantaneous) beam and the scanned pattern. A solution is shown to the problem of chromaticity in diffraction scanners.

129. Webb R.H., Hughes G.W., and Delori F.C., *Confocal scanning laser ophthalmoscope.* Appl.Opt. **26**, 1492–1499 (1987).

A confocal scanning imager moves an illumination spot over the object and a (virtual) detector synchronously over the image. In the confocal scanning laser ophthalmoscope this is accomplished by re-using the source optics for detection. The common optical elements are all mirrors—either flat or spherical—and the scanners are positioned to compensate astigmatism due to mirror tilt. A solid-state detector maybe at either a pupillary or retinal conjugate plane in the descanned beam and still have proper throughput matching. The 1-mm avalanche photodiode at a pupillary plane is preceded by interchangeable stops at an image (retinal) plane.

130. Welford W.T., *On the relationship between the modes of image formation in scanning microscopy and conventional microscopy.* J. Micros. **96**, 105–107 (1972).

131. White J.G., and Amos W.B., *Confocal microscopy comes of age.* Nature **328**, 183 (1987).

132. White J.G., Amos W.B., and Fordham M., *An evaluation of confocal versus conventional imaging of biological structures by fluorescence light microscopy.* J.Cell Biol. **105**, 41–48 (1987).

Scanning confocal microscopes offer improved rejection of out-of-focus noise and greater resolution than conventional imaging. In such a microscope, the imaging and condenser lenses are identical and confocal. These two lenses are replaced by a single lens when epi-illumination is used, making confocal imaging particularly applicable to incident light microscopy. We describe the results we have obtained with a confocal system in which scanning is performed by moving the light beam, rather than the stage. This system is considerably faster than the scanned stage microscope and is easy to use. We have found that confocal imaging gives greatly enhanced images of biological structures viewed with epifluorescence. The improvements are such that it is possible to optically section thick specimens with little degradation in the image quality of interior sections.

133. Wijnaendts van Resandt, R.W., H.J.B. Marsman, R. Kaplan, J. Davoust, E. H.K. Stelzer and R. Stricker. *Optical fluorescence microscopy in three dimensions: Microtomoscopy.* J.Micros. **138** 29–34, 1985.

134. Wijnaendts van Resandt, R.W. *Application of confocal beam scanning to the measurement of submicron structures.* Scanning Imaging Technology. **809** 101–106, 1987.

135. Stelzer, E.H.K., Marsman, H.J.B., Wijnaendts van Resandt, R.W. *A setup for a confocal scanning laser interference microscope* Optik **73** 30–3 (1986).

The interference mode installed on a CSLM is compared with that on a conventional microscope and high quality images are presented.

136. Wijnaendts van Resandt, R.W., H.J.B. Marsman, R. Kaplan, J. Davoust, E. H.K. Stelzer and R. Stricker, *Optical fluorescence microscopy in three dimensions: microtomoscopy* J.Micros. **138** 29–34 (1985).

The entire volume of the object is scanned mechanically through the well-defined focus of a laser illuminated, high numerical aperture objective. An identical optical path, arranged confocally, is used to detect the fluorescence emission from the focal volume. A pinhole in the image plane of the detection channel prevents fluorescence light, generated outside the focal volume, reaching the detector. Consequently a true resolution is obtained along the optical axis and three-dimensional imaging without the need for mathematical operations is possible.

137. Marsman, H.J.B., R. Stricker, R.W. Wijnaendts vanresandt, G.J. Brakenhoff, P., *Blom mechanical scan system for microscopic applications* Rev. Sci.Instrum. **54** 1047–52 (1983).

A high-speed mechanical scanning stage for microscopic applications has been designed and constructed. It is especially suitable for high- resolution confocal uv microscopy. It is a feedback design using electromagnetic actuators and piezoelectric sensors with motor-driven screws for coarse adjustment. Scanning of areas up to 1 mm square at up to 300 lines per second is possible with positional resolution of better than 0.01 mm. An exceptionally stable optical system is also described.

138. Wilke V., *Optical scanning microscopy—the laser scan microscope.* Scanning **7**, 88–96 (1985). The Zeiss CSLM.

139. Wilson T., and Sheppard C.J.R., *Imaging and super-resolution in the harmonic microscope.* Opt.Acta **26**, 761–770 (1979).

The imaging properties of harmonic microscopes which are either of the scanning or conventional form are considered. The scanning microscope exhibits super-resolution in that the spatial frequency cut-off is twice that for a microscope working at the fundamental wavelength, but the high spatial frequency response is not as good as for a microscope operating at the harmonic wavelength. The conventional harmonic microscope, if it uses a small condenser aperture to illuminate the specimen with coherent radiation, results in a spatial frequency cut-off half that of the scanning form, and coherent imaging characteristics such as fringes are to be expected.

140. Wilson T., Gannaway J.N., and Johnson P., *A scanning optical microscope for the inspection of semiconductor materials and devices.* J.Micros. **118**, 309–14 (1980).

A scanning optical microscope is described which exhibits a form of superresolution. Examples of its application to semiconductor device inspection are presented. The imaging properties of harmonic microscopes which are either of the scanning or conventional form are considered. The scanning microscope exhibits super-resolution in that the spatial frequency cut-off is twice that for a microscope working at the fundamental wavelength, but the high spatial frequency response is not as good as for a microscope operating at the harmonic wavelength. The conventional harmonic microscope, if it uses a small condenser aperture to illuminate the specimen with coherent radiation, results in a spatial frequency cut-off half that of the scanning form, and coherent imaging characteristics such as fringes are to be expected.

141. Wilson T., Gannaway J.N., and Sheppard C.J.R., *Optical fibre profiling using a scanning optical microscope.* Opt.and.Quantum.Electron. **12**, 341–345 (1980).

A scanning optical microscope is used to measure directly the refractive-index profile of an optical fibre. The effects of illuminating the fibre end with a highly convergent beam of light are considered.

142. Wilson T., *Imaging properties and applications of scanning optical microscopes.* Appl.Phys. (Germany.) **22**, 119–128 (1980).

This review paper, with 57 references, is concerned with the imaging properties and major uses of scanning optical microscopes. It is shown that the confocal scanning microscope exhibits a form of super-resolution and that the instrument in general has great application in nonlinear microscopy and the inspection of electronic devices.

143. Wilson T., Hamilton D.K., Shadbolt P.J. and Dodd B., *Scanning optical microscope as new metallographic tool.* Met.Sci. **14**, 144–146 (1980).

Micrographs are obtained for two standard metallurgical specimens and comparisons with conventional optical microscopes are made.

144. Wilson T., and Sheppard C.J.R., *The halo effect of image processing by spatial frequency filtering.* Optik **59**, 19–23 (1981).

In dark-field and phase contrast microscopy and also in coherent image processing techniques for edge enhancement a spatial frequency filter is used to obstruct or modify the zero spatial frequency component. The formation of haloes in images produced by these methods is discussed, and it is found that it is caused by the finite extent of the filter.

145. Wilson T., and Hamilton D.K., *Dynamic focusing in the confocal scanning microscopes.* J.Micros. **128**, 139–143 (1982).

The object is scanned axially, and the image built up as each section of the object passes through the focal plane.

146. Wilson T., and Sheppard C.J.R., *Imaging with finite values of fresnel number.* J.Opt.Soc.Am. **72**, 1639–1641 (1982).

A theory of imaging in the confocal scanning microscope that takes account of the finite fresnel number of the objectives is developed. It is shown that the coherent transfer function has no definite spatial frequency cutoff, the higher frequencies being enhanced in low-fresnel—number geometries accompanied by sign reversal and oscillation of the transfer function.

147. Wilson T. and Hamilton D.K., *Differential amplitude contrast imaging in the scanning optical microscope.* Appl.Phys.B (Germany) 187–191 (1983).

A split detector is used in a scanning optical microscope to produce high-quality differential amplitude contrast images. As light lateral offset in the detector position is shown to introduce information about object height variations to the image. These results are compared with images obtained by electrical differentiation.

148. Wilson T., and Hamilton D.K., *Difference confocal scanning microscopy.* Opt.Acta. 31, 453–465 (1984).

It is shown that an enhanced confocal image may be obtained by subtracting the type 1 from the confocal image. The resulting differential contrast image is found to be very sensitive to variations in object height.

149. T. Wilson and C.J.R. Sheppard, *Theory and Practice of Scanning Optical Microscopy,* Academic Press, London, 1984)

Reprints some of their early papers.

150. Wilson T., *Scanning optical microscopy.* Scanning 7, 79–87(1985).

Summary article.

151. Wilson T., Carlini A.R., and Sheppard, C.J.R., *Phase contrast microscopy by nearly full illumination.* Optik 70, 166–169 (1985).

The authors present a simple phase contrast technique where the two lenses in a scanning microscope are not equal. The method which is equally applicable to conventional and confocal scanning microscopes is demonstrated experimentally.

152. Wilson T., and Sheppard C.J.R., *Imaging of birefringent objects in scanning microscopes.* Appl.Opt. 24, 2081–2084 (1985).

The effective detector sensitivity function can be modified in a scanning optical microscope by placing a polarizer in front of a photodetector, in a divergent cone of light. Birefringent information from the specimen may be obtained simultaneously. Examples of amplitude and differential phase contrast images are presented.

153. Wilson T., and Hamilton D.K., *Dark-field scanning optical microscopy.* Optik 71, 23–26 (1985).

The additional properties of the dark-field confocal image are discussed and the advantages of electronic contrast enhancement illustrated.

154. Wilson T., McCabe E.M., and Hamilton D.K., *A new method for displaying low-contrast optical-beam-induced-contrast images in the scanning optical microscope.* J.Appl.Phys. 59, 702–703 (1986).

The new technique which displays the rectified, differentiated Obic signal, is insensitive to variations in the background signal level.

155. Wilson T., and Sheppard C.J.R., *Observations of dislocations and junction irregularities in bipolar transistors using the OBIC mode of the scanning optical microscope.* Solid-State. Electron. 291, 189–94 (1986).

By monitoring the appropriate junction current in a bipolar transistor in the OBIC mode of a scanning optical micro-scope dislocations in the emitter region or the spatial inhomogeneities of the emitter-base junction can be imaged. The method is very powerful as it does not cause specimen damage. Examples of scanning electron microscope induced damage are shown.

156. Wilson T., Carlini A.R., and Hamilton D.K., *Images of thick step objects in confocal scanning microscopes by axial scanning.* Optik (Germany.) 73, 123–126 (1986).

Scanned axially, theory agrees well with experiment.

157. Wilson T., and Carlini A.R., *The images of thick step objects in the confocal scanning optical microscope.* Optik 72, 109–114 (1986).

A method of calculating the images of thick step objects in confocal scanning optical microscopes. Images are presented of various step objects, including phase steps, in the extended focus, auto-focus and surface profilometry modes of the confocal microscope. Criteria for locating the geometrical position of the edge are also given.

158. Wilson T., and Carlini A.R., *Depth discrimination criteria in confocal optical systems.* Optik 76, 164–166 (1987).

Considers various depth discrimination criteria which describe the optical sectioning property of confocal optical systems. In particular the authors introduce a new criterion of sectioning property which applies to any arrangement including those operating under darkfield or differential conditions.

159. Wilson T., and Carlini A.R., *Size of the detector in confocal imaging systems.* Opt.Lett. 12, 227–229 (1987).

A criterion for detector size to give true confocal operation and demonstration that the lateral resolution is considerably more sensitive to detector size than is the axial resolution.

160. Wilson T., and Carlini A.R., *Three-dimensional imaging in confocal imaging systems with finite sized detectors.* J.Micros. 149, 51–66 (1988).

The effect of the finite size of the detector on both the lateral and axial resolution of the confocal system. The use of a finite sized detector means that the imaging is no longer truly coherent. The lateral resolution is considerably more sensitive to the detector size than is the axial response. The question of the rejection of flare light is also considered. Experimental results are shown and the authors find that acceptable extended-focus, auto-focus and height images may be obtained from non-truly-confocal systems. They also find that lens apodization has a far greater effect.

161. Wilson T., *Effect of detector displacement in confocal imaging systems.* Appl.Opt. 27, 3791–3799 (1988).

Confocal imaging systems rely on the use of an accurately positioned axial point detector. The authors discuss the effects of the various imaging modes of using a misaligned pinhole. They pay particular attention to the form of the transfer function and the depth discrimination property. A simple model of a thick edge type object is introduced, and it is found that in certain cases a degree of detector offset may be used to advantage in determining the position of the edge.

162. Wilson T., Carlini A.R., *The effect of aberrations on the axial response of confocal imaging systems.* J.Micros. **154** 243–256 (1989).

163. Xiao G.Q., Corle T.R., and Kino G.S., *Real-time confocal scanning optical microscope.* Appl.Phys.Lett. **53**, 716–718 (1988).

A real-time confocal scanning optical microscope is described. It is capable of generating 640 frames per second with 7000 lines per frame. It achieves this speed by simultaneously illuminating several thousand pinholes arranged in a spiral pattern on a rotating disk. An optical isolator is used to eliminate reflections from the surface of the disk. This type of microscope should have the same range and transverse definitions as a standard, single pinhole, confocal microscope.

164. Zapf Th., and Wijnaendts-van-Resandt R.W., *VLSI metrology using an automatic beam-scanning confocal laser microscope.* Scanning **10**, 157–162 (1988).

The authors present some of the technical details and possibilities of a fully automated beam scanning confocal microscope, designed especially for fully automated very large-scale integrated (VLSI) metrology, and to compare its basic properties with those of an object scanning system. In addition, a number of practical applications of the beam scanning system in the field of automated integrated circuit metrology are discussed.

PATENTS

165. Baer S.C., *Optical Apparatus providing focal-plane specific illumination.* U. S. Patent **3,547,512,** (1970).

166. Minsky M., *Microscopy Apparatus.* U.S. Patent **3,013,467** (1961).

167. Petran M., and Hadravsky M., *Zpusob a zarizeni proomezeni rozptylu svetla v mikrosckopu pro osvetleni shora.*

Czechoslovak Patent **128,936,** application 5–7–66, granted 15–2–68, published 15–9–68. (1966).

168. Petran M., and Hadravsky M., *Zpusob a zarizeni prozlepseni rozlisovaci schopnosti a kontrastu optickehomirkroskopu.* Czechoslovak Patent **128,937,** application 5–7–66, granted 15–2–68, published 15–9–68 (1966).

169. Petran M., and Hadravsky M., *Method and arrangement for improving the resolving power and contrast.* US Patent **3,517,980,** Filed 4–12–67, granted 30–6–70 (1967).

170. Pomerantzeff O., and Webb R.H., *Scanning ophthalmoscope for examining the fundus of the eye.* Patent **4,213,678** (1980).

Original SLO patent. Confocal (with Image Dissector) in Claim 12.

171. Webb R.H., and Wornson D.P., *Scanning Optical Apparatus and Method.* Patent **4,768,874,** (1988).

One dimension scanned, the other uses an array of pixel detectors.

172. Webb R.H., *Double Scanning Apparatus and Method.* Patent **4,765,730,** (1988).

Original double scanning patent Aug 23, 1988 filed Sept 17, 1985

173. Webb R.H., *Double Scanning Optical Apparatus and Method.* Patent **4,768,873,** (1988).

First update of double scanning patent Sept 6, 1988 filed June 19, 1986

Acknowledgements: Many people have helped with this update. Gordon Kino, Alan Boyde and Eric Hansen have actually sent long lists, much appreciated. I have not included some works in press, and may have cut off some journals which reach Boston slowly by ship, and I apologize for that.

INDEX

Note: page numbers in bold type refer to Chapters on the noted subject.